Blueprints **Notes & Cases**
Pathophysiology:
Cardiovascular, Endocrine, and Reproduction

D0622048

Blueprints Notes & Cases

Series Editor: Aaron B. Caughey MD, MPP, MPH

Blueprints **Notes & Cases**
Pathophysiology:
Cardiovascular, Endocrine, and Reproduction

Gordon Leung, MD
Cardiology Fellow
Division of Cardiology
University of California
San Francisco, California

Susan H. Tran, MD
Resident in Obstetrics and Gynecology
Kaiser Permanente Medical Center
San Francisco, California

Tina O. Tan, MD
Resident in Obstetrics and Gynecology
University of California
San Francisco, California

Aaron B. Caughey, MD, MPP, MPH
Clinical Instructor, Division of Maternal-Fetal Medicine
Department of Obstetrics & Gynecology
University of California, San Francisco
Division of Health Services and Policy Analysis
University of California, Berkeley
Berkeley & San Francisco, California

Series Editor: Aaron B. Caughey, MD, MPP, MPH

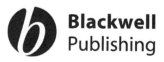

Blackwell
Publishing

© 2004 by Blackwell Publishing

Blackwell Publishing, Inc., 350 Main Street, Malden, Massachusetts 02148-5018, USA
Blackwell Publishing Ltd, 9600 Garsington Road, Oxford OX4 2DQ, UK
Blackwell Science Asia Pty Ltd, 550 Swanston Street, Carlton, Victoria 3053, Australia

All rights reserved. No part of this publication may be reproduced in any form or by any
electronic or mechanical means, including information storage and retrieval systems, without
permission in writing from the publisher, except by a reviewer who may quote brief passages in a
review.

03 04 05 06 5 4 3 2 1

ISBN: 1–4051-0350–7

Library of Congress Cataloging-in-Publication Data

Blueprints notes & cases : pathophysiology : cardiovascular, endocrine, and reproduction / authors, Gordon Leung . . . [et al.].
    p. ; cm. — (Blueprints notes & cases)
  Includes index.
  ISBN 1-4051-0350-7 (pbk.)
    1. Cardiovascular system—Pathophysiology—Case studies. 2. Endocrine glands—Pathophysiology—Case studies.
  3. Generative organs—Pathophysiology—Case studies.
    [DNLM: 1. Cardiovascular Diseases—physiopathology—Case Report. 2. Cardiovascular Diseases—physiopathology—
  Problems and Exercises. 3. Endocrine Diseases—physiopathology—Case Report. 4. Endocrine Diseases—physiopathology—
  Problems and Exercises. 5. Reproduction—Case Report. 6. Reproduction—Problems and Exercises.
  WG 18.2 B659 2004] I. Title: Pathophysiology : cardiovascular, endocrine, and reproduction. II. Title: Blueprints notes and
  cases. III. Leung, Gordon. IV. Series.
    RC669.9.B58 2004
    616.07—dc21   2003010571

A catalogue record for this title is available from the British Library

Acquisitions: Beverly Copland
Development: Selene Steneck
Production: Debra Lally
Cover design: Hannus Design Associates
Interior design: Janet Bollow Associates
Typesetter: Peirce Graphic Services in Stuart, in Florida
Printed and bound by Courier Companies in Westford, MA

For further information on Blackwell Publishing, visit our website: www.blackwellpublishing.com

Notice: The indications and dosages of all drugs in this book have been recommended in the
medical literature and conform to the practices of the general community. The medications
described do not necessarily have specific approval by the Food and Drug Administration for
use in the diseases and dosages for which they are recommended. The package insert for each
drug should be consulted for use and dosage as approved by the FDA. Because standards for
usage change, it is advisable to keep abreast of revised recommendations, particularly those
concerning new drugs.

Contents

I. CARDIOVASCULAR   Gordon Leung, MD

II. ENDOCRINE   Tina O. Tan, MD

III. REPRODUCTION   Susan H. Tran, MD

Contributors

Holbrook E. Kohrt
Class of 2004
Stanford University School of Medicine
Stanford, California

Elaine Yu
Class of 2004
University of California, San Francisco, School of Medicine
San Francisco, California

Reviewers

Tara Borghard
Class of 2004
Brown Medical School
Providence, Rhode Island

Valerie Julie Brousseau
Class of 2004
McGill University
Montreal, Quebec

Diane Lewis
Class of 2004
State University of New York at Stony Brook School
of Medicine
Stony Brook, New York

Rebecca Smith
Class of 2004
University of California, Irvine
Irvine, California

Mai Tran
Class of 2004
Western University of Health Sciences
Pomona, California

Tina Tran
Class of 2004
Medical College of Virginia
Richmond, Virginia

Preface

The first two years of medical school are a demanding time for medical students. Whether the school follows a traditional curriculum or one that is case-based, every student is expected to learn and be able to apply basic science information in a clinical situation.

Medical schools are increasingly using clinical presentations as the background to teach the basic sciences. Case-based learning has become more common at many medical schools as it offers a way to catalogue the multitude of symptoms, syndromes, and diseases in medicine.

Blueprints **Notes & Cases is a new series by Blackwell Publishing designed to provide students a textbook to study the basic science topics combined with clinical data.** This method of learning is also the way to prepare for the clinical case format of USMLE questions. The eight books in this series will make the basic science topics not only more interesting, but also more meaningful and memorable. Students will be learning not only the why of a principle, but also how it might commonly be seen in practice.

The books in the *Blueprints* Notes & Cases series feature a comprehensive collection of cases which are designed to introduce one or more basic science topics. Through these cases, students gain an understanding of the coursework as they learn to:

- Think through the cases
- Look for classic presentations of most common diseases and syndromes
- Integrate the basic science content with clinical application
- Prepare for course exams and Step 1 USMLE
- Be prepared for clinical rotations

This series covers all the essential material needed in the basic science courses. Where possible, the books are organized in an organ-based system.

Clinical cases lead off and are the basis for discussion of the basic science content. A list of **"thought questions"** follows the case presentation. These questions are designed to challenge the reader to begin to think about how basic science topics apply to real-life clinical situations. The **answers to these questions** are integrated within the **basic science review and discussion** that follows. This offers a clinical framework from which to understand the basic content.

The discussion section is followed by a high-yield **Thumbnail table and Key Points box,** which highlight and summarize the essential information presented in the discussion.

The cases also include two to four **multiple-choice questions** that allow readers to check their knowledge of that topic. Many of the answer explanations provide an opportunity for further discussion by delving into more depth in related areas. An **answer key** for these questions is at the end of the section for easy reference, and **full answer explanations** can be found at the end of the book.

This new series was designed to provide comprehensive content in a concise and templated format for ease in learning. A dedicated attempt was made to include sufficient art, tables, and clinical treatment, all while keeping the books from becoming too lengthy. We know you have much to read and that what you want is high-yield, vital facts.

The authors and series editor for these eight books, as well as everyone in editorial, production, sales and marketing at Blackwell Publishing, have worked long and hard to provide new textbooks to help you learn and be able to apply what you have learned. We engaged in multiple student email surveys and many focus groups to "hear what you needed" in new basic science level textbooks to meet the current curriculums, tests, and coursework. We know that you value this "student to student" approach, and sincerely hope you like what we have put together **just for you.**

Blackwell Publishing and the authors wish you success in your studies and your future medical career. Please feel free to offer us any comments or suggestions on these new books at blue@bos.blackwellpublishing.com.

Acknowledgments

With thanks and appreciation to the cardiology faculty and fellows at University of California, San Francisco, my family, and my wonderful wife, Cheryl.

—Gordon

For my dear friends and family (old and new), particularly my parents Lieu and Ngan, the residents and staff at Kaiser San Francisco, and my dearest Pi, whose infinite love, support, and hope make my life extraordinary.

—Susan

To my family, thank you for your never-ending love and support. To Susan and Aaron, thanks for your friendship, guidance, and this incredible opportunity. To Dr. Joel Schechter, thank you for all of your help and wisdom—you are a true teaching inspiration. To Jenn, Marisa, and Chanida, thanks for all the good times, the laughs, your ears to listen, and your shoulders to lean on. Finally, to Gallant, thank you for your love, your patience, and always being by my side.

—Tina

We would like to thank all of the staff at Blackwell, in particular Selene and Jen. I would also like to acknowledge the support I receive from my mentors at UCSF and UC Berkeley. I also want to thank my parents, Bill and Carol, my siblings Ethan and Samara, my closest friends Jim and Wendy, and my wife, Susan, for all of the support over the years.

—Aaron

Abbreviations

17-OHP	17-OH-progesterone	CK MB	creatine kinase myocardial band fraction
3βHSD	3β-hydroxysteroid dehydrogenase	CNS	central nervous system
Ab	antibody	CO	cardiac output
ABG	arterial blood gas	COPD	chronic obstructive pulmonary disease
ACE	angiotensin converting enzyme	CPM	central pontine myelinosis
ACS	acute coronary syndrome	CRH	corticotropin releasing hormone
ACTH	adrenocorticotropic hormone	CT	computed tomography
ADH	anti-diuretic hormone	CVA	cerebrovascular accident
ADP	adenosine diphosphate	CVS	chorionic villus sampling
AF	atrial fibrillation	CVS	cardiovascular system
AFP	alpha-fetoprotein	CXR	chest x-ray
AG	anion gap	ΔOD_{450}	spectrophotometric measurement of optical density at 450nm
AIDS	acquired immunodeficiency syndrome	D&C	dilatation and curettage
ALT	alanine aminotransferase	D&E	dilatation and evacuation
AR	aortic regurgitation	DDAVP	desmopressin
ARB	angiotensin receptor blockers	DES	diethylstilbestrol
AS	aortic stenosis	DHEA	dehydroepiandrosterone
ASCUS	atypical squamous cells of undetermined significance	DHEAS	dehydroepiandrosterone sulfate
ASD	atrial septal defect	DHT	dihydrotestosterone
AST	aspartate transaminase	DI	diabetes insipidus
ATP	adenosine triphosphate	DIC	disseminated intravascular coagulation
AV	atrioventricular	DKA	diabetic ketoacidosis
AVA	aortic valve area	DM	diabetes mellitus
AVNRT	atrioventricular nodal reentrant tachycardia	DMPA	depot medroxyprogesterone acetate
AVRT	atrioventricular reentrant tachycardia	DOPA	dihydroxyphenylalanine
BP	blood pressure	ED	emergency department
BUN	blood urea nitrogen	EF	ejection fraction
CAD	coronary artery disease	ECG	electrocardiogram
CAH	congenital adrenal hyperplasia	ESPVR	end-systolic pressure volume loop
CAT	computed axial tomography	ESR	erythrocyte sedimentation rate
CBC	complete blood count	ESS	endometrial stromal sarcoma
CCB	calcium channel blockers	ET	endothelin
CDI	central diabetes insipidus	EtOH	alcohol
CHF	congestive heart failure	FIGO	International Federation of Gynecology and Obstetrics
CIN	cervical intraepithelial neoplasia		
CK	creatine kinase	FSH	follicle stimulating hormone

G#	gravida (pregnancies)		KUB	kidneys, ureters, bladder
GA	gestational age		LA	left atrium
GAS	group A streptococcus		LAD	left anterior descending coronary artery
GFR	glomerular filtration rate		LDH	lactate dehydrogenase
GH	growth hormone		LDL	low density lipoproteins
GHRH	growth hormone releasing hormone		LGSIL	low-grade squamous intraepithelial lesion
GI	gastrointestinal		LH	luteinizing hormone
Glut-y	glucose transporter y		LMP	last menstrual period
GnRH	gonadotropin-releasing hormone		LSB	left sternal border
GTD	gestational trophoblastic disease		LV	left ventricle
H & E	hematoxylin and eosin		LVEDP	left ventricular end-diastolic pressure
HEENT	head, ears, eyes, nose, and throat		MEN	multiple endocrine neoplasia
H/N	head and neck		MI	myocardial infarction
Hb	hemoglobin		MIS	müllerian-inhibiting substance
HbA$_{1c}$	hemoglobin A$_{1c}$		MMT	mixed müllerian tumor
hCG	human chorionic gonadotropin		MR	mitral regurgitation
HCT	hematocrit		MRI	magnetic resonance imaging
HGSIL	high-grade squamous intraepithelial lesion		MS	mitral stenosis
HIV	human immunodeficiency virus		MSH	melanocyte stimulating hormone
HLA	human leukocyte antigen		Na$^+$/K$^+$ ATPase	sodium/potassium active transporter
HPV	human papilloma virus		NDI	nephrogenic diabetes insipidus
HR	heart rate		NIH	National Institutes of Health
HRT	hormone replacement therapy		NSAID	nonsteroidal anti-inflammatory drug
HTN	hypertension		NSTEMI	non-ST segment elevation myocardial infarction
HVA	homovanillic acid			
ICSI	intracytoplasmic sperm injection		OCP	oral contraceptive pills
IE	infective endocarditis		OS	opening snap
IGF-1	insulin-like growth factor 1		P#	para (total births after 20 wk GA)
IHD	ischemic heart disease		P2	pulmonic component to second heart sound
IUD	intrauterine device		Pap smear	Papanicolaou smear
IV	intravenous		Pco$_2$	pressure of carbon dioxide
IVC	inferior vena cava		PCOS	polycystic ovarian syndrome
IVDA	intravenous drug abuse		PDA	patent ductus arteriosus
IVF	in vitro fertilization		PDGF	platelet derived growth factor
JGA	juxtaglomerular apparatus		PFO	patent foramen ovale
JVD	jugular venous distention		PGE2	prostaglandin E2
JVP	jugular venous pressure		PID	pelvic inflammatory disease

PMI	point of maximum impulse	SRY	sex-determining region of the Y chromosome
PNMT	phenylethanolamine-N-methyltransferase	SSRI	selective serotonin reuptake inhibitor
Po_2	pressure of oxygen	SSS	sick sinus syndrome
PRL	prolactin	STD	sexually transmitted disease
PSTT	placental site trophoblastic tumor	STEMI	ST segment elevation myocardial infarction
PTH	parathyroid hormone	STI	sexually transmitted infection
PTHrP	parathyroid hormone related protein	SV	stroke volume
PTU	propylthiouracil	SVR	systemic vascular resistance
PUBS	percutaneous umbilical cord sampling	SVT	supraventricular tachycardia
PVC	premature ventricular contraction	T_3	tri-iodothyronine
PVN	paraventricular nucleus	T_4	thyroxine
QID	four times a day	TAH-BSO	total abdominal hysterectomy and bilateral salpingo-oophorectomy
RA	right atrium	TGA	transposition of great arteries
RAA	renin-angiotensin-aldosterone	TGF-α	transforming growth factor-α
RAI	radioactive iodine	TH	thyroid hormone
RBC	red blood cell	Tmax	maximum temperature
RCA	right coronary artery	TNF	tumor necrosis factor
RAS	renin-angiotensin system	TOF	Tetralogy of Fallot
RE	reticuloendothelial	TPO	thyroid peroxidase
RF	rheumatic fever	TR	tricuspid regurgitation
Rh	rhesus factor	TRH	thyroid releasing hormone
RR	respiratory rate	TSH	thyroid stimulating hormone
RRR	regular rate and rhythm	URI	upper respiratory infection
RUQ	right upper quadrant of abdomen	USA	unstable angina
RV	right ventricle	VF	ventricular fibrillation
RVH	right ventricular hypertrophy	VEGF	vascular endothelial growth factor
S1	first heart sound (closure of mitral and tricuspid valves)	VIP	vasoactive intestinal polypeptide
		VMA	vanillylmandelic acid
S2	second heart sound (closure of aortic and pulmonic valves)	VSD	ventricular septal defect
		VT	ventricular tachycardia
SA	sinoatrial	WBC	white blood cell count
SEM	systolic ejection murmur	WHI	women's health initiative
SERM	selective estrogen receptor modulator	WNL	within normal limits
SGOT	serum glutamic oxaloacetic transaminase	WPW	Wolff-Parkinson-White syndrome
SIADH	syndrome of inappropriate anti-diuretic hormone		
SON	supraoptic nucleus		

Normal Ranges of Laboratory Values

BLOOD, PLASMA, SERUM

Alanine aminotransferase (ALT, GPT at 30 C)	8–20 U/L
Amylase, serum	25–125 U/L
Asparatate aminotransferase (AST, GOT at 30 C)	8–20 U/L
Bilirubin, serum (adult) Total // Direct	0.1–1.0 mg/dL // 0.0–0.3 mg/dL
Calcium, serum (Ca^{2+})	8.4–10.2 mg/dL
Cholesterol, serum	Rec: < 200 mg/dL
Cortisol, serum	0800 h: 5–23 μg/dL // 1600 h: 3–15 μg/dL
	2000 h: ≤ 50% of 0800 h
Creatine kinase, serum	Male: 25–90 U/L
	Female: 10–70 U/L
Creatinine, serum	0.6–1.2 mg/dL
Electrolytes, serum	
Sodium (Na^+)	136–145 mEq/L
Chloride (Cl^-)	95–105 mEq/L
Potassium (K^+)	3.5–5.0 mEq/L
Bicarbonate (HCO_3^-)	22–28 mEq/L
Magnesium (Mg^{2+})	1.5–2.0 mEq/L
Ferritin, serum	Male: 15–200 ng/mL
	Female: 12–150 ng/mL
Follicle-stimulating hormone, serum/plasma	Male: 4–25 mIU/mL
	Female: premenopause 4–30 mIU/mL
	midcycle peak 10–90 mIU/mL
	postmenopause 40–250 mIU/mL
Gases, arterial blood (room air)	
pH	7.35–7.45
P_{CO_2}	33–45 mm Hg
P_{O_2}	75–105 mm Hg
Glucose, serum	Fasting: 70–110 mg/dL
	2-h postprandial: < 120 mg/dL
Growth hormone—arginine stimulation	Fasting: < 5 ng/mL
	provocative stimuli: > 7 ng/mL
Iron	50–70 μg/dL
Lactate dehydrogenase, serum	45–90 U/L
Luteinizing hormone, serum/plasma	Male: 6–23 mIU/mL
	Female: follicular phase 5–30 mIU/mL
	midcycle 75–150 mIU/mL
	postmenopause 30–200 mIU/mL
Osmolality, serum	275–295 mOsmol/kg
Parathyroid hormone, serum, N-terminal	230–630 pg/mL
Phosphate (alkaline), serum (p-NPP at 30 C)	20–70 U/L
Phosphorus (inorganic), serum	3.0–4.5 mg/dL
Prolactin, serum (hPRL)	< 20 ng/mL
Proteins, serum	
Total (recumbent)	6.0–7.8 g/dL
Albumin	3.5–5.5 g/dL
Globulin	2.3–3.5 g/dL
Thyroid-stimulating hormone, serum or plasma	0.5–5.0 μU/mL
Thyroidal iodine (^{123}I) uptake	8–30% of administered dose/24 h
Thyroxine (T_4), serum	5–12 μg/dL
Triglycerides, serum	35–160 mg/dL
Triiodothyronine (T_3), serum (RIA)	115–190 ng/dL
Triiodothyronine (T_3), resin uptake	25–35%
Urea nitrogen, serum (BUN)	7–18 mg/dL
Uric acid, serum	3.0–8.2 mg/dL

CEREBROSPINAL FLUID

Cell count	0–5 cells/mm^3
Chloride	118–132 mEq/L
Gamma globulin	3–12% total proteins
Glucose	40–70 mg/dL
Pressure	70–180 mm H_2O
Proteins, total	< 40 mg/dL

HEMATOLOGIC

Bleeding time (template)	2–7 minutes
Erythrocyte count	Male: 4.3–5.9 million/mm^3
	Female: 3.5–5.5 million/mm^3
Erythrocyte sedimentation rate (Westergren)	Male: 0–15 mm/h
	Female: 0–20 mm/h
Hematocrit	Male: 41–53%
	Female: 36–46%
Hemoglobin A$_{1C}$	≤ 6%
Hemoglobin, blood	Male: 13.5–17.5 g/dL
	Female: 12.0–16.0 g/dL
Leukocyte count and differential	
Leukocyte count	4500–11,000/mm^3
Segmented neutrophils	54–62%
Bands	3–5%
Eosinophils	1–3%
Basophils	0–0.75%
Lymphocytes	25–33%
Monocytes	3–7%
Mean corpuscular hemoglobin	25.4–34.6 pg/cell
Mean corpuscular hemoglobin concentration	31–36% Hb/cell
Mean corpuscular volume	80–100 μm^3
Partial thromboplastin time (activated)	25–40 seconds
Platelet count	150,000–400,000/mm^3
Prothrombin time	11–15 seconds
Reticulocyte count	0.5–1.5% of red cells
Thrombin time	< 2 seconds deviation from control
Volume	
Plasma	Male: 25–43 mL/kg
	Female: 28–45 mL/kg
Red cell	Male: 20–36 mL/kg
	Female: 19–31 mL/kg

SWEAT

Chloride	0–35 mmol/L

URINE

Calcium	100–300 mg/24 h
Chloride	Varies with intake
Creatine clearance	Male: 97–137 mL/min
	Female: 88–128 mL/min
Osmolality	50–1400 mOsmol/kg
Oxalate	8–40 μg/mL
Potassium	Varies with diet
Proteins, total	< 150 mg/24 h
Sodium	Varies with diet
Uric acid	Varies with diet

Part I

Cardiovascular

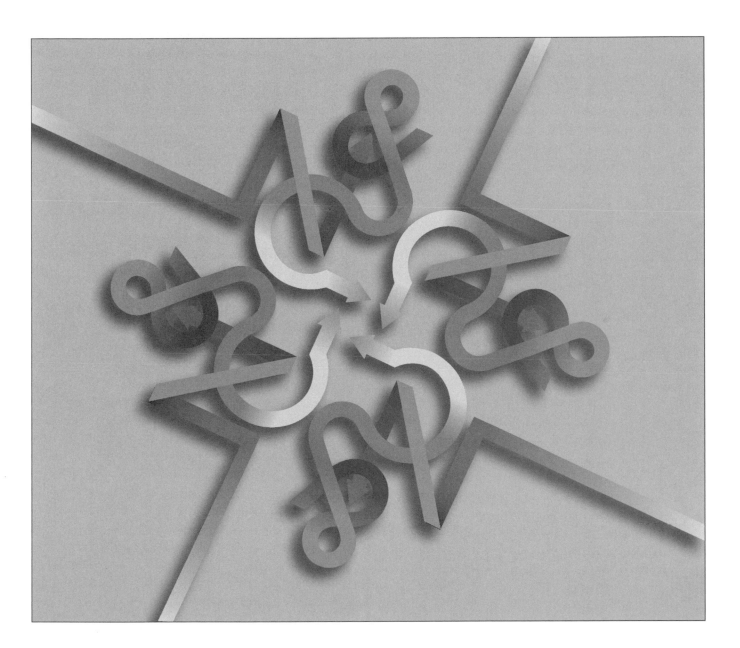

HPI: AHF is a 79-year-old man with a long-standing history of poorly controlled hypertension (HTN), stable coronary artery disease, and diabetes who presents to the emergency department with acute onset of shortness of breath but no chest pressure. He complains of increasing peripheral edema for several weeks, orthopnea, right upper quadrant (RUQ) pain, and increasing fatigue.

PE: **Vitals:** Blood pressure (BP) 160/50 mm Hg, heart rate (HR) 90 beats/min, respiratory rate (RR) 26 breaths/min, and maximum temperature (Tmax) 37°C. **General:** Tachypneic, uncomfortable appearing. **Head and Neck (H/N):** Jugular venous pressure (JVP) is 12 cm, pulses reduced in volume and upstroke. **Chest:** Crackles present one third of the way up bilaterally. **Cardiac:** Point of maximum impulse (PMI) displaced laterally and diffuse; S_3 and S_4 present. **Abdomen:** Mild pain in RUQ and mild hepatomegaly. **Extremity:** 3+ bilateral peripheral edema to knees.

Labs: Creatinine 1.6 mg/dL, blood urea nitrogen (BUN) 24 mg/dL, troponin I < 0.05 mg/dL. **Electrocardiography (ECG):** Normal sinus rhythm with nonspecific ST changes.

Thought Questions

- What is heart failure?

- What are the causes of heart failure?

- What are the key mediators of cardiac output?

- How are pressure volume loops affected in heart failure secondary to systolic dysfunction?

Basic Science Review and Discussion

Heart failure is defined as the inability of the heart to meet the metabolic demands of the tissues. The most common cause of heart failure is ischemic heart disease followed by dilated cardiomyopathy.

Cardiac output is the product of the heart rate times the stroke volume (CO = HR × SV). The stroke volume is determined by three parameters: (1) contractility, (2) preload, and (3) afterload. Contractility is the amount of force exerted at a given muscle fiber length. Preload is defined as the ventricular wall tension at the end of diastole and is quantified by the left ventricular (LV) end-diastolic pressure. Afterload is the ventricular wall tension during systole and is determined by the mean arterial pressure.

Another important equation is blood pressure equals cardiac output multiplied by the systemic vascular resistance (BP = CO × SVR).

Systolic dysfunction is the result of impaired LV contraction. The two major contributors to systolic dysfunction include impaired contractility and pressure overload (Table 1-1).

In systolic dysfunction, the normal pressure volume loop is changed in the following fashion: (1) the end-systolic pressure volume loop (ESPVR) is shifted downward and rightward, resulting in a decreased stroke volume; and (2)

the end-diastolic volume is increased with a resultant increase in the end-diastolic pressure. The decreased stroke volume precipitates a decreased cardiac output. The increased LV end-diastolic pressure is transmitted into the pulmonary bed, resulting in pulmonary edema (Figure 1-1).

Systolic dysfunction is compensated by three mechanisms:

1. *Ventricular hypertrophy:* Increased ventricular wall stress results in production of new myocardial sarcomeres and increased ventricular mass. Ventricular mass increases in two different patterns. **Pressure overload** causes synthesis of sarcomeres in parallel with previous sarcomeres, resulting in increased wall thickness without chamber dilatation. **Volume overload** stimulates sarcomere production in series with the previous sarcomeres, resulting in ventricular dilatation and enlargement.

Table 1-1 Major contributors to systolic dysfunction

Impaired contractility	Pressure overload
Ischemic heart disease	Uncontrolled hypertension
Myocardial infarction	Aortic stenosis
Chronic volume overload Aortic regurgitation Mitral regurgitation Ventricular septal defect Arteriovenous shunting	
Dilated cardiomyopathy Viral myocarditis Cocaine, alcohol abuse Toxins, chemotherapy Idiopathic	
Chronic high-output states Anemia Thyrotoxicosis Beri-beri	

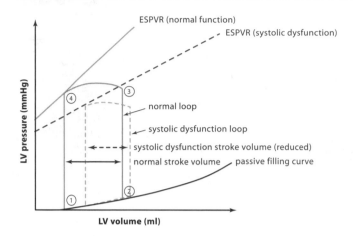

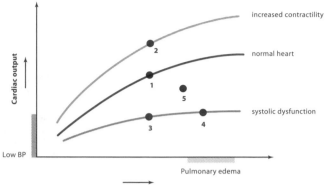

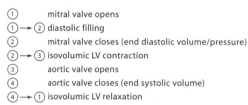

①   mitral valve opens

①→②   diastolic filling

②   mitral valve closes (end diastolic volume/pressure)

②→③   isovolumic LV contraction

③   aortic valve opens

④   aortic valve closes (end systolic volume)

④→①   isovolumic LV relaxation

1   normal patient
2   normal patient on dopamine (↑ cardiac output at same LVEDP)
3   systolic dysfunction patient with hypotension
4   systolic dysfunction patient with fluid overload (↑ LVEDP)
    but no ↑ in cardiac output: patient remains hypotensive with
    pulmonary edema
5   systolic dysfunction patient on positive inotropes and diuresis

Figure 1-1 A pressure volume loop is a plot of the LV pressure versus the LV volume and represents the cardiac cycle in a counter-clockwise direction. The width between the two vertical lines of the loop represents the stroke volume, and the area enclosed by the loop represents the cardiac output. In systolic dysfunction, the end-systolic pressure volume relationship is shifted downward and the end-diastolic volume as well as pressure (represented by point 2), increases. Both of these changes decrease the stroke volume as well as cardiac output.

Figure 1-2 The Frank-Starling response is the observation that the cardiac output increases as a function of the LV end-diastolic pressure. The response to an increase in preload is a greater stroke volume on the subsequent systolic contraction. Positive inotropes, such as dopamine, shift the Frank-Starling response curve upward so that a given LV end-diastolic pressure produces a greater cardiac output. In systolic dysfunction, the Frank-Starling curve is shifted downward so that a given LV end-diastolic pressure results in a lesser cardiac output.

2. *Neuroendocrine response:* When cardiac output declines, three neuroendocrine systems are activated to increase cardiac output. First, sympathetic tone increases, which then results in increased heart rate, increased contractility, and vasoconstriction. Second, the renin-angiotensin-aldosterone system is activated, which results in vasoconstriction and fluid retention to increase circulating volume and thereby **preload.** Third, increased antidiuretic hormone production promotes fluid retention.

3. *Frank-Starling response:* The increase in LV end-diastolic volume during systolic dysfunction results in an increase in preload. The **Frank-Starling response** to an increase in preload is a greater stroke volume on the subsequent systolic contraction. In effect, increased filling/preload causes an augmentation of cardiac output. In normal individuals, cardiac output increases as a function of end-diastolic volume. In systolic dysfunction, the cardiac output does not increase proportionally to an increase in end-diastolic volume. Pulmonary edema occurs as a result of the supranormal LV end-diastolic pressures necessary to maintain an adequate cardiac output (Figure 1-2).

Clinical Presentation

Symptoms

1. Fatigue: most common presenting symptom secondary to decreased cardiac output to skeletal muscle.

2. Dyspnea: secondary to pulmonary congestion when pulmonary venous pressure is greater than 20 mm Hg, which results in transudative leakage of fluid into the pulmonary parenchyma.

3. Decreased mental acuity and urine output: result of diminished forward flow to cerebral and kidney circulation.

4. Paroxysmal nocturnal dyspnea and orthopnea: fluid from gravity-dependent portions of body are redistributed into intravascular circulation when recumbent, resulting in increased intracardiac filling pressures.

5. Abdominal distension: elevated right-sided filling pressures cause hepatic swelling and intestinal edema.

6. Peripheral edema and weight gain: fluid retention due to neuroendocrine mechanisms and elevated right-sided pressures cause accumulation of interstitial fluid.

Physical Findings

Left-sided heart failure:

1. Enlarged point of maximal impulse in dilated cardiomyopathy.

2. Sustained point of maximal impulse in pressure overloaded states (aortic stenosis or HTN).

3. Cool extremities, mild cyanosis, and poor capillary refill secondary to poor cardiac output.

4. Tachycardia and tachypnea due to high sympathetic tone.

5. Cheyne-Stokes breathing: hyperventilation followed by temporary cessation of breathing due to increased circulation time between lungs and CNS respiratory centers.

6. Pulmonary ronchi and rales occur if left atrial pressure is greater than 20 mm Hg.

7. Third heart sound occurs during early diastole, during rapid ventricular filling phase: suggestive of pathologic increase in diastolic ventricular filling due to fluid overload.

8. Fourth heart sound: produced by contraction of atria in late diastole and occurs when the atrial-augmented filling enters a pathologically stiffened ventricle.

Right-sided heart failure:

1. Elevated jugular venous pulsation with prominent V wave and steep Y descent.

2. Peripheral edema.

3. Enlarged liver span from hepatic enlargement.

4. Ascites.

5. Hepatojugular reflux.

Treatment

1. Diuretics reduce intravascular volume, which results in a decreased LV preload. Decreased LV preload results in a lower LV end-diastolic pressure, which then falls below the range that can cause pulmonary congestion and edema.

2. Inotropes: Digoxin, beta-agonists (dopamine, dobutamine), and phosphodiesterase inhibitors (milrinone) increase the stroke volume, cardiac output, and actual contractility at any given preload.

3. Nitrates: Venous vasodilators decrease LV preload by increasing venous capacitance.

4. Angiotensin converting enzyme (ACE) inhibitors reduce systemic vascular resistance by inhibiting the formation of vasoconstrictor angiotensin II, and thereby decreasing LV afterload. Decreased afterload results in increased stroke volume at any given end-diastolic volume. ACE inhibitors also affect the neuroendocrine response by decreasing the formation of aldosterone, which then accelerates the elimination of sodium with a concomitant reduction in intravascular volume.

5. Angiotensin receptor blockers (ARBs) reduce systemic vascular resistance by blocking the angiotensin receptor, and thereby decreasing LV afterload.

6. Hydralazine and nitroprusside are both direct-acting arterial vasodilators that decrease LV afterload, resulting in an augmented stroke volume for a given preload.

Case Conclusion HF presents with systolic heart failure and dilated cardiomyopathy secondary to poorly controlled HTN. In addition, preexisting coronary artery disease contributes to decreased LV compliance and elevated diastolic filling pressures. His weight gain is secondary to fluid retention and his RUQ pain/hepatomegaly is the result of hepatic congestion from elevated right-sided filling pressures. His fatigue is the result of decreased cardiac output, and his orthopnea is secondary to redistribution of fluid from the extremities to the intravascular compartment. His elevated JVP is suggestive of a fluid-overloaded state. The elevated creatinine is secondary to inadequate renal perfusion secondary to poor cardiac output. His hyperadrenergic state leading to increased SVR and fluid overload contribute to his hypertensive presentation (remember BP = CO × SVR). His normal troponin and ECG without ischemia suggest that acute ischemia is an unlikely cause for his congestive heart failure (CHF) exacerbation. After aggressive diuresis and afterload reduction with ACE inhibitors, his symptoms markedly improve.

Thumbnail: Pharmacologic Management of CHF

Drug class	Examples
Renin-angiotensin-aldosterone inhibitors	ACE inhibitors → captopril Angiotensin receptor blockers → losartan Aldosterone antagonists → spironolactone
Beta-blockers	Cardioselective → metoprolol Nonselective with vasodilating properties → carvedilol
Digitalis	Digoxin
Vasodilators	Calcium channel blockers → amlodipine Nitrates Hydralazine Nitroprusside
Positive inotropic agents	Dobutamine, dopamine Phosphodiesterase inhibitors → milrinone
Diuretics	Thiazide diuretics → hydrochlorothiazide, metolazone Loop diuretics → furosemide Aldosterone antagonists → spironolactone

Key Points

▶ Cardiac output = heart rate × stroke volume.

▶ BP = cardiac output × systemic vascular resistance.

▶ Most common causes of systolic dysfunction in the United States are uncontrolled HTN, ischemic heart disease, and alcoholic cardiomyopathy.

▶ Three compensatory mechanisms for systolic dysfunction are ventricular hypertrophy, neuroendocrine response, and the Frank-Starling response.

Questions

1. Which of the following pathophysiologic processes results in a concentric hypertrophy rather than eccentric hypertrophy?
   A. Aortic regurgitation
   B. Mitral regurgitation
   C. Aortic stenosis
   D. Ventricular septal defect
   E. Atrial septal defect

2. The most effective agent for acutely decreasing LV preload is:
   A. ACE inhibitors
   B. Hydralazine
   C. Nitroprusside
   D. IV nitrates
   E. Angiotensin receptor blockers

HPI: DD is an 84-year-old man with a history of poorly controlled HTN and mild obesity who is evaluated in your clinic for subacute onset of shortness of breath. He has been admitted for similar episodes of dyspnea 4 times in the past 6 months. Although he is prescribed diltiazem and a diuretic, he admits to poor compliance with his medications.

PE: **Vitals:** BP 230/110 mm Hg, HR 130 beats/min, RR 28 breaths/min, Tmax 36.2°C, and pulse oximetry of 89% on room air. **General:** Tachypneic and using accessory muscles. **H/N:** JVP is 14 cm, pulses are hyperdynamic. **Chest:** Crackles are present half way up bilaterally. **Cardiac:** PMI is hyperdynamic with a palpable S_4, positive S_3 and S_4. **Abdomen:** No hepatosplenomegaly. **Extremity:** 2+/4 bilateral edema to mid-shins. **ECG:** LV hypertrophy. **Chest X-ray (CXR):** Normal-sized heart with moderate interstitial changes consistent with pulmonary edema.

Thought Questions

- What is diastolic heart failure?
- What are the differences between systolic and diastolic dysfunction?
- What are the different causes for diastolic heart failure?
- How are pressure volume loops affected in diastolic heart failure?

Basic Science Review and Discussion

Left ventricular diastolic dysfunction is present when there is clinical evidence of heart failure in the presence of normal ejection fraction. Up to one third of patients with heart failure symptoms have preserved systolic function and present with heart failure secondary to diastolic dysfunction.

Common pathophysiologic conditions associated with diastolic dysfunction include myocardial ischemia and LV hypertrophy secondary to HTN (refer to Thumbnail for full list). In diastolic heart failure, the LV has decreased compliance (increased chamber stiffness) and cannot fill at normal diastolic pressures. As a result, there is reduced LV volume, leading to decreased stroke volume and cardiac output. In addition, the greater than normal LV diastolic filling pressure results in pulmonary and systemic congestion (Figure 2-1).

Initial treatment of CHF secondary to diastolic dysfunction is similar to that of patients with systolic dysfunction. Treatments include supplemental oxygen, diuresis, IV nitroglycerin, and morphine. Long-term treatment of diastolic heart failure is aimed at (1) reducing afterload by controlling HTN, (2) prevention of myocardial ischemia, (3) avoiding tachycardia and promoting bradycardia, (4) improving ventricular relaxation, and (5) decreasing activation of the renin-angiotensin-aldosterone system.

Unlike systolic dysfunction, patients with heart failure secondary to diastolic dysfunction do not tolerate positive inotropic drugs such as milrinone, beta-agonists (dobutamine, dopamine), and digoxin. Because the ejection fraction is already preserved, positive inotropes have little benefit and may worsen underlying myocardial ischemia. In addition, beta-agonists promote tachycardia that can worsen diastolic dysfunction. The benefits of bradycardia include (1) increased coronary perfusion time, (2) decreased myocardial oxygen requirements, and (3) lower ventricular diastolic pressure and improved filling from more complete relaxation between beats.

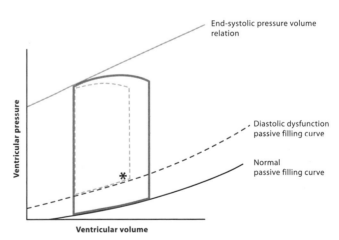

Figure 2-1 Diastolic dysfunction loop. Normal pressure volume loop is indicated by the thick black loop, while the pressure volume loop of diastolic dysfunction is indicated by the dotted loop. In diastolic dysfunction, the passive filling curve of the left ventricle is shifted upward so that at any diastolic volume, the ventricular pressure is greater than normal. As a result, the end-diastolic volume (star) is also reduced due to the reduced filling of the ventricle during diastole.

Case Conclusion   DD initially presents with diastolic heart failure secondary to poorly controlled HTN and poor medical compliance for his calcium channel blocker and diuretic. Bedside echocardiography documents LV hypertrophy and normal LV function. Although there are clinical symptoms and signs of left- and right-sided heart failure, the normal systolic function by echocardiography suggests that diastolic dysfunction is the major contributor to the patient's failure symptoms. The patient is treated with supplemental oxygen, IV lasix, morphine, and IV nitroglycerin, and subsequently improves.

Thumbnail: Etiology and Treatment of Diastolic Dysfunction

Causes of left ventricular diastolic dysfunction	
Pathophysiology	Specific examples
Left ventricular hypertrophy	Aortic stenosis Hypertensive heart disease
Infiltrative cardiomyopathies	Sarcoidosis, amyloidosis, hemochromatosis
Restrictive processes	Endocardial fibrosis, external radiation
Ischemia	Acute myocardial ischemia, chronic coronary artery disease
Miscellaneous	Hypertrophic cardiomyopathy, diabetes

Treatment of left ventricular diastolic dysfunction	
Goal of therapy	Therapeutic intervention
Prevent ischemia	Bypass surgery, angioplasty nitrates, beta-blockers
Reduce fluid overload	Diuretics, salt restriction, dialysis
Control HTN	Beta-blockers, ACE inhibitors, angiotensin II, receptor blockers, calcium channel blockers
Decrease neurohormonal activation	Beta-blockers, ACE inhibitors, spironolactone
Improve ventricular relaxation	Beta-blockers, calcium channel blockers
Prevent tachycardia	Beta-blockers, calcium channel blockers

Key Points

▶ Diastolic dysfunction is defined as clinical evidence of heart failure in patients with normal systolic ejection fraction.

▶ Decreased LV compliance in diastolic dysfunction is the underlying abnormality in diastolic dysfunction.

▶ Although the treatment for systolic dysfunction and diastolic dysfunction are similar, the major difference is the use of positive inotropes in diastolic dysfunction is relatively contraindicated.

Questions

1. A 74-year-old man with a history of hypertensive heart disease will be discharged today after a 2-day stay for management of his CHF secondary to presumptive diastolic dysfunction. Which one of the following treatments would be least effective in the long-term management of his heart failure?

   A. Furosemide
   B. Digoxin
   C. Verapamil
   D. Atenolol
   E. Lisinopril

2. Although beta-blockers are traditionally contraindicated in heart failure secondary to systolic dysfunction, this class of medications is considered beneficial in diastolic dysfunction. The modification of which parameter does not contribute to the beneficial effects of beta-blockers in diastolic dysfunction?

   A. Increasing diastolic filling time
   B. Decreasing myocardial oxygen demand
   C. Improved LV filling secondary to improved relaxation
   D. Decreasing risk of myocardial ischemia
   E. Increasing LV outflow gradient

HPI: JM is a 67-year-old man with cardiac risk factors of cigarette smoking, diabetes, and positive family history. He called 911 after 2 hours of prolonged chest pain associated with dyspnea and diaphoresis. In the emergency department, he is profoundly hypotensive and hypoxic. He is emergently intubated and started on IV dopamine for BP support.

PE: Vitals: BP 80/50 mm Hg, HR 130 beats/min, Tmax 38.1°C, RR 24 breaths/min (on ventilator). **General:** Cool, clammy, cyanotic, intubated. **H/N:** JVP 12 cm, markedly decreased carotid upstroke. **Chest:** Bilateral crackles diffusely. **Cardiac:** Dyskinetic apical impulse with positive S_3 and S_4, 4/6 systolic murmur at base radiating laterally. **Extremities:** Cool with decreased peripheral pulses, mild peripheral edema.

Labs: Hematocrit (HCT) 41.0, white blood cell count (WBC) 11K/mm³, total creatine kinase (CK) 40 U/L, creatinine kinase myocardial band fraction (CK MB) 1%, troponin I < 0.05 mg/mL. **CXR:** Endotracheal tube in good position, marked CHF, normal cardiac silhouette. **ECG:** 4 mm ST elevation in V_1 to V_4.

Thought Questions

- What are the differences between unstable angina, non-ST elevation myocardial infarction (MI), and ST elevation MI?

- What are the pathologic differences between non-ST elevation MI and ST elevation MI?

- What are nonatherosclerotic causes for myocardial ischemia and infarction?

- What are common complications of MI?

Basic Science Review and Discussion

Acute coronary syndrome (ACS) is a broad term that describes all conditions that result from a sudden impairment in blood flow leading to myocardial ischemia. ACS can be subdivided into three categories of increasing severity: (1) unstable angina (USA), (2) non-ST elevation myocardial infarction (NSTEMI), and (3) ST elevation myocardial infarction (STEMI). In contrast to NSTEMI and STEMI, biochemical markers (troponin, CK MB) remain negative in USA because no irreversible myocardial necrosis has occurred. STEMI is clinically differentiated from NSTEMI by the ECG pattern; STEMI is associated with ST elevation and/or new Q waves, while NSTEMI is associated with ST depressions and/or T-wave inversions (Figure 3-1).

NSTEMI and STEMI also relate pathologically to the degree of necrosis within the myocardial wall. NSTEMI is limited to subendocardial infarcts that involve the innermost layers of the myocardium. These inner layers of myocardium are the most susceptible to ischemia because they have the fewest collateral vessels and are subjected to the highest left ventricular wall pressure. STEMI is the most emergent ACS condition because persistent total occlusion results in transmural infarction spanning the entire thickness of the myocardium.

Although ACS is clinically subclassified into three categories, ACS also can be regarded as a clinical continuum, with all three syndromes sharing the underlying pathophysiology of compromised blood flow secondary to plaque disruption and thrombus formation. Over 85% of ACS is secondary to formation of an acute thrombus obstructing an atherosclerotic artery. The remaining 15% of ACS is secondary to nonatherosclerotic causes, including (1) coronary artery spasm (primary, such as Prinzmetal's angina or cocaine induced), (2) markedly increased myocardial oxygen

Nomenclature of Acute Coronary Syndrome (ACS)

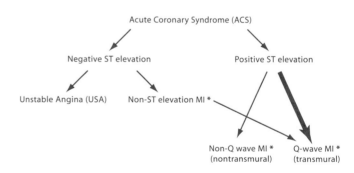

* = positive cardiac marker

Figure 3-1 Acute coronary syndrome (ACS) is divided into three categories: (1) unstable angina (USA), (2) non-ST elevation myocardial infarction (NSTEMI), and (3) ST-elevation myocardial infarction (STEMI). In USA, no myocardial necrosis has occurred and biochemical markers (troponin, CK MB) remain negative. In NSTEMI and STEMI, myocardial necrosis has occurred and biochemical markers are released. The majority of NSTEMI become non-Q wave MI, which is limited to partial myocardial thickness (nontransmural), but a minority of NSTEMI evolve into Q-wave MI, which involve the entire myocardial thickness (transmural). Conversely, the majority of STEMI become Q-wave MI involving the entire thickness of the myocardium, but a small fraction evolve into non-Q wave MI, which involve only a partial thickness of the myocardium.

Table 3-1 Cellular and histopathologic changes with the onset of oxygen deprivation

Feature	Time after MI
Onset of ATP depletion	seconds
Loss of contractility	< 2 min
Irreversible cell injury	20–40 min
Microvascular injury (seen in light microscope)	1–2 h
Beginning of coagulation necrosis, edema, focal hemorrhage	6 h
Hyperemic border with central yellow brown softening	3–7 days
Fibrosis and scarring	7 wk

demand (e.g., aortic stenosis), (3) increased blood viscosity (e.g., polycythemia vera), (4) vasculitis, and (5) anomalous coronary anatomy.

In atherosclerotic ACS, the 75% of thrombi are precipitated by mechanical rupture of the plaque, and 25% are secondary to superficial erosion of the endothelium covering the plaque. Once a plaque ruptures, subendothelial collagen activates platelet aggregation and the coagulation cascade via the extrinsic pathway. Activated platelets release (1) adenosine diphosphate (ADP), which promotes further platelet aggregation, and (2) thromboxane A_2, which can induce vasospasm and further decrease blood flow. Vasospasm is further potentiated by damaged endothelium that is unable to produce vasodilating substances such as nitric oxide and prostacyclin.

Cellular and histopathologic changes occur immediately with the onset of oxygen deprivation as outlined in Table 3-1.

Clinical Presentation and Diagnosis of Acute Coronary Syndrome The clinical presentation of ACS includes the typical substernal chest pressure that is often referred to as the C7-T4 dermatomes, which include the neck, shoulders, and arms. However, up to 20% of patients remain asymptomatic during ACS. Atypical or asymptomatic presentations are especially common in diabetics secondary to their periph-

eral neuropathy. Other symptoms and physical findings are summarized in Table 3-2.

In addition to the clinical signs/symptoms and ECG findings, serum biochemical markers are released into the circulation in STEMI and NSTEMI (but not USA). The two most widely used biochemical markers include (1) CK and the cardiac-specific isoenzyme CK MB and (2) troponin. Both markers begin to rise at 4 to 6 hours and peak at 24 hours, but troponin remains elevated for up to 10 days while CK returns to baseline after 48 hours. Other noncardiac-specific markers that are elevated in STEMI and NSTEMI include

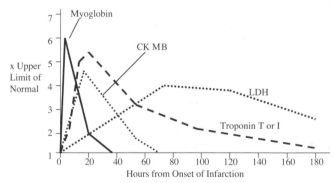

Figure 3-2 Serum markers of myocardial injury. Reprinted with permission from Awtry EH, Gururaj AV, Maytin M, et al. Blueprints in Cardiology. Malden, MA: Blackwell Science, 2003:69.

Table 3-2 Other symptoms and physical findings of ACS

Underlying pathophysiology	Signs and symptoms
Inflammatory response	Low grade fever, increased WBC count, increased erythrocyte sedimentation rate
Increased sympathetic tone	Tachycardia, diaphoresis, tachypnea, cool and clammy skin from vasoconstriction
Increased vagal tone (more common in inferior MI)	Nausea and vomiting, weakness, sinus bradycardia
Decreased LV contractility and compliance	Pulmonary rales and CHF Elevated jugular venous pressure Dyskinetic cardiac impulse S_4 from atrial contraction into noncompliant ischemic LV S_3 from rapid filling in failing LV
Ischemia-induced papillary muscle dysfunction	Ischemia-induced mitral regurgitation

Table 3-3 Complications of ACS

Arrhythmia	Pathophysiology
Ventricular fibrillation	Electrical instability secondary to ischemia
Ventricular tachycardia	
Sinus bradycardia	Excessive vagal output Ischemia of sinoatrial (SA) node
Sinus tachycardia	Increased sympathetic output, pain, CHF
Atrial fibrillation	Atrial ischemia, CHF-induced atrial stretch
1st, 2nd, or 3rd degree heart block	Ischemia of SA node Ischemia of atrioventricular (AV) node (usually seen in inferior MI with occlusion of right coronary artery) Excessive vagal output
Nonarrhythmic complication	**Pathophysiology**
Cardiogenic shock	Decreased cardiac output secondary to ischemia-induced decrease in contractility
CHF	Decreased contractility → systolic dysfunction Increased myocardial stiffness → diastolic dysfunction
Pericarditis	Occurs in 10% of patients post-MI Inflammation extending to peri- and epicardium
Mitral regurgitation	Ischemia-induced papillary muscle dysfunction
Ventricular septal defect	Myocyte necrosis/softening of ventricular septum
Rupture of LV free wall	Myocyte necrosis/softening of LV wall with hemorrhage into pericardial space and tamponade
Pseudoaneurysm of LV free wall	Myocyte necrosis/softening of LV free wall with incomplete rupture secondary to thrombus formation within transmural defect
Aneurysm of LV	Myocyte necrosis and fibrosis with bulging of LV wall Akinetic aneurysm predisposes patient to formation of mural thrombus and subsequent systemic embolization

serum glutamic oxaloacetic transferase (SGOT), lactate dehyrogenase (LDH), and myoglobin.

Complications of Acute Coronary Syndrome Complications of ACS can be subdivided into arrhythmic and nonarrhythmic categories as outlined in Table 3-3. Ventricular fibrillation is the most common reason for sudden cardiac death associated with myocardial infarction.

Treatment of Acute Coronary Syndromes Myocardial ischemia and infarction results from an imbalance of oxygen supply and demand. This imbalance is generated by interaction between five pathophysiologic processes that current treatments attempt to address. In general, the treatment for USA and NSTEMI is medical and includes beta-blockers, aspirin, nitrates, and heparin. However, in STEMI with complete and prolonged occlusion of a coronary artery, the goal of treatment is reperfusion by means of angioplasty or thrombolysis (Table 3-4).

Table 3-4 Etiology and treatment

Pathophysiologic etiology	Treatment
Mechanical obstruction	Angioplasty/stenting or coronary bypass surgery Thrombolysis
Dynamic obstruction/spasm (Prinzmetal's angina)	Nitrates Calcium channel blockers
Thrombosis	Heparin, low-molecular-weight heparin Direct thrombin inhibitors Aspirin, clopidogrel (ADP receptor inhibitor) IIbIIIa receptor antagonists
Increased oxygen demand	Beta-blockers, supplemental oxygen Nitrates, morphine, transfusion if anemic
Inflammation	Statins, aspirin

Case Conclusion   JM is in cardiogenic shock from an ST elevation MI secondary to an occlusion of his proximal left anterior descending (LAD) artery (ST elevation is in LAD distribution). His profound hypotension and CHF is secondary to two processes: (1) ischemic systolic dysfunction and (2) ischemia-induced papillary muscle rupture resulting in a flail mitral leaflet (4/6 murmur on examination). Although his clinical presentation, low-grade fever, leukocytosis, and ECG are consistent with ST elevation MI, the troponin and CK were negative on admission because 4 to 6 hours must elapse from infarction onset before significant elevation of these biochemical markers may be observed. JM subsequently developed ventricular fibrillation requiring electrical defibrillation before he was brought to the cardiac catheterization laboratory, where his LAD artery was successfully opened with angioplasty and stenting.

Thumbnail: Summary of Acute Coronary Syndromes

Syndrome	EKG findings	Biochemical markers	Treatment	Coronary lesion	Myocardial lesion
ST elevation MI	ST elevation New Q waves	Positive troponin or CK MB	Angioplasty Thrombolysis Aspirin Oxygen Beta-blockers Nitrates	Persistent thrombotic total occlusion	Transmural MI
Non-ST elevation MI	ST depression T-wave inversion No ST elevation No new Q wave	Positive troponin or CK MB	Aspirin Heparin Beta-blockers Oxygen Nitrates	Transient thrombotic total occlusion or thrombotic severe stenosis	Partial-thickness MI
Unstable angina	ST depression T-wave inversion No ST elevation No new Q wave	Negative troponin or CK MB	Aspirin Heparin Beta-blockers Oxygen Nitrates	Transient thrombotic total occlusion or thrombotic severe stenosis	Myocardium at ischemic risk

Key Points

▶ All three subcategories of ACS (USA, NSTEMI, and STEMI) share the same underlying pathophysiology (rupture or erosion of a vulnerable plaque).

▶ Biochemical markers (troponin and CK) are not elevated in USA but are elevated in MI (NSTEMI and STEMI).

▶ While the treatment for USA and NSTEMI is medical stabilization with aspirin, heparin, beta-blockers, oxygen, and nitrates, the management of STEMI is immediate reperfusion with angioplasty or thrombolysis.

▶ Ventricular fibrillation is the most common cause of sudden cardiac death within the first 24 hours of myocardial ischemia; therefore, telemetry (constant ECG monitoring) is essential for all patients admitted for acute coronary syndromes.

Questions

1. JF is an 80-year-old male diabetic who is a very poor historian. His family escorts him to your emergency room because he complained of an episode of acute dyspnea 8 days ago. His ECG is now normal but you are concerned that JF may have had an NSTEMI-induced CHF episode 8 days ago. Which biochemical test would be the most helpful to determine whether or not he had an infarct 8 days ago?

   A. CK
   B. SGOT
   C. Troponin I
   D. LDH
   E. Myoglobin

2. A 58-year-old man presents with chest pain, severe nausea, elevated JVP, pulsatile liver, severe bradycardia degenerating into third-degree heart block, with ST elevation in the inferior leads (II, III, aVF). Despite his severe hypotension with a blood pressure of 70/30 mm Hg, his lungs are clear and there is no evidence of heart failure. On angiography, which vessel is the most likely culprit vessel?

   A. LAD artery
   B. Circumflex artery
   C. Diagonal artery
   D. Right coronary artery
   E. Obtuse marginal artery

HPI: GS is a 76-year-old man with past medical history remarkable for diabetes, HTN, and smoking. He presents to your clinic with a chief complaint of transient monocular blindness, left lower extremity claudication, and new-onset chest pressure that begins after climbing two flights of stairs and resolves spontaneously with rest. He also notes his HTN has been difficult to control with multiple medications.

PE: **Vitals:** BP 180/90 mm Hg, HR 70 beats/min, RR 16 breaths/min, Tmax 37°C. **H/N:** Left carotid bruit, AV nicking on fundoscopic exam. **Chest:** Clear to auscultation. **Cardiac:** Mildly enlarged PMI, normal S_1, S_2, and positive S_3, no significant murmurs. **Abdomen:** Mid-abdominal bruit. **Extremities:** Bilateral femoral bruits with decreased left dorsalis pedis pulses. **ECG:** Anterior T-wave inversions.

Labs: Total cholesterol 300 mg/dL, LDL 190 mg/dL.

Thought Questions

- What are the three layers of the artery and what are their individual functions?

- What is the natural histopathologic progression of atherosclerosis?

- What is meant by the "response to injury" hypothesis for atherosclerosis initiation?

- Once an atherosclerotic plaque is established, what event triggers an MI?

- What are the common cardiac and extracardiac clinical manifestations of atherosclerosis?

Basic Science Review and Discussion

Atherosclerosis is the progressive infiltration of lipids and inflammatory cells within medium to large muscular arteries, leading to thickening and loss of elasticity of the arterial wall. This disease process is localized to the intimal layer of the arterial wall (Figure 4-1).

The wall of a muscular artery is composed of three distinct layers:

1. The **intima** is composed of the continuous, single-cell layered endothelium with underlying connective tissue and internal elastic lamina. The internal elastic lamina separates the intima from the media. The endothelial layer has three important functions: (a) regulate vascular tone, (b) establish blood-tissue permeability, (c) and determine vascular response to hemostasis and inflammation.

2. The **media** is the thickest of the three layers and is composed primarily of concentric layers of smooth muscle cells and their associated extracellular matrix (elastic and collagen fibers). Smooth muscle cells are the most prevalent cell type in arteries, constituting more than 95% of all cells. The smooth muscle layer allows the intima to constrict and dilate the artery. Smooth muscle tone is modulated both by local mechanisms (nitric oxide → relaxation, endothelin/angiotensin II → contraction) as well as systemic factors (sympathetic tone).

3. The **adventitia** is the outermost layer and is composed of the external elastic lamina, fibroblasts, sympathetic nerve terminals, and adipocytes. The adventitia also carries lymphatics and a blood supply (vaso vasorum), which penetrate the outer one third of the media. The external elastic lamina demarcates the media from the adventitia. The adventitia is a connective tissue structure that integrates the vessel into the surrounding tissue.

Three types of atherosclerotic plaques representing different stages of atherosclerosis have been described based on histopathologic studies: (1) **fatty streaks** are intimal accumulation of lipid-laden macrophages (**foam cells**) that do not affect blood flow, (2) **fibrous plaques** are heterogeneous structures with a smooth muscle/extracellular matrix cap covering a lipid/inflammatory cell core within the

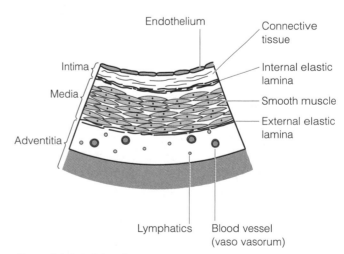

Figure 4-1 Arterial wall.

deeper part of the plaque, and (3) complicated lesions are plaques that also contain hematoma or thrombi in addition to the lipids, fibrous issue, and inflammatory cells. Complicated lesions result from rupture of a fibrous plaque and are the primary structures underlying the morbidity and mortality associated with atherosclerosis.

A "response to injury" underlies the pathogenesis of atherosclerosis. The primary event is injury to the endothelium by factors such as diabetes mellitus, hyperlipidemia, HTN, smoking, and other risk factors for atherosclerosis. After the endothelium is damaged, low-density lipoprotein (LDL) particles accumulate within the intima and become oxidized.

Oxidized LDL leads to the release of leukocyte adhesion molecules (VCAM-1) and chemotactic cytokines (chemokines), which recruit monocytes and T-cell lymphocytes into the intima. Activated T cells within the intima produce proinflammatory cytokines [interferon-γ and tumor necrosis factor-α (TNF-α)], which activate macrophages and smooth muscle cells. The monocytes then differentiate into macrophages with a capacity to internalize oxidized LDL via cell surface scavenger receptors. The lipid-laden macrophage is then transformed into a foam cell as oxidized LDL builds up within the inflammatory cell. The accumulation of foam cells results in a fatty streak.

Although fatty streaks may disappear spontaneously, some streaks become fibrous plaques, especially at sites subject to hemodynamic stress. Macrophages release (1) platelet-derived growth factor (PDGF), which promotes smooth muscle cell proliferation, and (2) vascular endothelial growth factor (VEGF), which promotes endothelial cell proliferation. Cell migration/proliferation and synthesis of collagen and proteoglycans occur, leading to the formation of a fibrous cap that separates the lipid-filled core from the injured endothelium.

Once the luminal size of the vessel has been reduced to 60% to 70% in cross-sectional area by a fibrous plaque, exertional angina develops. A decrease in resting coronary blood flow (rest angina) does not occur until the stenosis is greater than 90%. However, acute clinical events such as MI or thrombotic/embolic cerebrovascular accidents occur when a thrombus forms on the fibrous plaque. Plaque rupture results when macrophages within the plaque release matrix metalloproteinases that can digest the collagen within the cap. Although plaque rupture and thrombus formation often precipitate an acute coronary syndrome, the endogenous fibrinolytic system can counteract complete lumen obstruction by thrombus.

Although atherosclerosis is the underlying process in coronary artery disease, there are many clinically relevant extracardiac manifestations of atherosclerosis. Atherosclerotic disease of the peripheral arteries can manifest as claudication in peripheral vascular disease or acute limb ischemia with total occlusion of the vessel. Emboli from atherosclerotic disease in the aortic arch or carotid arteries can result in cerebral vascular accidents.

Case Conclusion GS presents to your clinic with severe peripheral vascular disease and coronary artery disease secondary to aggressive atherosclerosis secondary to multiple risk factors. His transient monocular blindness is secondary to atheroembolic disease from his critical left carotid stenosis (left carotid bruit). The refractory HTN is secondary to renal artery stenosis (abdominal bruits). His chest pressure is secondary to stable angina and significant coronary artery stenosis. His reduced left lower extremity pulses and left leg claudication are secondary to severe stenosis of his left common femoral artery.

Thumbnail: Risk Factors for Atherosclerosis and End-Organ Damage Secondary to Atherosclerosis

Risk factors for atherosclerosis		
Nonmodifiable factors	Modifiable factors	Other factors
Increased age	Smoking	Diabetes
Male sex	Blood pressure	Obesity
Ethnic group	Hyperlipidemia	Increased homocysteine
Family history	Sedentary lifestyle	Elevated C-reactive protein
End-organ damage secondary to atherosclerosis		
Organ system	Manifestation	
Cardiac	Coronary artery disease and myocardial ischemia	
CNS	Embolic stroke from carotid or aortic arch atheroembolism	
Renal	Refractory hypertension from renal artery stenosis	
Gastrointestinal	Mesenteric ischemia from mesenteric artery stenosis	
Musculoskeletal	Claudication from atherosclerosis-induced arterial insufficiency	
Vascular	Atherosclerosis-induced aortic dissection or abdominal aneurysm Acute limb ischemia from atheroembolic phenomenon	

Key Points

▶ The atherosclerotic process is a "response-to-injury" process that is initiated by endothelial damage.

▶ The histopathologic sequence of atherosclerosis is (1) fatty streak, (2) fibrous plaque, (3) complicated lesion.

▶ The rupture of the complicated lesion with subsequent occlusion of the artery by thrombus formation is the underlying event in acute coronary syndromes and thrombotic/embolic cerebrovascular events.

Questions

1. What percentage of the arterial lumen must be occluded with atherosclerotic plaque before stable angina develops?

   A. 20%
   B. 40%
   C. 70%
   D. 80%
   E. 90%

2. Which of the following developmental drugs would be unlikely to pass efficacy testing in the prevention of atherosclerosis progression?

   A. Oxidized LDL scavenger
   B. Matrix metalloproteinase inhibitor
   C. Monoclonal anti-PDGF antibody
   D. TNF-α epitope analogue
   E. Enhanced aspirin

HPI: JL is a 52-year-old woman who recently emigrated from Southeast Asia. She presents to the clinic with chief complaints of palpitations, coughing, and dyspnea on exertion. Her past medical history is notable for severe febrile illness as a child associated with sore throat and a heart murmur since childhood.

PE: **Vitals:** T 37.0°C, HR 106 beats/min (irregular), BP 110/80 mm Hg, RR 22 breaths/min. **H/N:** Malar erythema, JVP 12 cm with positive hepatojugular reflex. **Chest:** Bilateral crackles one third of the way up. **Cardiac:** NL PMI with right ventricular (RV) heave, accentuated P_2 with opening snap (OS), 2/6 diastolic decrescendo murmur. **Extremities:** 2+/4 peripheral edema. **CXR:** Mild pulmonary edema. **ECG:** Atrial fibrillation with right ventricular hypertrophy (RVH).

Thought Questions

- What are the most common causes of mitral stenosis and mitral regurgitation (MR)?

- How do the physical findings change over time with progression of mitral stenosis?

- What maneuvers can be performed to increase/decrease MR?

- What are common causes of secondary triscuspid regurgitation?

Basic Science Review and Discussion

Mitral Stenosis Over 90% of mitral stenosis cases are secondary to rheumatic fever. Other rare causes include systemic lupus erythematosus and carcinoid tumors. Complications of untreated mitral stenosis include systemic embolism from thrombus, severe pulmonary HTN, endocarditis, and pulmonary edema.

Pathophysiology The normal mitral valve can open 4 to 6 cm² in cross-sectional area. The onset of clinical symptoms occurs when the mitral valve area is less than 2.5 cm². Narrowing of the mitral valve results in increased left atrial (LA) pressure, which is then transmitted retrograde to the pulmonary and right heart circulation. LA HTN results in several pathophysiologic effects:

1. LA enlargement, which increases the risk of atrial fibrillation.

2. The reduced ability of the LA to empty during diastole results in increased stasis of blood within the LA. Low-velocity flow, compounded with atrial fibrillation, increases the risk of intracardiac thrombus formation and systemic thromboembolism. Twenty percent of patients diagnosed with mitral stenosis and not on anticoagulation present with a LA thrombus.

3. Cardiac output is reduced in severe mitral stenosis. The degree of cardiac output impairment is inversely related to the heart rate. The long diastole that occurs with relative bradycardia allows for decompression of the overfilled LA and reduction of the mean LA pressure. Conversely, relative tachycardia shortens the time period for diastolic emptying and results in a dramatically increased mitral valve gradient and higher mean LA pressure.

4. Reduced ejection fraction (EF) is noted in one third of patients with mitral stenosis. The reduced EF is secondary to (a) reduced preload of the left ventricle, (b) scarring of the LV secondary to the rheumatic carditis, and (c) increased afterload from vasoconstriction and neurohormonal activation.

5. In the initial phases of severe mitral stenosis, elevated pulmonary pressures result in pulmonary edema from transudation of fluid once LA pressures exceed 25 to 28 mm Hg. With chronic pulmonary HTN, there is reactive narrowing and intimal hyperplasia of the pulmonary circulation. Although this thickening of capillaries decreases the risk of pulmonary edema (so that LA pressures must be much higher than 28 mm Hg in order to induce pulmonary edema), prolonged pulmonary HTN results in RVH, RV dilatation, and right-heart failure.

History Although severe mitral stenosis can appear as early as 5 years after an acute rheumatic fever episode, symptomatic mitral stenosis usually does not present until several decades after. The major symptoms are dyspnea and fatigue secondary to pulmonary edema and decreased cardiac output, respectively. Chest fullness or atypical chest pain may result from pulmonary HTN. RVH and RV failure can lead to peripheral edema. LA enlargement can compress the left main bronchus and induce a cough. Systemic embolization from intra-atrial thrombus and atrial fibrillation are additional presentations. If the above symptoms persist despite maximal medical therapy, percutaneous mitral valve valvotomy or mitral valve surgery should be considered (Table 5-1).

Physical examination

1. RV heave associated with pulmonary hypertension, RVH, and RV dilatation.

Table 5-1 Severity of mitral stenosis

Stage	Cross-sectional area (cm²)	Symptoms
Minimal	> 2.5 cm	None
Mild	1.4–2.5	Minimal dyspnea on exertion, mild fatigue
Moderate	1.0–1.4	Moderate dyspnea on exertion, orthopnea
Severe	< 1.0	Dyspnea at rest

2. Peripheral edema from right-sided heart failure.

3. Malar flush, otherwise known as "mitral valve facies" secondary to systemic vasoconstriction and decreased cardiac output.

4. Characteristic auscultation findings include (a) accentuated P_2 associated with pulmonary HTN; (b) loud S_1 secondary to abrupt closure of the mitral valve leaflets that were held wide open by the prolonged transmitral pressure gradient; (c) OS after S_2 secondary to abrupt deceleration of the mitral valve leaflets (the S_2-OS interval shortens with progression of mitral stenosis, and the OS may be inaudible in severe mitral stenosis); (d) diastolic, rumbling, decrescendo murmur starting with the OS. As the mitral stenosis becomes more severe, the longer it takes for the LA to empty during diastole, and the longer the murmur lasts.

Management

Medical treatment

1. Minimize the hemodynamic consequences of stenosis by limiting exercise and starting beta-blockers, calcium channel blockers, and/or digoxin to maintain relative bradycardia, maximize diastolic filling period, and minimize trans-mitral valve gradient.

2. Anticoagulation for patients with history of recurrent atrial fibrillation or recurrent atrial fibrillation.

3. Antibiotic prophylaxis to prevent endocarditis and recurrent rheumatic fever.

4. Percutaneous mitral balloon valvotomy in patients who are suitable candidates (absence of severe MR, severe mitral valve calcification, and/or thickening).

Surgical treatment   Surgical options include commissurotomy or mitral valve replacement. Mitral valve replacement is indicated for patients with mitral stenosis compounded with MR and patients with severely deformed valves.

Mitral Regurgitation   MR is the second most common valvular lesion in the United States. The mitral valve apparatus includes not only the valve itself but also the chordae tendineae, papillary muscles, and the mitral valve annulus.

As a result, malfunction of any of these components can lead to mitral valve regurgitation. The most common cause of MR is myxomatous degeneration mitral valve prolapse followed by ischemic heart disease. Other causes of MR include endocarditis, rheumatic heart disease, collagen vascular disease, chordal rupture, and dexfenfluramine and fenfluramine use.

Pathophysiology   The pathophysiologic response of the heart depends on whether the MR is acute or chronic. In acute-onset MR, there is an acute increase in LV preload from both the pathologic regurgitant fraction and the physiologic pulmonary venous inflow. With increased preload, stroke volume is increased by the Frank-Starling mechanism, but because a large fraction of the stroke volume is retrograde, the effective forward cardiac output is decreased. The sudden volume overload within the LV also increases LV end-diastolic pressure, which in turn raises LA pressure and pulmonary artery pressure. Pulmonary edema and dyspnea ensue when LA pressures exceed 25 to 28 mm Hg.

In chronic, compensated MR, the left ventricle adapts to the volume overload by eccentric LV hypertrophy. The lengthening of individual cardiomyocytes causes the LV to dilate, and the total mass is increased. Because contractile function remains the same, a larger diastolic volume can be accommodated with a resultant increase in stroke volume and forward cardiac output. The thinning of the LV wall also increases LV compliance, permitting the dilated LV to fill during diastole while maintaining a relatively normal LV end-diastolic pressure (which will prevent pulmonary edema). LA dilatation also occurs in response to MR. The dilated LA is also more compliant and allows for increased regurgitant volume without a rise in pulmonary artery pressures, which could cause pulmonary congestion. However, a chronically dilated LA is predisposed to atrial fibrillation.

Over time, chronic, compensated MR can degenerate into decompensated MR. With prolonged LV dilatation (which increases the radius) and decreased LV wall thickness, the LV transmural stress increases (remember LaPlace's law: stress = (pressure × radius)/thickness) to the point where the LV systolic function declines. With the decline in systolic function, the LV end-diastolic volume and pressure increase, with resultant pulmonary congestion and dyspnea.

History   Mild to moderate MR or chronic severe MR may not be symptomatic. On the other hand, in acute MR or chronic decompensated MR there is a rise in pressures within the left-sided heart chambers, and patients present with symptoms of CHF (dyspnea, orthopnea, and fatigue) secondary to pulmonary congestion and decreased cardiac output.

Physical examination   An apical holosystolic murmur radiates to the axilla and is usually accompanied by a third

Table 5-2 Provocative maneuvers

Maneuver	Hemodynamic effect	Effect on murmur intensity
Handgrip	Increases afterload	MR increases but no change in aortic stenosis (AS)
Premature ventricular contractions	Increased stroke volume	AS increases but no change in MR

heart sound. In acute, severe MR the systolic murmur is short and soft because the pressure in the small, noncompliant atrium rises quickly and reduces/shortens the pressure gradient between the LV and LA during systole. The provocative maneuvers outlined in Table 5-2 can be performed to differentiate between aortic stenosis versus MR (both systolic murmurs).

Management In the hemodynamically stable patient, the medical treatment of choice for acute MR is sodium nitroprusside. As a vasodilator, nitroprusside lowers the afterload, which improves forward cardiac output and decreases the regurgitant fraction. In the hemodynamically unstable patient with severe MR, an intra-aortic balloon counterpulsation is the treatment of choice. Counterpulsation decreases afterload and helps maintain the diastolic blood pressure.

In chronic MR, vasodilator therapy (ACE inhibitors, angiotensin receptor blockers) is also used to augment forward cardiac flow. With the onset of heart failure symptoms, standard CHF therapy is initiated (diuretics and digoxin).

Surgical treatment Surgical treatment includes three alternatives: (1) mitral valve repair, (2) mitral valve replacement with conservation of the mitral valve apparatus, and (3) standard mitral valve replacement with no conservation of the mitral valve apparatus. Mitral valve repair is the preferred method of treatment since repair preserves the mitral valve apparatus and obviates the need for anticoagulation or a prosthetic valve. Mitral valve replacement with chordal preservation is preferred if mitral valve function cannot be restored by repair alone (severely deformed rheumatic mitral valve). The standard mitral valve replacement with removal of the mitral apparatus is avoided when possible. Although valve competence is ensured, removal of the subvalvular structures damages the LV, with a resultant decrease in LV performance. Surgery should be considered in acute, severe MR. In chronic, stable MR, surgery is indicated in the following situations:

1. Patient becomes symptomatic.
2. LV EF falls below 60%.
3. Dilatation of the LV so that the end-systolic dimension is greater than 45 mm.
4. Development of pulmonary HTN.

Tricuspid Stenosis Tricuspid stenosis is a rare condition caused by rheumatic heart disease or carcinoid syndrome.

Pathophysiology and history The stenotic tricuspid valve results in right atrial (RA) HTN and right-sided failure signs and symptoms (ascites, peripheral edema). A gradient of greater than 5 mm Hg is considered severe, and therapy is required.

Physical examination

1. Diastolic rumble across left sternal border: murmur increases with inspiration because of increase right heart flow.
2. Distended neck veins with a large "a" wave because of the RA contraction against a stenotic tricuspid valve.
3. Ascites and peripheral edema.

Management If diuretics are not effective in relieving the right-sided failure symptoms, tricuspid valvulotomy or surgical valve replacement should be considered.

Tricuspid Regurgitation The etiologies for **tricuspid regurgitation (TR)** are divided between primary causes and secondary causes (Table 5-3). The most common cause of tricuspid regurgitation is secondary to pulmonary HTN. The most common cause of primary tricuspid regurgitation is bacterial endocarditis.

Pathophysiology In tricuspid regurgitation, systemic venous pressures are elevated, resulting in right-sided heart failure symptoms (peripheral edema, elevated jugular venous pressure, and ascites). In response to chronic volume or pressure overload, the right-sided heart chambers hypertrophy and dilate.

Table 5-3 Causes of tricuspid regurgitation

Primary etiologies	Secondary etiologies
Bacterial endocarditis	Pulmonary HTN
Trauma	Mitral stenosis
RV infarction	Atrial septal defect/intracardiac shunts
Myxomatous degeneration	LV failure/RV dilation

History Although no specific history or symptoms are directly attributable to tricuspid regurgitation, the constellation of symptoms are similar to generalized right-sided heart failure (fatigue, dyspnea, edema, ascites, RUQ tenderness from hepatic congestion).

Physical Examination

1. Distended neck veins with a prominent V wave (secondary to the regurgitant fraction of blood during systole that is transmitted retrograde from the RV to RA and then to jugular veins).
2. RUQ tenderness and increased liver span from hepatic congestion.
3. Ascites and peripheral edema.

4. RV heave/lift on palpation of precordium secondary to the enlarged RV.
5. Accentuated P_2 if pulmonary HTN is present.
6. TR murmur is a soft, holosystolic murmur located over the left sternal border and increases with inspiration.

Management Because tricuspid regurgitation is most often secondary to another cause [pulmonary HTN secondary to chronic obstructive pulmonary disease (COPD), pulmonary embolism, connective tissue disease, etc.], treating the underlying cause is the mainstay of therapy. Medical therapy with vasodilators for primary tricuspid regurgitation has minimal effect since the pulmonary vascular resistance is already low. Tricuspid valve replacement/repair should be considered if the patient has RV failure.

Case Conclusion JL presents with mitral stenosis secondary to rheumatic fever as a child. As a result of long-standing, undiagnosed mitral stenosis, she presents with coughing due to compression of the left mainstem bronchus by LA enlargement. Increased LA filling pressures have caused pulmonary congestion and pulmonary HTN (accentuated P_2) with resultant RV hypertrophy. Elevated right-sided filling pressures have caused right-sided heart failure with an elevated JVP and peripheral edema. The atrial fibrillation secondary to LA enlargement and the "mitral valve facies" are also associated with mitral stenosis.

Thumbnail: Auscultation and Physical Findings of Mitral and Tricuspid Valve Disease

Valvular abnormality	Physical Findings	Auscultation
Mitral stenosis	Malar erythema Atrial fibrillation RV lift Peripheral edema	Loud S_1 and OS Diastolic rumble S_2–OS interval shortens with progression of MS Accentuated P_2 in pulmonary HTN
MR	if acute → pulmonary edema if chronic → PMI enlarged and displaced	Holosystolic murmur at apex radiating to axilla S_3 present
Tricuspid stenosis	Ascites Peripheral edema	Diastolic rumbling at LSB Murmur increased, with inspiration
Tricuspid regurgitation	Prominent V waves of neck veins Enlarged, pulsatile liver Possible ascites and edema RV sternal lift	Holosystolic murmur at LSB Murmur increased with inspiration

---

Key Points

- In addition to the hemodynamic consequences, mitral stenosis places the patient at much higher risk for endocarditis and systemic thromboembolic disease.
- MR can result not only from a defect of the valve itself, but also from any other components of the mitral valve apparatus (chordae, papillary muscles, or mitral valve annulus).
- The pathophysiologic response to MR depends on whether the onset of MR is acute or chronic.
- The most common cause of tricuspid regurgitation is pulmonary HTN.

Questions

Please refer to Figures 5-1 through 5-5 with regard to the following questions:

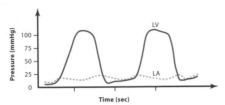

Figure 5-1 Tracing 1.

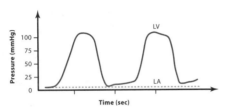

Figure 5-2 Tracing 2.

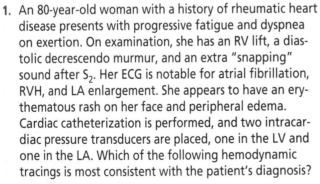

Figure 5-3 Tracing 3.

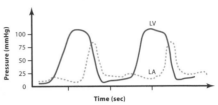

Figure 5-4 Tracing 4.

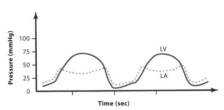

Figure 5-5 Tracing 5.

1. An 80-year-old woman with a history of rheumatic heart disease presents with progressive fatigue and dyspnea on exertion. On examination, she has an RV lift, a diastolic decrescendo murmur, and an extra "snapping" sound after S_2. Her ECG is notable for atrial fibrillation, RVH, and LA enlargement. She appears to have an erythematous rash on her face and peripheral edema. Cardiac catheterization is performed, and two intracardiac pressure transducers are placed, one in the LV and one in the LA. Which of the following hemodynamic tracings is most consistent with the patient's diagnosis?

   A. Tracing 1
   B. Tracing 2
   C. Tracing 3
   D. Tracing 4
   E. Tracing 5

2. The patient above underwent a percutaneous procedure to repair the affected valve. After 2 days, she becomes more short of breath and a holosystolic murmur radiating laterally is detected. Cardiac catheterization with two transducers, one in the LV and one in the LA, is performed again. Which of the following hemodynamic tracings is consistent with the patient's diagnosis?

   A. Tracing 1
   B. Tracing 2
   C. Tracing 3
   D. Tracing 4
   E. Tracing 5

HPI: AB is a 76-year-old Asian man who presents with new-onset syncope. He denies palpitations or angina but experiences dyspnea with mild exertion and early fatigue. His past medical history is notable for diabetes, HTN, and a severe childhood febrile illness with associated sore throat. AB has also experienced a persistent cardiac murmur since the childhood illness.

PE: **Vitals:** T 37.0°C, HR 70 beats/min, BP 160/80 mm Hg, RR 16 breaths/min, JVP 7 cm with slow carotid upstroke and decreased carotid volume. **Chest:** Clear to auscultation. **Cardiac:** Sustained enlarged, PMI with late-peaking 4/6 systolic murmur at right sternal border radiating into the neck and single second heart sound. OS present after S_2 with a 2/4 diastolic decrescendo murmur. **Extremities:** No edema. **CXR:** Mild cardiomegaly. **ECG:** Normal sinus rhythm with LV hypertrophy.

Thought Questions

- How is the diagnosis of rheumatic fever established?

- What are the three symptoms typically associated with aortic stenosis (AS)?

- How does the LV adapt to AS versus aortic regurgitation (AR)?

- What physical findings are associated with severe AR?

- What are the hemodynamic consequences of acute versus chronic mitral regurgitation?

Basic Science Review and Discussion

Rheumatic Heart Disease   Rheumatic fever (RF) is secondary to untreated group A streptococcus (GAS) pharyngitis. RF is an inflammatory condition involving primarily the connective tissue of the heart, joints, and CNS. The pathogenesis is unclear but is thought to be secondary to an autoimmune response between rheumatogenic streptococcal antigens and human tissue epitopes. The diagnosis of an acute initial attack is summarized in Table 6-1. After establishing evidence of a previous GAS infection by throat culture or rising GAS antibody titers, the presence of two major manifestations or one major and two minor manifestations suggests diagnosis of RF.

RF carditis involves all three layers of the heart (endocardium, myocardium, and pericardium) and is almost always associated with a valvulitis involving the **mitral** and **aortic** valves. The median age for RF is 9 to 11 years. During the initial RF attack, mitral regurgitation is the most common valvular manifestation, with AR the second most common. The pulmonic and tricuspid valves are rarely involved. The symptoms of rheumatic valve scarring do not usually become apparent until 10 to 30 years after the initial RF episode. After the initial RF episode, 40% of patients will develop mitral stenosis and 25% will develop AR or AS in addition to mitral stenosis.

Although the prevalence is only 0.6 per 1000 U.S. school-aged children, it is the most common acquired heart disease in children and young adults worldwide (up to 21 per 1000 Asian school-aged children). Treatment of GAS pharyngitis virtually eliminates the risk for progression to RF, but up to 3% of untreated GAS pharyngitis may progress to RF after a 3-week latency period. Treatment of the acute RF episode is largely supportive, with salicylates or steroids to decrease inflammation and penicillin to treat residual GAS. After the initial attack of RF, the patient is at risk for recurrent RF attacks and therefore requires long-term continuous antibiotic prophylaxis (10 years to lifelong depending on residual valvular disease).

Aortic Stenosis

Etiology and pathogenesis   AS is the most common valve lesion in the United States. There are three forms of AS: (1) congenital/bicuspid, (2) rheumatic/postinflammatory, and (3) senile/degenerative. The etiology of AS depends on the patient's age group (Table 6-2). Among patients under age 70, the most common cause is a congenitally bicuspid aortic valve. Over age 70, the most common cause is degenerative/senile AS. Both diabetes and hypercholesterolemia are risk factors for degenerative AS, and degenerative AS is associated with HTN and smoking.

Pathophysiology   The normal aortic valve area (AVA) is greater than 3.0 cm². In AS, the increased resistance across the aortic valve imposes a chronic pressure overload on the

Table 6-1 Diagnosis of an acute initial attack

Major manifestations	Minor manifestations
Carditis	Arthralgias
Polyarthritis	Fever
Chorea Erythema marginatum	Increased acute phase reactants (ESR, C-reactive protein)
Subcutaneous nodules	Prolonged PR interval

Table 6-2 Causes of aortic stenosis

Under 70 years old		Over 70 years old	
50%	Bicuspid	48%	Degenerative
25%	Postinflammatory	27%	Bicuspid
18%	Degenerative	23%	Postinflammatory
3%	Unicommisural	2%	Unknown
2%	Hypoplastic		
2%	Unknown		

LV. To compensate for the pressure overload, the LV hypertrophies in order to decrease LV wall stress according to the law of Laplace. The law of Laplace states that stress across the ventricular wall generated by increasing pressure or increasing LV dimensions is inversely proportional to the wall thickness:

$$\text{Stress} = \frac{\text{Pressure} \times \text{Radius}}{2 \times \text{Thickness}}$$

However, with progressive LV hypertrophy, abnormal pathophysiologic mechanisms set in with:

1. Reduced LV compliance and resultant increased left ventricular end-diastolic pressure (LVEDP).

2. Left atrial hypertrophy secondary to increased LVEDP and increased atrial contribution to diastolic filling.

3. Decreased coronary blood flow.

4. Increased myocardial oxygen demand from three pathophysiologic processes: (a) increased muscle mass, (b) increased wall stress, and (c) a decreased perfusion pressure gradient between the aorta and subendocardium; as a result of the increased oxygen demand, angina occurs.

5. Eventual CHF secondary to insurmountable afterload and subsequent LV dilatation and systolic dysfunction.

History AS presents as a gradual disease and, unlike mitral stenosis, patients usually remain well compensated and asymptomatic for many years. When symptoms develop, the valve area is usually 0.6 cm². The four common AS-associated clinical presentations are:

1. Angina—50% of patients with severe AS have concomitant significant coronary artery disease (CAD). In patients without CAD, angina is due to increased oxygen demand.

2. Syncope—secondary to reduced cerebral perfusion during exercise when systemic blood pressure declines as a result of a fixed cardiac output and an increase in systemic vasodilatation.

3. Heart failure—secondary to LV dilatation and decreased systolic function.

4. GI bleeding—either idiopathic or angiodysplasia of the right colon.

The latency period from the onset of severe symptoms to the average age of death is approximately 5 years for angina, 3 years of syncope, and 2 years for CHF.

Physical examination Arterial pulse rises slowly, is sustained, and is small in volume. Cardiac impulse is sustained and will become inferolaterally displaced with LV dilatation and failure. A systolic thrill may be appreciated upon palpation of the precordium. Upon auscultation, S_1 is normal, and S_2 may be single for three reasons: (1) immobility of the aortic valve makes A_2 inaudible, (2) P_2 is buried in the prolonged ejection murmur, or (3) A_2 coincides with P_2 because of the prolonged LV systolic phase. S_4 may also be present because atrial contraction is increased. A prolonged LV systolic phase may also result in paradoxical splitting with P_2 before A_2. The systolic AS murmur is mid-peaking, loudest at the base, and transmitted cranially along both carotid vessels. Occasionally, high-frequency components radiate to the apex and may be confused for mitral regurgitation (Gallavardin phenomenon). As the stenosis becomes more severe, the murmur peaks later in systole and becomes longer in duration. Finally, as the LV fails and cardiac output declines, the systolic murmur becomes softer.

Management

Medical treatment Symptomatic candidates with severe AS should be referred to surgery because medical management has little influence on the disease course. Patients with severe AS should also avoid vigorous physical activity. In asymptomatic patients (or in nonoperative candidates), the three components of medical therapy include:

1. Digoxin—if LV filling is increased or EF is reduced.

2. Diuretics—for fluid overload from LV dysfunction but must not overdiurese. Over diuresis may result in hypovolemia, leading to decreased LV end-diastolic pressure, leading to decreased cardiac output, and in turn leading to hypotension.

3. Beta-blockers—must be used judiciously because they can depress cardiac output.

Surgical treatment Indications for surgery include:

1. Severe AS with AVA 0.9 cm² or less with symptoms secondary to AS.

2. Asymptomatic patients with progressive LV dysfunction or hypotensive response to exercise.

Aortic Regurgitation

Etiology and pathogenesis The etiology of AR can be classified into acute versus chronic processes (Table 6-3).

Table 6-3 Etiology of aortic regurgitation

Causes of acute AR	Causes of chronic AR
Bacterial endocarditis	Connective tissue disorders (most common cause of chronic AR: Marfan's, Ehlers-Danlos, osteogenesis imperfecta)
Blunt chest trauma	Blunt chest trauma
Aortic dissection	Aortic dissection Bacterial endocarditis Congenital (bicuspid aortic valve, coarctation) Degenerative calcific disease of aortic valve Antiphospholipid syndrome Drugs (Dexfenfluramine/phentermine)

Pathophysiology   In acute-onset AR, the LV is unable to adapt to the sudden increase in volume. As a result, there is an immediate rise in LVEDP and premature mitral valve closure. Premature mitral valve closure prevents left atrial emptying, and the increased LVEDP is transmitted to the atrium and pulmonary vasculature, resulting in dyspnea and pulmonary edema.

In chronic AR, the LV must adapt to volume as well as pressure overload. The LV therefore undergoes both dilatation (in response to volume overload) and hypertrophy (in response to pressure overload). Dilatation increases LV compliance and permits the LV to accommodate a large regurgitant fraction and increasing preload. With the increased LV stroke volume and large regurgitant fraction, patients with AR have a large difference between their systolic and diastolic pressures. In addition, because AR occurs during diastole, relative bradycardia, which increases the diastolic filling period, can exacerbate AR. After prolonged exposure of the LV to pressure and fluid overload, myocardial fibrosis and dysfunction develops, leading to CHF symptoms.

History   Chronic AR is well tolerated and asymptomatic. By the time patients present with dyspnea or angina, LV dilatation and systolic dysfunction is usually present. Angina is secondary to decreased aortic perfusion pressure and increased myocardial oxygen demand. Nocturnal angina is secondary to relative bradycardia while sleeping, which increases the diastolic filling period and regurgitant volume and decreases diastolic coronary perfusion.

Physical examination   Physical findings are notable for the following:

1. Auscultation—diastolic high-pitched murmur loudest over third intercostal space along the left sternal border (LSB). The murmur radiates apically and is loudest with the patient in an upright position. The more severe the AR, the longer the murmur lasts in diastole. A high intensity also corresponds to severe AR, but the intensity can decrease in decompensated AR with decreased cardiac output. The Austin-Flint murmur is a mid- to late-diastolic rumble that is observed in moderate to severe chronic AR and can mimic mitral stenosis. The murmur is secondary to vibration of a prematurely and partially closed mitral valve by rapid left atrial inflow.

2. "Waterhammer" or Corrigan's pulse—widened pulse pressure.

3. Traube's sign—auscultation of femoral artery reveals "pistol shot" sounds secondary to arterial wall vibrations.

4. Duroziez's sign—auscultation of partial compressed femoral artery reveals a systolic and diastolic "to and fro" murmur secondary to the regurgitant volume.

5. Quincke's sign—alternating capillary filling and emptying of the nailbeds with partial compression.

6. Bisferens morphology of carotid pulse—a slight dip during the carotid upstroke secondary to a Venturi effect-induced temporary depression of the systolic pressure.

7. Hyperdynamic LV apical impulse.

Management

Medical treatment   In chronic asymptomatic AR, the goal of treatment is to decrease afterload with vasodilators such as hydralazine, nifedipine, or ACE inhibitors. Adjunctive therapy for CHF symptoms includes digitalis, nitrates, and diuretics. Bradycardia is poorly tolerated because prolonged diastole increases the regurgitant fraction. Atrial fibrillation is also poorly tolerated due to the importance of atrial systole.

Surgical treatment   Aortic valve replacement should be considered for the following indications: (1) onset of angina or dyspnea, (2) objective evidence of decreased exercise tolerance, and (3) in asymptomatic patients, evidence of LV dysfunction at rest (decreased LV EF or progressive LV chamber dilatation).

Pulmonic Stenosis   Pulmonic stenosis is usually a congenital malformation or secondary to carcinoid syndrome.

Pathophysiology and history   The stenotic pulmonic valve causes RV pressure overload and hypertrophy. Associated symptoms include angina, dyspnea, and syncope (if forward flow is severely impeded). Patient usually become symptomatic with gradients of > 50 mm Hg.

Physical examination

1. RV lift is present secondary to RVH.

2. Loud systolic ejection murmur preceded by an ejection click.

3. Ejection click of pulmonic valve decreases with inspiration because the valve is passively opened.

Management   Percutaneous balloon valvotomy is the procedure of choice in the symptomatic patient or when the gradient exceeds 75 mm Hg.

Pulmonic Regurgitation   Pulmonic regurgitation is often present in severe pulmonary HTN. The classic murmur is a decrescendo murmur at the LSB that is similar to an AR murmur. Treatment is directed toward the underlying cause of pulmonary HTN.

Case Conclusion   AB was admitted, and transthoracic echocardiography documented severe AS with a calculated valve area of 0.6 cm² and a peak gradient of 80 mm Hg. Mild mitral stenosis was also present with a calculated valve area of 1.4 cm². Severe LV hypertrophy and mild LV enlargement was also noted. Further questioning determined that he most likely had an episode of acute RF that resulted in both aortic and mitral stenosis. Syncope is one of the three symptoms of critical AS and predicts a 3-year survival period. AB underwent successful aortic valve replacement and mitral valve repair.

Thumbnail: Physical Findings in Aortic and Pulmonic Valvular Disease

Valvular abnormality	Physical findings	Auscultation
AS	Sustained apical impulse Nondisplaced apical impulse Delayed upstroke, low volume	Mid-systolic murmur Murmur radiates to neck Single or paradox, split S_2 3rd or 4th heart sounds 2nd right intercostal space Late peaking → more severe
AR	Corrigan's/Waterhammer pulse "Pistol shot" femoral arteries Duroziez's sign (femoral murmur) Quincke's sign (capillary pulsations) Widened pulse pressure	Diastolic regurgitant murmur LSB Radiates to xiphoid Intensity of murmur varies directly with BP Longer murmur lasts in diastole → more severe Best heard with patient upright
Pulmonic stenosis	RVH → RV heave over sternum	Loud systolic ejection click Systolic murmur over LSB
Pulmonic regurgitation	RVH → RV heave over sternum	Decrescendo murmur over LSB

Key Points

▶ Rheumatic heart disease is the most common acquired heart disease in children and young adults worldwide.

▶ Rheumatic heart disease primarily affects the aortic and mitral valves.

▶ In aortic stenosis, latency period from the onset of severe symptoms to the average age of death is approximately 5 years for angina, 3 years for syncope, and 2 years for CHF.

▶ Acute AR presents as a volume overload phenomenon, while chronic AR is a volume as well as pressure overload situation.

Questions

Please refer to Figures 6-1 through 6-5 for question 1.

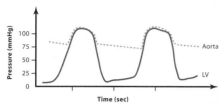

Figure 6-1 Tracing 1.

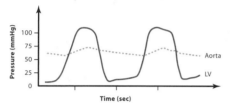

Figure 6-2 Tracing 2.

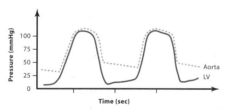

Figure 6-3 Tracing 3.

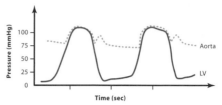

Figure 6-4 Tracing 4.

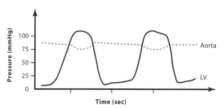

Figure 6-5 Tracing 5.

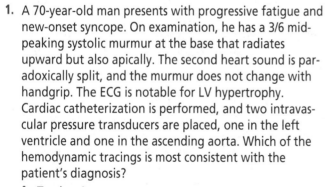

1. A 70-year-old man presents with progressive fatigue and new-onset syncope. On examination, he has a 3/6 mid-peaking systolic murmur at the base that radiates upward but also apically. The second heart sound is paradoxically split, and the murmur does not change with handgrip. The ECG is notable for LV hypertrophy. Cardiac catheterization is performed, and two intravascular pressure transducers are placed, one in the left ventricle and one in the ascending aorta. Which of the hemodynamic tracings is most consistent with the patient's diagnosis?

   A. Tracing 1
   B. Tracing 2
   C. Tracing 3
   D. Tracing 4
   E. Tracing 5

2. An 84-year-old patient has increasing CHF symptoms, angina, and a diastolic, decrescendo murmur. A widened pulse pressure and a "Waterhammer" pulse are detected on examination. A transthoracic echocardiogram reveals severe aortic insufficiency with moderate LV enlargement and moderate systolic dysfunction. A recent cardiac catheterization revealed no significant epicardial coronary disease. Which of the following interventions would worsen the patient's condition?

   A. ACE inhibitors
   B. Diuresis
   C. Digoxin
   D. Hydralazine
   E. Beta-blockers

HPI: JC is a 26-year-old man with a history of hepatitis C and IV drug use who was in good health until 3 days ago when he noted the acute onset of fevers, chills, and myalgias. Three hours prior to admission, he became increasingly short of breath and was unable to move his right arm.

PE: **Vitals:** T 39.4°C, HR 110 beats/min, BP 90/50 mm Hg, RR 22 breaths/min. **H/N:** Small retinal hemorrhages, JVP 7 cm. **Chest:** Few basilar crackles. **Cardiac:** Hyperdynamic PMI with III/VI systolic murmur at apex radiating laterally. **Abdomen:** Splenomegaly. **Extremities:** IV needle markings, painless erythematous macules on palms. **ECG:** Sinus tachycardia with nonspecific changes. **CXR:** Multiple 1 cm opacifications throughout both lung fields.

Labs: WBC 16K/mm^3, HCT 29.0, platelets 400K/mm^3. **Urinalysis:** 3+ red blood cells (RBCs), 3+ WBC, > 100,000 bacteria all per high power field.

Thought Questions

- What are the common organisms that cause infective endocarditis (IE)?

- What criteria are used for the diagnosis of IE?

- What are the sequelae of IE?

- What preexisting medical conditions and procedures require antibiotic prophylaxis for IE?

Basic Science Review and Discussion

Infective endocarditis (IE) is an infection of the endocardium by microorganisms. Despite the decrease of rheumatic heart disease, IE has been stable or increasing because of (1) the increase of age-related degenerative valve disease, (2) increase in nosocomial endocarditis in the elderly, and (3) increased diagnosis with echocardiography. IE is a major cause of severe valvular lesions and is responsible for 10% to 25% of mitral and aortic regurgitation requiring surgical intervention. Despite early medical and surgical therapy, the **mortality rate for IE remains 20%.**

IE usually affects the left-sided heart chambers and valves (85% of total) over the right-sided heart chambers and valves (15% of total). The aortic valve alone is affected in 60% of cases, the mitral valve alone is affected in 35% of cases, and simultaneous involvement of both valves occurs in 10% of cases.

Although bacteremia is found in up to 70% of IE cases, the undamaged endothelium is resistant to infection. In addition to bacteremia, two other prerequisites for IE include (1) an aseptic, fibrinoplatelet thrombus formation or (2) damaged endothelium. The damaged endothelium may be secondary to rheumatic heart disease or valvular heart disease which can lead to aberrant blood flow traumatizing the endothe-

lium. Preexisting rheumatic/valvular/congenital disease is detected in up to 75% of cases of left-sided endocarditis.

IE manifests as valvular vegetations, valvular degeneration, myocardial abscesses, and extracardiac embolic phenomena. After the formation of the aseptic, fibrinoplatelet thrombus, transient bacteremia infects the thrombus to form a valvular vegetation. The **vegetation** is a sessile lesion composed of fibrin, platelets, WBCs, and microorganisms.

After localized valvular infection and vegetation formation, the affected valve can degenerate and cause severe regurgitation and heart failure. The valvular infection can then spread locally to form fistulae, aortic aneurysms, conduction disease, and septic pericarditis. Embolization of vegetations to other organs such as kidneys, spleen, liver, coronary arteries, and brain can cause septic infarction of the target organ (e.g., brain emboli leading to stroke, coronary artery emboli leading to MI) and distant abscesses. Finally, stimulation of the immune system can result in glomerulonephritis and arthritis.

Clinical Presentations   The clinical symptoms and signs of IE are fairly nonspecific, but the most common finding is fever. Other associated symptoms included sweating, chills, fatigue, and arthralgias. On examination, a murmur is detected in 30% to 50% of patients. Other signs include splenomagaly, hematuria, proteinuria, anemia, and retinal hemorrhages (**Roth spots**). Other peripheral signs include **Janeway lesions** (small, nontender, erythematous macules on the palms and soles) and **Osler's nodes** (painful 1- to 3-mm, erythematous nodules on the fingertips or toe pads). The majority of IE cases (90%) present subacutely, with symptoms occurring within 2 weeks of the initial bacteremia. Ten percent of cases present acutely with a sudden onset of high fever. Acute-onset IE is usually associated with beta-hemolytic streptococcus, *Staphylococccus aureus,* or *Pseudomonas aeruginosa.*

Although IE predominantly affects the left-sided cardiac structures, 15% of IE involves the right-sided valves. Right-sided IE is associated with IV drug use, and the tricuspid valve is the most frequently affected valve (80% of cases). In addition to traditional symptoms, right-sided IE is complicated by septic pulmonary emboli. The most common cause of right-sided IE is *Staphylococcus aureus* or *Staphylococcus epidermidis.*

The diagnosis of IE is based on the **Duke criteria** (Box 7–1). Endocarditis is diagnosed when a patient's clinical presentation fulfills two major criteria, one major and three minor criteria, or five minor criteria.

Given that endocarditis usually follows bacteremia, **antibiotic prophylaxis** is justified for several clinical procedures. All patients with prosthetic heart valves, congenital heart disease [ventricular septal defect (VSD), bicuspid aortic valve, patent ductus arteriosus (PDA)], valvular heart disease (AS, AR, MR, mitral valve prolapse), and previous history of IE require antibiotic prophylaxis. Procedures that require antibiotic prophylaxis for the aforementioned patients include all dental, GI, urologic, upper respiratory tract, and genital procedures.

Box 7-1 Duke criteria

Major criteria
1. Positive blood cultures
2. New murmur, positive echo finding

Minor criteria
1. Fever
2. Presdisposing cardiac condition, IV drug abuse (IVDA)
3. Vascular phenomena (emboli, petechiae)
4. Immunologic findings (Roth spots, Osler nodes, glomerulonephritis)
5. Echo findings consistent with endocarditis but not meeting major criteria
6. Positive blood cultures not meeting major criteria

Medical therapy for endocarditis is long-term IV antibiotics for 2 to 6 weeks. The particular regimen and duration of antibiotic therapy depends on the particular microorganism and location of the IE. **Indications for surgery** include CHF secondary to valve dysfunction, persistent sepsis, recurrent embolism, intracardiac abscess, or fungal endocarditis.

Case Conclusion   JC presents with acute-onset endocarditis secondary to his IV drug use. His IV drug use has resulted in right-sided endocarditis involving the tricuspid valve with septic pulmonary emboli as detected by chest x-ray. His shortness of breath is secondary to acute MR from mitral valvular degeneration. His hypotension and tachycardia are secondary to sepsis syndrome. The small retinal hemorrhages, glomerulonephritis, and neurologic complications are the result of systemic arterial embolization of vegetations to the eyes, kidneys, and brain.

Thumbnail: Microbiology of Infectious Endocarditis

Causes of bacteremia	Percentage of cases	Microbiology
Dental procedures	20	Penicillin-sensitive streptococcus
Respiratory tract infection Respiratory/oropharyngeal surgery	5	Penicillin-sensitive streptococcus
GI interventions/GI tumors/GI disease	15	Enterococci, *Streptococcus bovis*, gram-negative bacilli, staphylococcus
Urosepsis	10	Enterococci, gram-negative bacilli, *S. aureus*
Gynecologic infection/surgery	5	Streptococci, enterococci
Other causes: wound infections, in-dwelling catheters, IV drug use, osteomyelitis, cardiac procedures	25	*S. aureus, S. epidermidis*, gram-negative bacilli Fungi

Key Points

- IE predominantly affects the left-sided heart chambers and valves, and the aortic valve is the most commonly affected valve.
- The two precipitating factors for endocarditis are transient bacteremia and damaged endothelium leading to aseptic, fibrinoplatelet thrombus formation.

- Right-heart valve endocarditis is predominantly the result of IV drug use.
- Heart failure is the principal cause of mortality in IE, and systemic embolization is the major cause of extracardiac complications.

Questions

1. A 68-year-old man is admitted with 3 weeks of abdominal pain, fevers, chills, sweats, and a new systolic murmur. A transthoracic echocardiogram shows mitral valve vegetations, and 3/3 blood cultures are subsequently positive for *Streptococcus bovis*. After successfully completing his 4 weeks of IV penicillin treatment, he undergoes a whole body computed tomography (CT) scan to evaluate his 25-pound weight loss. Which of the following tumors is most likely to be found?

   A. Thyroid carcinoma
   B. Squamous cell lung cancer
   C. Adenocarcinoma of the colon
   D. Transitional cell carcinoma of the bladder
   E. Small cell lung cancer

2. A 24-year-old woman complains of palpitations and occasional dyspnea on exertion. Which one of the following conditions would not require antibiotic prophylaxis for dental procedures?

   A. Mitral valve prolapse with mitral regurgitation
   B. Bicuspid aortic valve
   C. Mitral valve prolapse without mitral regurgitation
   D. Patent ductus arteriosus
   E. Prosthetic heart valve

> **HPI:** JK is a 67-year-old man with multiple cardiac risk factors, including smoking, HTN, hyperlipidemia, and diabetes. His chief complaint is substernal chest pressure on exertion occurring once a week. He referred himself to the emergency department after his chest pressure started occurring several times a day since last week, and he presents with 3/10 chest pain at rest that started 1 hour ago.
>
> **PE:** **Vitals:** BP 160/90 mm Hg, HR 110 beats/min, RR 24 breaths/min, Tmax 37.2°C. **General:** Diaphoretic and tachypneic. **H/N:** JVP is 12 cm. **Chest:** Bilateral rales one fourth of the way up. **Cardiac:** Dyskinetic apical impulse with 2/6 systolic murmur radiating laterally, positive S_4. **Extremities:** Decreased radial pulse volume and mild peripheral edema. **ECG:** 2 mm ST depressions in V_4 to V_6.
>
> After treatment with supplemental oxygen, aspirin, and sublingual nitroglycerin, his chest pain as well as his ECG changes resolved. JK was admitted to the telemetry unit for further evaluation.

Thought Questions

- What physiologic parameters regulate myocardial oxygen supply and demand?

- What is the underlying pathophysiology for the three different types of angina?

- How do the available treatments of stable angina influence myocardial oxygen supply and demand?

Basic Science Review and Discussion

Ischemic heart disease (IHD) is a condition where there is inadequate blood supply relative to the metabolic needs of the myocardium. IHD is a major consequence of coronary artery atherosclerosis and can manifest as stable angina, unstable angina (USA), silent ischemia, and MI. Myocardial ischemia is the result of a myocardial oxygen supply and demand imbalance.

Myocardial Oxygen Supply Myocardial oxygen supply is dependent on three factors: (1) oxygen carrying capacity/ coronary blood flow, (2) diastolic perfusion pressure, and (3) coronary vascular resistance. **Oxygen carrying capacity** is determined by systemic oxygenation and the hematocrit. Since there is systolic compression of the subendocardial vessels, coronary blood flow is phasic, and most flow occurs during diastole. The perfusion pressure is similar to aortic diastolic pressure. Therefore, shortening of the diastolic filling period (tachycardia), decrease of the pressure difference between the coronary arteries and LV (coronary or aortic stenosis), or reduction of the aortic diastolic pressure (aortic insufficiency) can all decrease myocardial oxygen supply.

The left ventricular myocardium has a limited oxygen extraction reserve because it normally extracts 75% of the oxygen delivered (two to three times that of other organs).

In addition, the anaerobic metabolic capacity myocardium is limited. Therefore, in order to avoid ischemia, an increase in myocardial oxygen demand must be accompanied by an increase in coronary blood flow.

Coronary vascular resistance is the third major determinant of myocardial oxygen supply. Changes in coronary vascular resistance autoregulate coronary flow so that flow is relatively constant despite changes in coronary blood pressure. As perfusion pressure changes, active changes in the coronary vascular resistance maintain constant flow. However, autoregulation is lost below perfusion pressures of 60 mm Hg and flow becomes pressure dependent. With severe coronary stenosis, a fall in perfusion pressure below 60 mm Hg results in the loss of autoregulation and maximal vessel dilatation.

Coronary vascular resistance is regulated by local metabolic and neurohormonal factors. **Metabolic factors** include oxygen, adenosine, and nitric oxide. Adenosine, nitric oxide, hypoxia, and hypercapnia serve as vasodilators, and oxygen serves as a vasoconstrictor. **Neurohormonal factors** include sympathetic innervation to the alpha- and β_2-receptors on the coronary vessels. Stimulation of alpha-receptors on the larger epicardial vessels causes vasoconstriction, while stimulation of β_2-receptors on the subendocardial vessels promotes vasodilatation. Although coronary artery vasoconstriction during periods of high sympathetic output may seem paradoxical, this effect may actually promote improved subendocardial perfusion and reduce the amount of retrograde flow with systole at higher heart rates.

Extrinsic compression of the coronary vasculature is greatest during systole, and coronary blood flow is therefore limited during the systolic ejection period. As the heart rate increases, the systolic ejection period remains relatively constant while the diastolic filling period shortens. With a shortened diastolic filling period, the amount of time for coronary blood flow is reduced.

Myocardial Oxygen Demand   Myocardial oxygen demand is determined by **heart rate, contractility,** and **wall tension.** The cardiac oxygen requirement increases with accelerating heart rate since the myocardium has a limited potential for anaerobic metabolism. **Cardiac contractility** is the second determinant of myocardial oxygen demand. Increasing force of contraction under catecholaminergic or inotropic stimulation increases oxygen utilization. **Wall tension** is the third determinant of myocardial oxygen demand. Wall tension is the force that counteracts the stretching of cardiac myocytes and is approximated by Laplace's formula (wall tension = transmural pressure × radius/(2 × wall thickness). As a result, increases in LV diameter (dilated LV in chronic aortic/mitral regurgitation or long-standing HTN) or increases in systolic ventricular pressure (HTN or aortic stenosis) will increase wall tension, and thereby increase oxygen demand. Although LV hypertrophy develops with HTN or aortic stenosis, increasing wall thickness may actually be compensatory by decreasing wall tension and myocardial oxygen demand per gram of tissue.

Consequences of Myocardial Ischemia   When cardiac flow falls below metabolic requirements, adenosine triphosphate (ATP) stores are rapidly depleted, myocardial pH decreases, and extracellular potassium concentration rises. These pH and electrolyte imbalances increase the risk for ventricular arrhythmias. Angina and the subsequent stimulation of the sympathetic and parasympathetic pathways are precipitated by the products of anaerobic metabolism, including lactate, adenosine, and xanthine. Autonomic nervous system activation causes diaphoresis, tachycardia, and nausea.

Systolic function and contractility rapidly decline, resulting in a decrease in cardiac output. Diastolic relaxation is also impaired, which contributes to an elevation in LV filling pressure. This ischemia-induced systolic and diastolic dysfunction can precipitate dyspnea and tachypnea secondary to pulmonary edema and heart failure.

Clinical Features of Myocardial Ischemia

Stable angina   Stable angina is the chronic predictable occurrence of chest pressure or pain caused by myocardial ischemia in association with physical exertion or emotional stress. Stable angina occurs when the arterial lumen is narrowed by more than 70%. The classic presentation of stable angina is retrosternal chest pressure or pain that may radiate to the neck or left arm, which is precipitated by exertion/stress and relieved with discontinuation of effort or sublingual nitroglycerin. During an anginal episode, the ECG may demonstrate transient **ST depression** or **T-wave inversions.** Treatment is usually with risk factor modification and antianginal drug therapy (refer to Thumbnail section).

Variant angina   Variant angina, also known as **Prinzmetal's angina,** is described as angina at rest associated with transient ST elevation, which resolves either spontaneously or with nitrate administration. **Coronary artery spasm** is the most common cause of variant angina and often occurs in the context of atherosclerotic disease, but spasm may also occur in the complete absence of atherosclerotic plaques or focal stenoses. Vascular hyperreactivity and endothelial dysfunction are hypothesized to play a major pathogenic role in variant angina. Although variant angina may cause severe ischemia, it is rarely fatal and is usually treatable with calcium channel blockers and nitrates. Patients who use cocaine are at especially high risk for variant angina. Vasospasm in cocaine users can sometimes be so severe that myocardial necrosis occurs with resultant MI.

Unstable angina   USA is described as angina increasing in frequency or severity or angina at rest. USA is a much more serious clinical situation than stable angina and often is a precursor of MI. Although USA is similar to stable angina in that both manifest when there is an imbalance between myocardial oxygen supply and demand, USA has a different underlying pathophysiology. While a fixed stenosis is the critical lesion in stable angina, the rupture of the fibrous plaque with subsequent platelet aggregation, thrombosis, and vasospasm is the precipitant in USA. Therefore, in addition to the standard anti-ischemic regimen used for stable angina (see Thumbnail), USA requires aggressive antiplatelet (aspirin), antithrombosis (heparin, IIbIIIa blockade), and antivasospasm (IV nitroglycerin) therapy.

Diagnosis of Myocardial Ischemia   Although the history and physical exam are the most important factors in the diagnosis of myocardial ischemia, additional diagnostic studies to confirm or exclude CAD can be helpful. The standard 12-lead ECG is helpful, especially if obtained with and without chest pain. ST-segment depression or elevation and T-wave abnormalities can frequently be observed, although the absence of ECG changes does not exclude myocardial ischemia. The subsequent workup and diagnosis of the three different types of angina are different.

Stable angina   The workup of stable angina includes **treadmill stress testing** or **pharmacologic stress testing.** With treadmill stress testing, a continuous ECG is obtained while a patient increases his or her myocardial oxygen demand by walking on a treadmill. If a flow-limiting stenosis is present, the increased myocardial oxygen demand will induce myocardial ischemia and ECG changes. The sensitivity of the treadmill test can be increased by intravascular injection of a radioactive tracer (thallium, sestamibi) that is then imaged under a camera to visualize coronary perfusion. Pharmacologic stress testing involves administration of a vasodilatation agent (persantine, adenosine) followed by intravascular injection of a radioactive tracer. If a flow-limiting stenosis is present, the affected vessel will not be able to vasodilate to a similar degree, and a reduced amount of tracer will perfuse that coronary distribution. When images of the heart are acquired, the relatively underperfused territory will appear "cold."

Variant angina   The diagnosis of variant angina can be difficult because the vasospastic events are usually too transient and unpredictable to record. One method is 24-hour ambulatory ECG monitoring for transient ECG changes. A second method is cardiac catheterization with intracoronary vessel ergonovine challenge (ergonovine is a pro-vasospastic substance) in an attempt to precipitate vasospasm. Nevertheless, the diagnosis of variant angina is usually made by history alone because the vasospastic events are usually too transient and unpredictable. The relief of symptoms with a therapeutic trial of antivasospastic agents such as nitrates or calcium channel blockers supports the diagnosis of variant angina.

Unstable angina   Because USA is a much more serious clinical situation and places the patient at high risk for progression to MI, the diagnostic test of choice is diagnostic cardiac catheterization and possible angioplasty.

Case Conclusion   The patient's clinical course has progressed from stable angina to USA. Myocardial ischemia precipitates systolic and diastolic dysfunction, which is subsequently followed by pulmonary congestion and elevated JVP. A decline in systolic function results in a dyskinetic apical impulse. Decreased diastolic compliance and increased wall stiffness contribute to the formation of an S_4. Ischemia-induced LV wall motion abnormalities and papillary muscle dysfunction result in mitral regurgitation and worsening of pulmonary congestion. Finally, increased sympathetic tone increases HR and BP and promotes diaphoresis. The patient subsequently was evaluated by cardiac catheterization and underwent angioplasty of a 90% middle LAD stenosis.

Thumbnail: Medical Treatment of Myocardial Ischemia

Medication	Mechanism of action
Beta-blockers	1. Decrease contractility and HR 2. Increase diastolic filling period 3. Blunt rise in BP with exercise
Calcium channel blockers	1. Decrease contractility and HR 2. Decrease vasospasm and coronary vasodilator 3. Increase diastolic filling period 4. Decrease peripheral vascular resistance
Nitrates	1. Decrease preload → decreased ventricular volume and wall stress 2. Increase coronary perfusion as coronary vasodilator 3. Decrease coronary vasospasm

---

Key Points

▶ Myocardial ischemia is due to an imbalance between myocardial oxygen supply and demand.

▶ Coronary blood flow occurs during diastole. Tachycardia therefore not only increases myocardial oxygen demand but also decreases diastolic perfusion time.

▶ Stable angina is the result of a flow-limiting stenosis and can usually be treated medically.

▶ USA is the result of a ruptured fibrous plaque with overlying thrombus. USA often evolves into a myocardial infarction and is a medical emergency.

▶ Variant/Prinzmetal's angina is coronary artery vasospasm secondary to vascular hyperreactivity.

Questions

1. A 48-year-old woman with a history of migraines experiences occasional chest pressure at rest various times during the day. She is very active and does not associate her episodes with physical exertion. What type of angina is she experiencing?

   A. Stable angina

   B. Variant angina

   C. USA

   D. Silent ischemia

   E. Gastrointestinal angina

2. A 23-year-old woman with recurrent chest pain and a normal coronary angiogram and negative ergonovine challenge 1 month prior presents with recurrent chest pain. A repeat angiogram would most likely demonstrate which finding?

   A. Normal arteries

   B. 80% LAD stenosis

   C. Coronary artery vasospasm

   D. Muscle bridge causing extrinsic compression of the coronary artery

   E. Anomalous coronary takeoff

3. A 57-year-old patient with renal failure on dialysis presents with chest pain. On examination a friction rub is present and the substernal chest pain is pleuritic in nature. No point tenderness is present and the pain is not relieved with antacids. A coronary angiogram is performed because of significant ECG changes (diffuse ST elevation) consistent with ischemia. The coronary angiogram is normal. Which of the following diagnoses is most likely?

   A. Aortic dissection

   B. Esophageal spasm

   C. Pericarditis

   D. Costochondritis

   E. Duodenal ulcer

HPI: JF is a 73-year-old woman with a history of morbid obesity and diabetes mellitus. She presents to your clinic with 1 week of increasing dyspnea, blurry vision, and headache.

PE: **Vitals:** BP 220/150 mm Hg, HR 100 beats/min, RR 24 breaths/min, Tmax 37.4°C. **H/N:** JVP 13 cm, blurring of optic disc. **Chest:** Crackles one third of the way up bilaterally. **Cardiac:** Normal S_1, S_2, with positive S_3 and S_4, hyperdynamic PMI. **Abdomen:** Soft, nontender, no ascites. **Peripheral:** 2+/4 pulses, mild peripheral edema. **ECG:** Sinus tachycardia with 2 mm ST depression anterolaterally. **CXR:** Mild CHF.

Labs: Potassium 2.9 mEqL, sodium 150 mEqL, creatinine 2.3 mg/dL.

Thought Questions

- What physiologic parameters determine systemic BP?

- What systems are involved in the regulation of BP?

- Which organ systems are affected by long-term HTN and how?

- What general classes of drugs are available for treatment of HTN?

- What are causes of secondary HTN?

Basic Science Review and Discussion

Pathophysiology A normal BP is defined as a systolic BP of less than 140 mm Hg and a diastolic BP of less than 90 mm Hg. **Essential or primary HTN** is defined as elevated BP in which secondary causes such as pheochromocytoma or hyperaldosteronism (Conn's syndrome) have been excluded. **Secondary HTN** is defined as high BP attributed to a definable cause. Essential HTN accounts for 95% of HTN cases, and 25% to 40% of HTN is genetically determined.

Systemic BP is governed by several principles:

Systemic BP = cardiac output × peripheral resistance

Cardiac output = stroke volume × heart rate

Peripheral resistance is related to the **viscosity of the blood, length of the artery,** and **inversely related to the fourth power of the luminal radius.** Because the blood viscosity and arterial length is not usually changed, peripheral resistance is primarily determined by small distal arteries measuring 1 mm or less.

Although the primary mechanism for essential HTN has not been fully elucidated, several potential theories have been suggested. The three major systems involved in the regulation of BP are the heart, kidney, and vascular system. Increased sympathetic tone is thought to contribute to the pathophysiology of essential HTN. Activation of the sympa-

thetic nervous system raises BP by stimulating the three systems to increase cardiac output, fluid retention, and vascular resistance. Norepinephrine is the primary transmitter in the sympathetic nervous system, and circulating levels of norepinephrine are elevated in hypertensive patients.

Elevated levels of circulating norepinephrine increase cardiac output by increasing the heart rate and stroke volume of the heart. Increased sympathetic tone also results in vascular hypertrophy, which decreases luminal radius and leads to a rise in peripheral resistance and BP.

The renin-angiotensin-aldosterone (RAA) system is another important regulator of BP (Figure 9-1). Renin is produced by the juxtaglomerular cells of the kidney and catalyzes the formation of angiotensin I from liver-synthesized angiotensinogen. Angiotensin I is then converted into angiotensin II by ACE, which is produced in the lungs. Angiotensin II induces vasoconstriction, increases aldosterone production, and increases renal sodium reabsorption. Similar

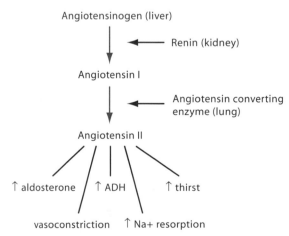

Figure 9-1 Angiotensinogen from the liver is catalyzed by renin into angiotensin I. Angiotensin I is then catalyzed by ACE into angiotensin II. ACE inhibitors block conversion of angiotensin I into angiotensin II. Angiotensin receptor blockers prevent binding of angiotensin II to its specific receptor.

to norepinephrine, angiotensin II also induces vascular hypertrophy.

Two other regulators of HTN include nitric oxide and endothelin. Nitric oxide, released by the endothelial cells, (1) functions as a vasodilator, (2) decreases vascular hypertrophy, and (3) decreases platelet adhesion. Endothelin is a peptide produced by the endothelium, which can act as a vasoconstrictor or vasodilator, depending on whether endothelin binds to (1) ET_a receptors on vascular smooth muscle cells, resulting in vasoconstriction, or to (2) ET_b receptors on endothelial cells, causing release of nitric oxide and prostacyclin and subsequent vasodilation. Preliminary evidence suggests that endothelin is an important pathophysiologic factor in HTN. For example, bosentan, a recently approved endothelin receptor antagonist approved for treatment of pulmonary HTN, has also been shown to decrease BP in patients with essential HTN.

Major risk factors associated with HTN include (1) obesity, (2) physical inactivity, (3) high salt intake, (4) excess alcohol consumption, (5) genetic predisposition, and (6) African-American ethnicity.

Complications of Hypertension   Sustained elevation in BP triggers a variety of hemodynamic, cardiac, vascular, and neurohormonal pathogenic processes:

1. Hemodynamic—increased total peripheral resistance and increased vessel and cardiac wall stress.
2. Cardiac—myocyte hypertrophy, LV remodeling, alterations in extracellular matrix.
3. Vascular—endothelial dysfunction, coronary and peripheral atherosclerosis, decreased vascular compliance, and increased vascular reactivity.
4. Neurohormonal—increased catecholamine secretion and activation of the RAA system.

HTN can also result in end-organ complications and damage:

Cardiovascular system   HTN accelerates coronary atherosclerosis and increases myocardial oxygen demand, with both factors increasing the risk of ischemic heart disease. Heart failure related to HTN is secondary to ventricular remodeling. Heart failure can progress from diastolic dysfunction secondary to abnormal ventricular relaxation to symptomatic systolic dysfunction. HTN-induced chamber dilatation also increases the risk for arrhythmias and sudden cardiac death.

Peripheral vascular system   High BP promotes endothelial dysfunction, atherosclerosis, and degeneration of the aortic media. In addition, the increased wall stress predisposes hypertensive patients to aortic dissection and abdominal aortic aneurysm.

Renal system   HTN can result in glomerular damage, hypertensive nephrosclerosis, and end-stage renal disease. Hypertensive nephrosclerosis is the most common cause of end-stage renal disease in the United States and Europe. Although the exact mechanism is unclear, the histologic changes associated with hypertensive nephrosclerosis include (a) hyaline arteriolar sclerosis (vessel walls become thickened with hyaline infiltrate), (b) myointimal hypertrophy and hyperplasia (smooth muscle proliferation), and (c) fibrinoid necrosis (necrosis of capillary walls).

Central nervous system   HTN is the major treatable risk factor for both hemorrhagic and thrombotic cerebrovascular accidents (CVAs). Hemorrhagic CVAs result from the rupture of cerebral parenchymal vessels subjected to increasing wall stress. Thromboembolic CVAs are a complication of HTN-induced atherosclerotic plaque that has embolized to distal vessels.

Visual system   Severe and acute BP elevation (malignant HTN) can cause the retinal vessels to rupture, with resultant hemorrhages and retinal infarction. Papilledema, or swelling of the optic disc, can also result from high intracranial pressure. With chronically elevated HTN, hypertensive retinopathy can develop. Physical findings on fundoscopic exam include "copper wire" arterioles secondary to light reflected off sclerosed arteries and arteriovenous "nicking" caused by indentation of crossing veins by medial hypertrophy of the small retinal arteries.

Hypertensive Crisis   Hypertensive crisis is a life-threatening situation that occurs when there is an abrupt rise in BP above baseline. In general, the diastolic BP exceeds 120 mm Hg. This rise in BP can cause rapid-progression end-organ damage, including renal failure, myocardial ischemia, pulmonary edema, retinopathy, CVA, and hypertensive encephalopathy. Hypertensive encephalopathy is the result of cerebral edema that overwhelms the autoregulatory capacities of the brain. The goal of treatment is immediate and controlled reduction of BP with agents such as sodium nitroprusside, labetolol, nitroglycerin, or hydralazine.

Treatment of Hypertension   Management of HTN can be divided into nonpharmacologic and pharmacologic strategies.

Nonpharmacologic treatments

1. Diet. Restriction of sodium intake decreases the activation of the RAA system; the greater the compensatory stimulation of the RAA system, the less the reduction in BP. As a result, the effect of sodium restriction is more apparent among hypertensive patients and the elderly because their slow response of the RAA axis allows for a greater decline in BP. Potassium supplementation is beneficial for potassium-deficient hypertensives, but the exact mechanism is unclear. High potassium levels may

promote sodium excretion and increase nitric oxide-dependent vasodilatation. Excessive alcohol intake is a well-defined risk factor for HTN, but the exact mechanism is unclear.

2. Obesity. Weight loss is recommended because there is a strong association between body weight and BP. Insulin resistance in obese patients may result in compensatory hyperinsulinemia, which in turn increases catecholamine secretion, promotes renal sodium retention, and alters vascular reactivity.

3. Exercise. BP decline associated with exercise is explained by (a) a decrease in peripheral vascular resistance and resting cardiac output, (b) decreases in plasma norepinephrine levels, and (c) reduction in the RAA axis activity.

Pharmacologic treatments

1. Diuretics. The major action of diuretics in reducing BP is the sustained loss of extracellular salt and water. The three classes of diuretics include thiazide diuretics (hydrocholorthiazide), potassium-sparing diuretics (spironolactone), and loop diuretics (furosemide). Thiazide diuretics are especially effective in African-American patients and the elderly.

2. Adrenergic modifiers. Adrenergic inhibitors diminish the activity of the sympathetic nervous system, either centrally or peripherally. Beta-blockers (metoprolol, atenolol) decrease BP by decreasing renin secretion and by reducing heart rate and contractility. Alpha$_1$-adrenergic receptor antagonists (prazosin, terazosin) decrease BP by relaxing vascular smooth muscle and lowering total peripheral vascular resistance. Centrally acting α_2-adrenergic agonists (clonidine and methyldopa) reduce sympathetic outflow to the heart, peripheral vascular system, and kidneys.

3. Calcium channel blockers (CCBs). The dihydropyridine CCBs (amlodipine, felodipine, nifedipine) decrease BP primarily by decreasing systemic vascular resistance. The nondihydropyridine CCBs, verapamil and diltiazem, reduce cardiac contractility, sinus node conduction, and atrioventricular conduction and vasodilate arterioles.

4. ACE inhibitors. ACE inhibitors (captopril, lisinopril) decrease BP by inhibiting ACE and thereby preventing the formation of angiotensin II. The reduced levels of angiotensin II prevent vasoconstriction and decrease afterload. ACE inhibitors also prevent degradation of the kinins, which have a vasodilator effect. However, accumulation of kinins can result in a cough as a side effect.

5. ARBs. ARBs decrease BP by displacing angiotensin II from its receptor, resulting in a decrease in systemic vascular resistance. Because ARBs do not increase kinin levels, cough is not a common side effect.

Case Conclusion   JF presents in hypertensive emergency with a diastolic BP of greater than 120 mm Hg and evidence of end-organ damage, including papilledema, renal insufficiency, and myocardial ischemia. A brain CT scan revealed no CVA, and her BP was reduced by 25% over 6 hours with IV labetolol and IV sodium nitroprusside. Her ECG changes and pulmonary edema secondary to diastolic dysfunction resolved with lowering of her BP.

Thumbnail: Secondary Causes of Hypertension

Clinical finding with HTN	Potential secondary cause
Hypokalemia	Primary aldosteronism
Abdominal mass	Polycystic kidney disease
Obesity, snoring, daytime somnolence	Obstructive sleep apnea
Elevated serum creatinine, proteinuria	Chronic renal insufficiency
Headache, palpitations, volatile BP, perspiration	Pheochromocytoma
Truncal obesity and striae	Cushing's syndrome
Radial-femoral pulse delay or asymmetric pulse	Coarctation of aorta
Abdominal bruit with refractory HTN	Renal artery stenosis
Organ transplant patient	Cyclosporine
Pregnancy	Eclampsia, pre-eclampsia
Miscellaneous drug-induced HTN	Oral contraceptives, cold remedies (neosynephrine), cox-inhibitors

Key Points

▶ BP is equal to cardiac output × peripheral resistance. Cardiac output is equal to heart rate × stroke volume. Peripheral resistance is increased by angiotensin and stimulation of the α_1-adrenoreceptors on vascular smooth muscle.

▶ Essential HTN accounts for the majority of HTN (95%), but clinical findings may suggest secondary causes of HTN. Consider secondary causes of HTN if the BP is not easily controlled.

▶ Risk factors for essential HTN include (1) obesity, (2) physical inactivity, (3) high salt intake, (4) excess alcohol consumption, (5) genetic predisposition, and (6) African-American ethnicity.

Questions

1. A 48-year-old patient with insulin-dependent diabetes mellitus presents to your clinic with essential HTN. Which antihypertensive would be your first choice?

   A. Metoprolol
   B. Diltiazem
   C. Lasix
   D. Clonidine
   E. Lisinopril

2. A 67-year-old woman presents with refractory HTN despite multiple medications. Her examination is notable for an abdominal bruit. Which antihypertensive could potentially cause the most harm to the patient?

   A. Clonidine
   B. Verapamil
   C. Hydrochlorothiazide
   D. Lisinopril
   E. Atenolol

HPI: JS is a 48-year-old woman with no significant past medical history who notes 3 months of palpitations, weight loss, and heat intolerance. The palpitations occur once or twice per week, last several minutes before self-terminating, and are not associated with chest pain or presyncope. A Holter monitor records several episodes of a regular narrow complex tachycardia at 160 beats/min. Review of the event monitor diary is notable for the association between coffee intake and tachycardia initiation. The patient is instructed to splash cold water on her face with palpitations. When she does so, the palpitations promptly terminate.

PE: **Vitals:** T 37.8°C, HR 110 beats/min, BP 90/50 mm Hg, RR 22 breaths/min. **H/N:** JVP 6 cm, 1-cm nodule in left thyroid lobe. **Chest:** Clear to examination. **Cardiac:** Tachycardic with normal impulse, normal S_1 and S_2 with no murmurs. **Abdomen:** Soft, no masses. **Extremities:** Hyperreflexic in upper and lower extremities. **ECG:** Sinus tachycardia with non-specific changes.

Thought Questions

- What are the two basic mechanisms that result in supraventricular tachycardias?

- How do antiarrhythmics suppress abnormal automaticity and re-entry?

- Which supraventricular tachycardias are terminated with adenosine or vagal maneuvers and why?

- What are the five phases of the cardiac action potential and how are they modified by antiarrhythmics?

- What are the different classes of antiarrhythmics and what are their mechanisms of action?

Basic Science Review and Discussion

Whenever the HR is greater than 100 beats/min for three beats or more, a tachyarrhythmia is present. Tachyarrhythmias can originate either above the ventricles (supraventricular) or within the ventricles (ventricular). A supraventricular tachycardia (SVT) is any tachycardia that originates in the atria or that uses the atrium or AV junction and involves the tissue above the bifurcation of the bundle of His to propagate the tachycardic circuit.

SVTs are classified into whether the tachycardia circuit involves the AV node or not. AV node-dependent tachycardias include AV nodal re-entrant tachycardia (AVNRT), AV re-entrant tachycardia (AVRT), and junctional tachycardia. AV node-independent tachycardias include sinus tachycardia, sinus node re-entry tachycardia, atrial tachycardia, atrial flutter, and atrial fibrillation (AF). An SVT can be classified as AV node dependent if the tachycardia can be terminated by blocking the AV node with a vagal maneuver such as a carotid sinus massage or use of an AV node-blocking agent (adenosine). Although normal conduction and all supraventricular arrhythmias (both AV node-dependent and AV node-independent) all propagate through the AV node, AV node-dependent tachycardias specifically incorporate the AV node as an essential component of the re-entrant circuit.

The cardiac action potential is divided into five phases and is detailed in Table 10-1 and Figure 10-1.

All SVTs result from either a disorder of impulse formation or impulse conduction. Normal impulse formation depends on the intrinsic automaticity that is present in the SA node, some areas of the atria, the AV node, and the bundle of His. Intrinsic automaticity depends on unique pacemaker channels that open to Na^+ or K^+ when the membrane potential increases to -60 mV. The slow influx of cations during

Table 10-1 Depolarization phases

Phase	Description	Mechanism
0	Upstroke/rapid depolarization	Opening of Na^+ channels
1	Early rapid repolarization	Inactivation of Na^+ channels and activation of K^+ and Ca^{2+} outward currents
2	Plateau	Conductance decreases for all ions
3	Final rapid repolarization	Inactivation of Ca^{2+} inward current and activation of K^+ outward current
4	Resting membrane potential/ diastolic depolarization	Membrane potential maintained -50 to -80 mV due to inward K^+ current: if tissue has pacemaker channels, slow influx of cations can cause diastolic depolarization and automaticity

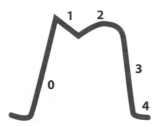

Figure 10-1 Depolarization phases.

phase 4 depolarization drives the membrane potential closer to zero. When the membrane reaches the -40 mV threshold potential, voltage gated Ca^{2+}/Na^+ channels open (phase 0 of the action potential), creating the upstroke of the action potential. Potassium efflux is then responsible for the repolarization of the pacemaker cell.

Abnormal Impulse Formation Secondary to Abnormal Automaticity   Altered impulse formation manifesting as increased automaticity can result in sinus tachycardia or ectopic atrial tachycardia. In ectopic (unifocal/multifocal) atrial tachycardia, foci of increased automaticity external to the SA node can override the intrinsic SA node pacemaker, resulting in an ECG with multiple P-wave morphologies. Each P-wave morphology corresponds to a different focus of increased automaticity.

Antiarrhythmics suppress automaticity by one of three mechanisms:

1. Decreasing the slope of phase 4 spontaneous depolarization
2. Shifting the threshold voltage at which Na^+/Ca^{2+} influx occurs to a more positive level
3. Hyperpolarizing the resting membrane potential

Abnormal Impulse Formation Secondary to Reentry   The second mechanism contributing to SVTs is aberrant impulse conduction manifested as re-entry. A re-entrant loop is a self-sustaining electrical pathway that repeatedly depolar-

izes the surrounding myocardium. In order for a re-entrant circuit to be established, both a unidirectional block and slowed retrograde conduction are necessary. Re-entry is the underlying mechanism for AVNRT, AVRT, re-entrant atrial tachycardia, atrial flutter, and AF.

In AVNRT, the re-entrant circuit is localized in the AV node. Once re-entry is established, the impulse not only depolarizes the ventricle via the bundle of His in an anterograde direction, but also depolarizes the atrium via retrograde conduction. Because these depolarizations occur nearly simultaneously, the small P wave occurs at the same time as the much larger QRS depolarization, and the P wave therefore may not be visible on the ECG. AVRT is similar to AVNRT except that in AVRT, one limb of the re-entrant circuit is an accessory bypass tract external to the AV node (Figure 10-2).

In typical atrial flutter, the re-entrant circuit is usually localized within the right atrium and propagates in a counterclockwise fashion when viewed from the cardiac apex. Atypical atrial flutter re-entrant circuits can also be established in other parts of the atrium or localized around scar tissue. In AF, the exact pathophysiologic mechanism is unclear, but one widely accepted theory suggests that multiple wave fronts of electrical activity sweep through the atria in a re-entrant but random fashion.

Antiarrhythmics suppress re-entry by slowing conduction or increasing refractoriness enough to essentially convert unidirectional block to bidirectional block.

Clinical Presentations   All supraventricular tachycardias present with a narrow complex QRS pattern by ECG (unless aberrant conduction of the supraventricular impulse is present). Typical manifestations of SVT include recurrent palpitations, chest fullness, "skipped" beats associated with lightheadedness, or presyncope. It is difficult to clinically differentiate between the different types of SVT based on clinical symptoms. The termination of the SVT with adenosine or vagal maneuvers suggests that the arrhythmia is AV node dependent.

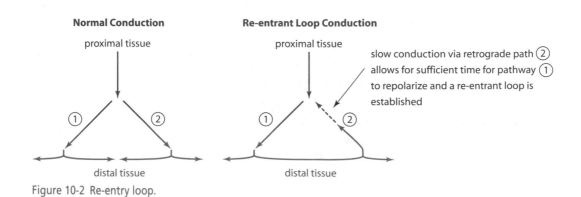

Figure 10-2 Re-entry loop.

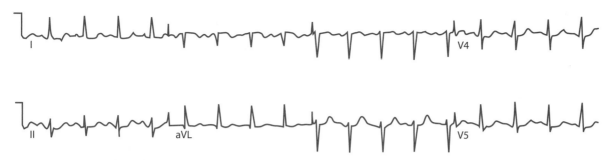

Figure 10-3 Sinus tachycardia.

Sinus tachycardia ECG demonstrates normal P waves followed by QRS complex (Figure 10-3). Sinus tachycardia is defined as an HR of 100 beats/min or greater. Sinus tachycardia is usually secondary to increased sympathetic tone from physiologic (exercise) or pathophysiologic (fever, stress, pain, hyperthyroidism, hypovolemia, hypoxemia, anemia, etc.) causes. Addressing the precipitating stressor is the focus of treatment.

AVNRT/AVRT ECG demonstrates a very regular, narrow complex QRS tachycardia of 100 to 250 beats/min. P waves may or may not be present (Figure 10-4). In general, AVRT presents in adolescents and young adults, while AVNRT is more common in middle-aged adults with no history of structural heart disease. Because these SVTs involve the AV node, adenosine or vagal maneuvers are effective at terminating AVNRT/AVRT. Pharmacologic treatment is with CCBs (class IV), beta-blockers (class II), digoxin, and class Ia and Ic medications. However, catheter-based radiofrequency (RF) ablation is the mainstay of therapy for these arrhythmias.

Atrial tachycardia This term refers to a number of different types of tachycardia that originate in the atria. The P-wave axis or morphology is different, and the QRS is usually the same as sinus rhythm. Because these tachycardias do not involve the AV node, vagal maneuvers or AV

nodal blockers are usually ineffective at terminating the tachycardia. Most atrial tachycardias, with the exception of multifocal atrial tachycardia, are treated using RF ablation. Therapy for multifocal atrial tachycardia is directed at the underlying pulmonary illness. The subclassification of atrial tachycardia is based on mechanism.

Increased automaticity Multifocal atrial tachycardia is associated with chronic pulmonary disease and presents with an atrial rate of 100 to 130 beats/min and the P wave has three or more morphologies (Figure 10-5). Treatment is based on the underlying pulmonary process. Unifocal atrial tachycardia is often seen in younger patients. Catheter-based radiofrequency ablation is the treatment of choice.

Re-entry Intra-atrial re-entry atrial tachycardia is associated with underlying heart disease or atrial arrhythmia history, such as AF or flutter.

Atrial fibrillation AF is the chaotic depolarization of the atrium with loss of synchronized mechanical contraction of the atrium during ventricular diastole. AF is associated with multiple conditions, including advanced age, low potassium or magnesium levels, postsurgical state, CHF, hyperthyroidism, and hyperadrenergic states. Because the atrial rate is so elevated at 350 to 600 depolarizations per minute, dis-

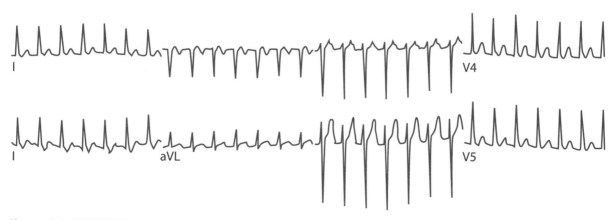

Figure 10-4 AVNRT/AVRT.

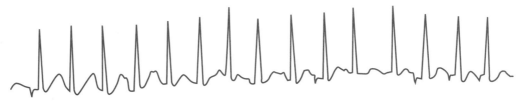

Figure 10-5 Multifocal atrial tachycardia.

tinct P waves are not discernable (Figure 10-6). The ventricular response (QRS complex) is "irregularly irregular" and usually 140 to 160 beats/min for untreated AF because the AV node can only conduct a fraction of the incoming atrial depolarizations. The clinical consequences of AF include (1) increased risk of stroke due to thrombus formation within the fibrillating atrium, and (2) hypotension and CHF secondary to a reduced diastolic filling period with sustained rapid ventricular response. Treatment includes decreasing the ventricular rate by further blocking the AV node with beta-blockers, CCBs, or digoxin. Class Ic (propafenone, flecainide) and class III agents (sotalol, amiodarone) can also be used to suppress and terminate AF. If medications are not successful, electrical cardioversion can be applied to restore normal sinus rhythm.

Atrial flutter   Atrial flutter is secondary to a re-entrant circuit usually within the right atrium but can also originate as a re-entry circuit in other parts of the atrium. The classic ECG pattern is a "sawtooth" P-wave pattern at a rate of 300 beats/min with a slower ventricular rate that is usually an even multiple of the atrial rate (e.g., atrial flutter with 2:1 block has a ventricular rate of 150 beats/min) (Figure 10-7). Atrial flutter often degenerates into AF. The treatment of choice for atrial flutter is RF ablation of the re-entrant circuit. The pharmacologic treatment for atrial flutter is similar to that for AF, and electrical cardioversion can also be applied to restore normal sinus rhythm. The clinical consequences of increased risk for stroke secondary to intra-atrial thrombus formation and CHF are also elevated for prolonged atrial flutter.

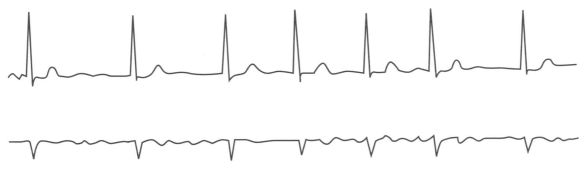

Figure 10-6 Atrial fibrillation.

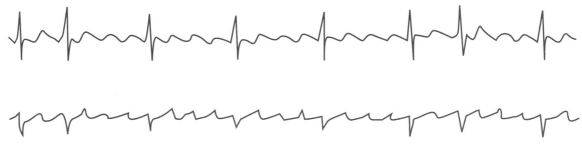

Figure 10-7 Atrial flutter.

Case Conclusion   JS is experiencing an AV nodal-dependent SVT precipitated by her hyperthyroidism (low-grade fever, baseline sinus tachycardia, hyperreflexia, and thyroid nodule) and caffeine intake. The termination of the tachycardia by vagal stimulation (cold water stimulus) suggests that the tachycardia involves the AV node. The regular nature of the tachycardia excludes AF, which is usually irregularly irregular. Given her middle age, her diagnosis is most likely AVNRT. After her hyperthyroidism was treated and her caffeine intake was reduced, her tachycardia resolved.

Thumbnail: Classification of Antiarrhythmic Mechanisms

Class	General mechanism	Examples
I	Sodium channel blockade	See subclasses (Ia, Ib, Ic) below
Ia	Decreases phase 0 upstroke rate	Quinidine, procainamide, disopyramide
Ib	Little effect on phase 0 in normal tissue Decreases phase 0 upstroke rate in abnormal tissue Shortens repolarization or little effect	Lidocaine, mexiletine, phenytoin
Ic	Markedly decreases phase 0 upstroke rate Markedly slows conduction	Flecainide, propafenone, encainide, moricizine
II	Beta-blockade	Metoprolol, esmolol, atenolol, propranolol
III	Potassium channel blockers Prolongation of repolarization	Amiodarone, sotalol, ibutilide, dofetilide, bretylium
IV	Calcium channel blockade	Verapamil, diltiazem

Key Points

▶ AV node-dependent tachycardias (AVNRT and AVRT) usually terminate with administration of an AV node-blocking agent or increased vagal tone.

▶ AV node-independent tachycardias (sinus tachycardia, atrial flutter, AF, atrial tachycardias) do not usually terminate with AV node-blocking agents (adenosine) or vagal stimulus (carotid sinus massage).

▶ SVTs are secondary to two basic mechanisms: (1) abnormal impulse formation secondary to abnormal automaticity, and (2) abnormal impulse formation secondary to re-entry.

Questions

1. FD is a 74-year-old man postoperative day 1 from a radical prostatectomy for prostate cancer. After breakfast, he develops palpitations and lightheadedness. The surgical intern administers 6 mg IV adenosine, which promptly resolves the tachycardia. The tachycardia recurs 2 hours later and an ECG obtained during the second episode would most likely reveal:

A. AF
B. Multifocal atrial tachycardia
C. Atrial flutter
D. Sinus tachycardia
E. AV nodal re-entry tachycardia

2. SH is a 18-year-old woman who complains of palpitations, and her workup is still pending. She was wondering whether RF ablation could be the appropriate treatment for her palpitations. Which diagnosis would be the most suitable and straightforward for RF ablation?

A. Multifocal atrial tachycardia
B. AF
C. Typical atrial flutter
D. Atypical atrial flutter
E. Sinus tachycardia

HPI: GT is a 76-year-old man with a history of HTN and diabetes with a chief complaint of two recent episodes of syncope. He also complains of increasing fatigue, weight gain, and cold intolerance. His current medications include lisinopril, glyburide, and hydrochlorothiazide.

PE: Vitals: BP 90/60 mm Hg, HR 46 beats/min, RR 14 breaths/min, Tmax 34.5°C. **H/N:** JVP 6 cm. **Chest:** Clear to auscultation. **Cardiac:** Normal PMI, normal S_1, S_2, no murmurs. **Abdomen:** Soft, nontender, no bruits, no pulsatile masses. **Extremities:** Diffusely hyporeflexic. **ECG:** Sinus bradycardia with first-degree AV block.

Labs: Normal electrolytes and complete blood count (CBC).

Thought Questions

- What are the two mechanisms responsible for brady-arrhythmias?

- What are the two main categories of sinus node dysfunction?

- What is the difference between second-degree Mobitz I and Mobitz II AV block?

- What are the classic ECG findings of each bradyarrhythmia?

Basic Science Review and Discussion

Bradyarrhythmias are abnormal heart rhythms when the HR is less than 60 beats/min. Bradyarrhythmias are the result of either decreased impulse formation from the SA node or impaired conduction.

Cardiac Conduction System   Cardiac conduction originates at the SA node, which is a collection of pacemaker cells located in the RA between the superior vena cava and right atrial appendage. In 60% of patients, the SA node blood supply is the SA nodal artery from the proximal right coronary artery (RCA). In 40% of patients, the SA node blood supply is a branch of the circumflex artery. Although the SA node receives innervation from both the parasympathetic and sympathetic nervous system, the SA node is predominantly under the influence of the parasympathetic system at rest. As a result, a denervated SA node in a transplanted heart (which does not receive autonomic stimuli) signals at 90 to 100 beats/min, which is significantly higher than usual normal resting heart rate of 60 to 80 beats/min.

After the spontaneous formation of an electrical signal in the SA node, the impulse is conducted in a delayed fashion to the AV node. This intrinsic delay allows for atrial contraction to be completed before the contraction of the ventricles. In 90% of people, the AV node receives its blood supply from a branch of the RCA (10% from the LAD artery). Since the majority of the blood supply to the SA and AV nodes is from the RCA, ischemia of this coronary vessel often causes bradyarrhythmias The impulse then leaves the AV node and enters the bundle of His. After 1 cm, the bundle of His bifurcates into the right and left bundles. The left bundle bifurcates again into an anterior and posterior fascicle (Figure 11-1). A common ECG finding is a left or right bundle branch block pattern, which corresponds to a conduction disturbance in the corresponding bundle branch.

SA Node Dysfunction   SA node dysfunction is the result of intrinsic or extrinsic factors. Intrinsic factors are structural changes within the node itself. The most common pathologic finding is replacement of the pacemaker cells with fibrous tissue. Intrinsic causes of SA node dysfunction include connective tissue disorders, infiltrative disease (amyloid), inflammation (myocarditis), chronic ischemia, and idiopathic degeneration.

Extrinsic causes temporarily inhibit SA node automaticity but do not physically modify the node. The most common extrinsic cause is drugs, including beta-blockers, CCBs, digoxin, lithium, and antiarrhythmic drugs. Autonomically

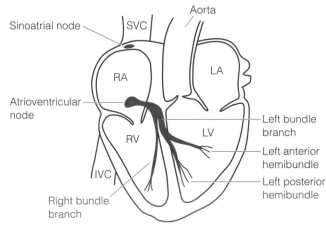

Figure 11-1 Cardiac conduction system.

mediated syndromes such as carotid SA hypersensitivity, situational (coughing, vomiting), and neurocardiogenic syncope can also cause transient SA node dysfunction. Other extrinisic causes include hypothermia, hypothyroidism, and electrolyte disorders.

Mild SA node dysfunction can result in sinus bradycardia, which is secondary to decreased automaticity of the SA node. Some well-conditioned athletes or older patients have intrinsically high vagal tone and have asymptomatic and benign sinus bradycardia. More severe SA node dysfunction can result in sick sinus syndrome (SSS). In SSS, the automaticity of the sinus node is highly variable, and sinus pauses can be followed by atrial tachyarrhythmias. Treatment usually requires an electronic pacemaker for the bradycardia and antiarrhythmic drug therapy for the tachyarrhythmia.

When SA node activity is suppressed for a prolonged period in severe sinus node dysfunction, pacemaker foci in the AV node or ventricle generate escape rhythms to maintain an adequate heart rate. Junctional escape beats from the AV node are characterized by QRS complexes at a rate of 60 beats/min and are not preceded by P waves since there is no intrinsic atrial activity. Ventricular escape beats are characterized by wide QRS complexes at 30 to 40 beats/min and also are not preceded by P waves. Treatment for extreme intrinsic sinus node dysfunction is implantation of a permanent pacemaker.

Impaired Conduction   Impaired conduction can be classified as three types: first-degree AV block, second-degree AV block, and third-degree AV (complete) block. Impaired conduction is usually the result of degeneration of the conduction pathway, MI, or drug toxicity.

First-degree AV block is a lengthening of the normal delay between atrial and ventricular depolarization so that the PR interval is greater than 0.2 second. The cause of first-degree AV block is similar to the causes for sinus node dysfunction. First-degree AV block usually occurs at the level of the AV node, and most patients remain asymptomatic and require no intervention.

Second-degree AV block is due to intermittent failure of AV conduction so that not every P wave (atrial depolarization) is followed by a QRS complex (ventricular depolarization). Second-degree AV block is further subclassified as Mobitz type I (Wenckebach) or Mobitz type II block. In Mobitz type I block the conduction delay between the atria and ventricles lengthens with each beat until an atrial impulse is not conducted to the ventricle. On an ECG, the PR interval progressively lengthens until a P wave does not generate a QRS depolarization. Mobitz type I block occurs at the level of the AV node and usually does not require treatment. In Mobitz type II block, the PR interval remains constant before the sudden loss of AV conduction manifested by a P wave not followed by a QRS depolarization. Mobitz type II block is more serious and more likely to occur distal to the AV node in the His' bundle. Since Mobitz type II block is much more likely to progress to third-degree AV block, the treatment of choice is electronic pacemaker implantation.

Third-degree block is complete absence of conduction between the atria and ventricles with no fixed relationship between the P waves and QRS complexes. While the atria depolarize at the intrinsic SA node rate (60–80 beats/min), the ventricles independently depolarize at the ventricular escape rate of 30 to 40 beats/min. Because third-degree AV block can severely compromise heart rate and cardiac output, emergent pacemaker therapy is necessary.

Case Conclusion   GT's syncope evaluation included a transthoracic echocardiogram that revealed normal LV function and normal valve morphology and function. Subsequent 24-hour Holter testing revealed several symptomatic 5-second sinus pauses, and an electronic pacemaker was placed. Further workup revealed severe hypothyroidism, and GT was started on synthroid. Since he has been taking synthroid, his hypothyroid symptoms have resolved and pacer interrogation has revealed no additional sinus pauses. His clinical course is suggestive of extrinsic SA nodal dysfunction secondary to hypothyroidism.

Thumbnail: ECG Tracings of Common Bradyarrhythmias

A

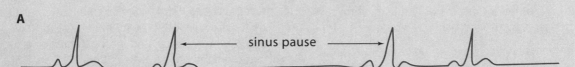

sinus pause

B

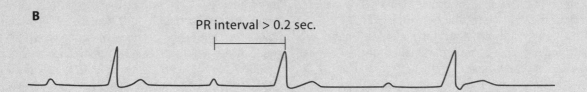

PR interval > 0.2 sec.

C

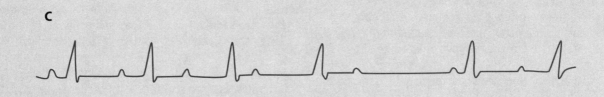

D

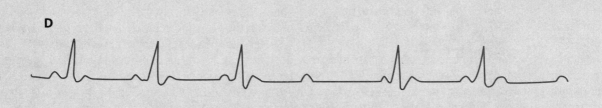

E

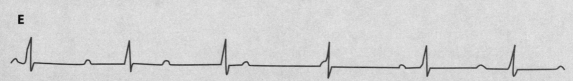

A: Sinus pause.

B: First-degree AV block.

C: Second-degree AV block type I.

D: Second-degree AV block type II.

E: Third-degree AV block.

Key Points

- ▶ Bradyarrhythmias are the result of either sinus node dysfunction or impaired conduction.

- ▶ Sinus node dysfunction can be secondary to either intrinsic or extrinsic causes.

- ▶ First-degree AV block and second-degree Mobitz type I block usually need no further intervention, whereas second-degree Mobitz type II block and third-degree heart block require electronic pacemaker placement.

- ▶ Bradyarrhythmias present with symptoms of lightheadedness, fatigue, exercise intolerance, and syncope.

Questions

1. Myocardial infarction of which coronary artery is most likely complicated by severe bradycardia?
   A. Circumflex coronary artery
   B. Obtuse marginal coronary artery
   C. LAD coronary artery
   D. Right coronary artery
   E. Ramus intermedius

2. A patient with which ECG finding is most likely to receive a pacemaker within the next year?
   A. Left bundle branch block
   B. Right bundle branch block
   C. Right bundle branch block and left posterior hemiblock
   D. Right bundle branch block with left anterior hemiblock
   E. Right bundle branch block with alternating anterior and posterior left hemiblock

HPI: JF is a 64-year-old man with a history of chronic renal insufficiency and heart failure secondary to idiopathic dilated cardiomyopathy. He presents to the emergency department with 3 days of nausea, vomiting, and occasional palpitations associated with lightheadedness. His medications included an ACE inhibitor, a low-dose beta-blocker, and a loop diuretic, and spironolactone had recently been started.

PE: Vitals: BP 90/60 mm Hg, HR 100 beats/min, RR 16 breaths/min, Tmax 37.0°C. **H/N:** JVP 6 cm. **Chest:** Clear to auscultation. **Cardiac:** Diffuse PMI with positive S_3 and 3/6 systolic murmur at base radiating laterally. **Abdomen:** No hepatosplenomegaly, good bowel sounds, no focal masses or tenderness. **Extremities:** Minimal peripheral edema with 1+/4 symmetric radial pulses. **ECG:** Normal sinus rhythm with peaked T-waves. **CXR:** Normal.

While an IV is placed in his arm, he immediately become unconscious and is found to be pulseless and without spontaneous respirations. Advanced cardiac life support protocol is initiated.

Thought Questions

- What is the relationship between premature ventricular contractions (PVCs) and ventricular fibrillation (VF) and ventricular tachycardia (VT)?

- What is the difference between monomorphic and polymorphic VT?

- What is the most common cause of VF and VT?

- What are other causes of VF and VT?

Basic Science Review and Discussion

Ventricular arrhythmias originate from ventricular tissue and are classified as VT or VF. VT and VF are the major causes of sudden cardiac death. PVCs are common, benign, and usually asymptomatic. PVCs are the result of ectopic ventricular foci generating an action potential independent of the SA and AV nodal conduction system. PVCs appear as wide QRS depolarizations because the electrical activity travels slowly through myocardium rather than through the normal conduction system. In people with no significant structural heart disease, PVCs do not progress to VT or VF.

Ventricular Tachycardia   VT is a rapid rhythm greater than 100 beats/min originating in the ventricle and is caused either by re-entry, triggered activity, or enhanced automaticity. If three PVCs occur in a row, a diagnosis of VT is established. VT is subclassified as nonsustained (<30 seconds) or sustained (≥30 seconds). In VT, the QRS complexes are very broad and occur at a rate of 100 to 200 beats/min (Figure 12-1).

VT can also be subclassified by morphology as monomorphic versus polymorphic. All the QRS complexes are the same shape in monomorphic VT because the tachycardia evolves from a single arrhythmogenic focus. The most common cause of monomorphic VT is re-entry in scarred

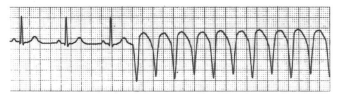

Figure 12-1 Ventricular tachycardia: a wide-complex tachycardia defined as three or more premature ventricular contractions in a row.

myocardium created after MI. In polymorphic VT, the QRS complexes are different shapes because the tachycardia evolves from several ventricular foci. Polymorphic VT is usually associated with active ischemia rather than re-entry from myocardial scarring.

Patients with VT usually complain of palpitations, chest fullness, and lightheadedness. If VT is sustained, hypotension occurs and loss of consciousness ensues from decreased cardiac output. The treatment of choice for symptomatic VT is electrical cardioversion. Electrical cardioversion produces a transient electrical field over the entire heart to re-establish organized electrical activity and contractile function. Although VT is a life-threatening arrhythmia, degeneration of VT into VF is even more lethal.

Ventricular Fibrillation   VF is the most lethal arrhythmia and is the result of multiple disorganized circulating wavefronts of electrical activity (Figure 12-2). The most common etiology of VF is ischemia from MI. As a result of the chaotic depolarizations, no coordinated contractile function can occur, and cardiac output suddenly declines. VF presents with sudden loss of consciousness with subsequent sudden cardiac death if electrical defibrillation is not emergently performed.

Wolff-Parkinson-White Syndrome   Wolff-Parkinson-White (WPW) syndrome is ventricular depolarization by an anomalous conduction pathway before the ventricle is depolar-

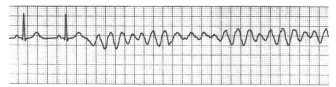

Figure 12-2 Ventricular fibrillation: the most common cause of sudden cardiac death.

ized by the normal AV conduction pathway (Figure 12-3). As a result, WPW syndrome is considered a pre-excitation syndrome (ventricle is prestimulated) by an accessory conduction pathway. Although only half the cases of WPW syndrome are symptomatic, patients with symptomatic

WPW syndrome usually present as young adults with either a supraventricular tachycardia or AF. The diagnostic test of choice is a short PR interval and a delta wave. Treatment of choice for WPW syndrome is catheter-based ablation of the accessory pathway.

Rarely, AF in WPW can induce ventricular fibrillation because of rapid ventricular stimulation via the accessory pathway. Therefore, treatment of AF with AV node-blocking agents (CCBs and digoxin) is contraindicated because these agents can precipitate VF by diverting the atrial impulses from the AV node into the accessory pathway. Procainamide is the treatment of choice for AF in the setting of WPW.

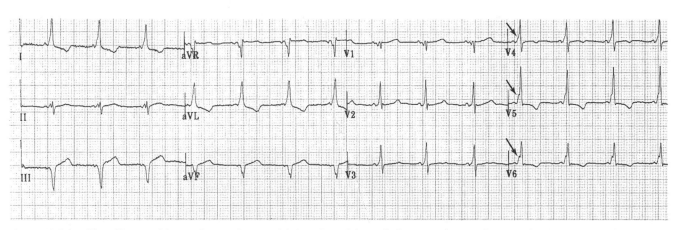

Figure 12-3 Wolff-Parkinson-White syndrome: the ventricle is activated through the AV node as well as via a bypass tract. Conduction via the bypass tract occurs earlier than via the AV node, and this earlier activation produces the delta wave (arrows in V4–V6) and shortens the PR interval.

Case Conclusion   JF was found to be in VF but electrical cardioversion was unsuccessful. Given that his ECG findings were consistent with hyperkalemia, treatment for high potassium was initiated with insulin, glucose, and sodium bicarbonate. He was then successfully defibrillated and returned to normal sinus rhythm. His systolic murmur is attributed to mitral regurgitation secondary to mitral annular dilatation associated with dilated cardiomyopathy.

His VF arrest was secondary to his spironolactone-induced hyperkalemia in conjunction with his dilated cardiomyopathy. Spironolactone is a potassium-sparing diuretic, and hyperkalemia is a potentially life-threatening side effect, especially in the setting of concomitant renal insufficiency and ACE inhibitor use. His VF was initially refractory to electrical defibrillation because of the high potassium. Only after the high potassium was corrected was electrical defibrillation successful. His potassium level was 7.4 mEq/L.

Thumbnail: Causes of VT and VF

Nonischemic causes of VT and VF

Although ischemic heart disease accounts for 80% of VF and VT, there are several other causes of these life-threatening arrhythmias. Causes of VF/VT can be subdivided into structural nonischemic heart disease and nonstructural heart disease.

Ischemia	Structural nonischemic disease	Nonstructural heart disease
Myocardial ischemia	Aortic stenosis	Electrolyte abnormalities
Coronary spasm	Amyloidosis	WPW syndrome
Coronary anomaly	Sarcoidosis	Long QT syndrome
	Hemochromatosis	Drug-induced long QT
	Dilated cardiomyopathy	Brugada syndrome*
	Hypertrophic cardiomyopathy	
	Pulmonary HTN	
	RV dysplasia	
	Chagas' disease	

*Brugada syndrome: association of right bundle branch block and nonischemic ST elevation and sudden death in otherwise healthy patients, usually young Asian males.

Key Points

▶ PVCs are common and do not progress to VT or VF in people with no significant heart disease.

▶ Monomorphic VT is most often caused by re-entry within preexisting scar tissue after MI while polymorphic VT suggests active ischemia.

▶ Treatment of symptomatic VT of VF is emergent electrical cardioversion.

▶ WPW syndrome is premature ventricular depolarization by an accessory conduction pathway.

Questions

1. A 69-year-old man with a history of two prior MIs presents with recurrent polymorphic VT requiring multiple electrical cardioversions. What would be the next clinical step in his management?
   A. Automatic implantable cardiac defibrillator (AICD) implantation
   B. IV magnesium replacement
   C. IV antiarrhythmics
   D. Thrombolysis
   E. Emergent cardiac catheterization and possible angioplasty

2. A 54-year-old woman is undergoing diuresis for CHF and blood transfusion for lower GI bleeding. While a nurse is assessing her vitals she loses consciousness. Her pulse is 140 beats/min and faint. Her morning labs include a potassium of 2.1 mEq/L and a calcium of 6.2 mEq/L. What would be her most likely arrhythmia on ECG?
   A. AF
   B. Atrial flutter
   C. Atrioventricular re-entry tachycardia (AVRT)
   D. Torsade de pointes VT
   E. VF

HPI: JS is a 56-year-old man who presents with the inability to move his right arm and leg for 6 hours. He is otherwise healthy but on review of systems he notes he has been increasingly fatigued and short of breath. An ECG demonstrates RVH, and his chest x-ray reveals RV enlargement and prominent pulmonary arteries. Brain magnetic resonance imaging (MRI) is consistent with an embolic left middle cerebral stroke. Heparin is started and cardiology is consulted for further evaluation.

PE: **Vitals:** T 37.0°C, HR 70 beats/min, BP 110/60 mm Hg, RR 16 breaths/min. **H/N:** JVP elevated at 12 cm. **Chest:** Clear to auscultation. **Cardiac:** RV lift, accentuated P_2, fixed split S_2, no significant murmur. **Extremities:** Mild cyanosis. **Neurologic:** Decreased strength and fine motor control of right upper and lower extremities with associated hyperreflexia.

Thought Questions

- What is the anatomic difference between an atrial septal defect and patent foramen ovale (PFO)?

- What pathophysiologic changes occur with left-to-right versus right-to-left shunts?

- What is Eisenmenger's syndrome?

- What are the common physical findings and clinical presentations of the common congenital cardiac abnormalities?

Basic Science Review and Discussion

Congenital heart disease is defined as a cardiac abnormality in structure and function present a birth. About 0.8% of live births are complicated by a congenital heart abnormality. Normal cardiovascular embryologic development will be reviewed in Case 14 since congenital abnormalities are usually the result of altered embryonic development of a cardiac structure.

Atrial Septal Defects and Patent Foramen Ovale

Anatomy and pathology   An atrial septal defect (ASD) is an opening within the atrial septum, allowing for flow of blood from the LA to the RA. It is relatively common, representing 6% to 10% of all cardiac anomalies, and is twice as common in females as in males. Although ASDs can occur anywhere along the interatrial septum, the most common is the ostium secundum defect, accounting for 69% of all ASDs. An ostium secundum defect is actually a developmental defect of the septum primum.

A PFO is an open conduit between the superior portion of the septum secundum on the RA side and the septum primum on the LA side. Postnatally, the foramen is normally held shut by overlapping of the two septa and the higher pressure in the LA. However, high RA pressures can cause the two septa to separate, allowing paradoxical embolization from right to left to occur.

Pathophysiology   In the setting of a large ASD, a chronic left-to-right shunt imposes a volume overload on the RV and RA, resulting in right-sided chamber hypertrophy and dilatation. The volume overload also causes dilatation of the pulmonary vascular bed and hypertrophy/luminal narrowing of the pulmonary arteries. As a result, 10% of patients with large ASDs can develop severe and irreversible pulmonary HTN secondary to increased pulmonary vascular resistance. With the elevated right-sided pressures, the left-to-right shunting eventually decreases (with a resultant decrease in the murmur), and may even reverse from right-to-left. The elevation of pulmonary artery pressure to systemic level causing a bidirectional or shunt reversal is known as Eisenmenger's syndrome. Shunt reversal results in systemic hypoxia, because deoxygenated blood from the RA mixes with the oxygenated blood in the LA.

Clinical presentation   Most ASDs are asymptomatic and may never be detected if very small. Large left-to-right shunts can result in fatigue and dyspnea. On physical exam, an RV precordial lift may be present due to dilatation of the RV. A widely and fixed split S_2 (composed of an aortic component followed by a pulmonary component) is present because the RV volume overload results in prolonged emptying of the RV and a subsequent delay in pulmonic valve closure. The ASD itself does not generate a murmur because there is little pressure gradient across the ASD. However, the increased blood flow through the cardiac chambers can result in two different types of murmurs: (1) a soft systolic murmur at the second intercostal space secondary to increased blood flow across the pulmonic valve, or (2) an early- to mid-diastolic murmur secondary to increased blood flow across the tricuspid valve. Chest radiographs demonstrate a cardiac enlargement and RVH. The ECG shows RVH.

Management   Elective surgical repair is the preferred treatment for major ASD. If major ASDs are left untreated, CHF can develop, especially in patients over 40. If left untreated, (1) CHF is quite common in patients over 40, (2) atrial arrhythmia incidence increases by up to 62% by age 60, and (3) pulmonary HTN can develop in 10% of patients. A percutaneous double umbrella device can also be used to close major ASDs less than 22 mm in diameter with adequate edges around the lumen.

Ventricular Septal Defects

Anatomy and pathology A ventricular septal defect (VSD) is an opening within the interventricular septum, allowing flow of blood from the LV to the RV. VSDs are slightly more common in females than in males. Although VSDs are the most common congenital cardiac anomaly associated with chromosomal abnormalities, 95% of VSDs are not associated with a chromosomal defect.

Although VSDs can occur anywhere along the ventricular septum, the most common type is a defect in the membranous septum, which is beneath the septal leaflet of the tricuspid valve and extends up to the aortic valve.

Pathophysiology Similar to ASDs, VSDs initially result in shunting of blood from a high pressure LV to a lower pressure RV. With right-sided volume overload, narrowing of the pulmonary arteries occurs and pulmonary HTN develops in 10% to 20% of patients (Eisenmenger's syndrome—refer to ASD section for description). LA dilatation, secondary to increased venous return from the lungs, can also cause the foramen ovale to open, creating an additional left-to-right shunt.

Unlike ASDs, there is bidirectional shunting of blood across VSDs with left-to-right shunting during isovolumetric contraction and right-to-left shunting during isovolumetric relaxation. This bidirectional shunting results in LV volume overload, LV hypertrophy, and eventually LV systolic dilatation and dysfunction.

Clinical presentation VSD presentation depends on the size of the VSD and the severity of the left-to-right shunt. A VSD may not be detected in newborns because pulmonary vascular resistance is high at birth, which minimizes the amount of left-to-right shunting. Several weeks after birth, as the pulmonary vascular resistance decreases, the amount of left-to-right shunting and associated signs and symptoms increase. Most VSDs are diagnosed in children when they are referred for a cardiac murmur.

With small VSDs, patients are asymptomatic and present with a high-pitched, lower left sternal border, holosystolic murmur extending past the S_2 with an associated palpable thrill. As the VSD becomes moderate in size, patients present with tachycardia and mild tachypnea. A mid-diastolic rumble may be present secondary to increased blood flow across the mitral valve, and the precordium is hyperdynamic. When the VSD is large, severe volume overload of the LV and LA occurs, with findings of pulmonary edema (tachypnea, rales) and an S_3.

If secondary pulmonary HTN develops, the holosystolic murmur of the VSD may disappear due to the decline in the pressure gradient between the RV and LV. Pulmonary HTN also causes (1) an accentuated pulmonic component of S_2, (2) RV lift secondary to RV hypertrophy, and (3) an early diastolic decrescendo murmur from pulmonic insufficiency. The increased shunting of deoxygenated blood from the RV to the systemic circulation within the LV (Eisenmenger's syndrome) results in cyanosis and systemic hypoxia.

Management Small asymptomatic VSDs require only periodic follow-up and antibiotic prophylaxis for endocarditis because many of them may spontaneously close. As VSDs become larger and patients become symptomatic, diuretics and digoxin are usually administered to alleviate right heart failure symptoms. Surgical therapy is recommended if there is increasing pulmonary pressure or if the amount of blood flow within the pulmonary circulation exceeds the amount of blood flow with the systemic circulation by a factor of 2 (both determined by cardiac catheterization).

Tetralogy of Fallot

Anatomy and pathology Tetralogy of Fallot (TOF) is composed of four anatomic features:

1. Pulmonic stenosis
2. RVH
3. VSD
4. Overriding of the aorta (aorta is displaced anteriorly and receives blood from both ventricles)

TOF is the most common cyanotic congenital heart disease in both children and adults and accounts for 4% to 10% of all congenital heart disease. TOF is the result of abnormal anterior and cephalad displacement of infundibular septum during embryonic development, resulting in unequal division of the conus. This unequal division results in the anterior aortic displacement, VSD, and pulmonic stenosis (which then induces RVH).

Pathophysiology Cyanosis and hypoxemia are present in TOF because deoxygenated blood returning to the RV encounters increased resistance from the pulmonic stenosis. This deoxygenated blood is routed through the VSD and into the aorta. Hypoxemia is induced by situations where systemic vascular resistance is lowered, systemic venous return is increased, or pulmonic stenosis is worsened. For example, crying or exposure to cold air can precipitate cyanosis because venous return increases and systemic vascular resistance decreases. Severe cases of hypoxemia can induce unconsciousness and convulsions. Compensation for the hypoxemia includes collateral circulation and polycythemia.

Clinical presentation   Cyanosis beginning at 3 to 6 months and a pulmonic stenosis murmur is a classic presentation. Cyanosis often induces clubbing of the nails. An RV precordial lift secondary to RVH is also present. Squatting is a characteristic position for these children. In this posture, the systemic vascular resistance increases (compression of abdominal aorta) and systemic venous return decreases (from compression of leg veins) with a resultant improvement in aortic oxygenation.

Management   Medical management includes iron supplementation to prevent anemia, antibiotics for endocarditis prophylaxis, and beta-blockers to decrease the degree of infundibular/RV outflow contraction during systole. Definitive treatment is surgical and includes RV outflow tract reconstruction and closure of the VSD.

Transposition of the Great Arteries (TGA)

Anatomy and pathology   TGA occurs when the origin of the aorta and main pulmonary artery are reversed, with the aorta arising from the RV and the main pulmonary artery arising from the LV. TGA is often associated with VSD, pulmonic stenosis, PDA, and coarctation. It occurs with a 2:1 male-female ratio.

Pathophysiology   With TGA, there are two separate circulations. The RV acts as the systemic ventricle and recirculates deoxygenated blood back into the systemic circulation. The LV acts as the pulmonic ventricle and recirculates oxygenated blood back to the lungs. Because there is no mixing of the oxygenated LV circuit with the deoxygenated RV circuit, TGA is lethal if not corrected

However, TGA is compatible with life in utero. In the TGA fetus, oxygenated blood from the placenta enters the RA and then passes into either the RV or LA via the PFO (Figure 14-1). Due to the transposition, LA blood then enters the LV and is pumped into the pulmonary artery (instead of the aorta). However, due to the high pulmonary vascular resistance, the majority of the oxygenated blood in the pulmonary artery flows into the aorta/systemic circulation via the ductus arteriosus instead of into the pulmonary vasculature.

Oxygenated blood that has passed from the RA to the RV is also pumped into the aorta (instead of the pulmonary artery). After birth, the physiologic closure of the ductus arteriosus and the foramen ovale do not permit shunting of oxygenated blood from the right-sided circulation into the deoxygenated left-sided circulation. Without a communication between the two parallel circuits, the infant becomes hypoxic and cyanotic.

Clinical presentation   The most common presentation of TGA is severe cyanosis. Unlike most other congenital cardiac abnormalities, no murmur is appreciated.

Management   Medical management includes immediate infusion of prostaglandin E to maintain patency of the ductus arteriosus, which will permit continued mixing of deoxygenated blood in the right-sided circulation with oxygenated blood in the left-sided circulation. Palliative interventional therapy includes balloon atrial septostomy to permit mixing of systemic and pulmonary blood at the atrial level. All patients will eventually need definitive surgical therapy, which includes an atrial baffle procedure (Mustard or Senning procedure) or arterial switch procedure.

Case Conclusion   A transesophageal echocardiogram demonstrated that JS has a 2.7-cm ASD. His stroke was most likely secondary to a paradoxical embolism that migrated from the lower extremities into the right-sided heart chambers, through the ASD, into the LA and LV, and then to his cerebral circulation. As a result of the chronic left-to-right volume overload, he has developed RV enlargement/hypertrophy (RV lift detected on exam and RV enlargement by CXR and ECG), pulmonary HTN, and reversal of flow via the ASD (Eisenmenger's syndrome). His accentuated P_2 on exam is secondary to pulmonary HTN, and the fixed split S_2 is the result of delayed pulmonic valve closure from increased RV flow. Although his initial shunt was left to right, the flow is now right to left secondary to Eisenmenger's sydrome, with resultant systemic hypoxia, fatigue, cyanosis, and clubbing. Because the ASD was greater than 22 mm in diameter, he was referred for open heart surgical repair.

Thumbnail: Diagrams of Common Congenital Cardiac Abnormalities

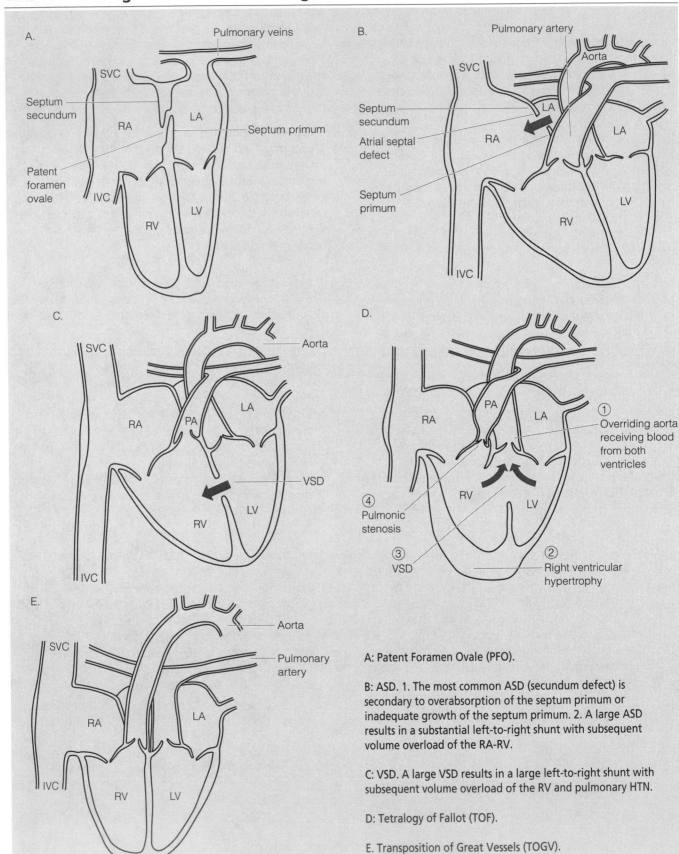

A: Patent Foramen Ovale (PFO).

B: ASD. 1. The most common ASD (secundum defect) is secondary to overabsorption of the septum primum or inadequate growth of the septum primum. 2. A large ASD results in a substantial left-to-right shunt with subsequent volume overload of the RA-RV.

C: VSD. A large VSD results in a large left-to-right shunt with subsequent volume overload of the RV and pulmonary HTN.

D: Tetralogy of Fallot (TOF).

E. Transposition of Great Vessels (TOGV).

Key Points

▸ PFO/ASD: A PFO or ASD can result in paradoxical embolization (thrombus from leg can shunt across PFO/ASD into left heart chambers and cause a stroke if the thrombus lodges within the brain).

▸ VSD: Eisenmenger's complex is defined as pulmonary HTN at the systemic level caused by high pulmonary vascular resistance with reversed or bidirectional shunt through a VSD. Eisenmenger's syndrome is identical to Eisenmenger's complex, but the shunt is secondary to a congenital defect other than VSD (e.g., ASD or PDA).

▸ TOF: The tetralogy is pulmonic stenosis, RVH, VSD, and overriding aorta.

▸ TGA: TGA is compatible with life in the fetus due to right-to-left shunting of oxygenated blood at the ductus arteriosus and PFO. After birth, the ductus arteriosus and PFO close, resulting in life-threatening hypoxia.

Questions

1. A newborn infant is noted to be increasingly cyanotic after birth and an immediate echocardiogram confirms the diagnosis of transposition of the great arteries. Which of the following interventions would be most helpful in reversing the pathophysiologic process?

   A. Supplemental oxygen
   B. Inotropic support with dobutamine
   C. Indomethacin administration
   D. Prostaglandin infusion
   E. Blood transfusion

2. A 6-month-old girl presents with cyanosis and a pulmonic stenosis murmur. Further evaluation of the patient reveals she has TOF. Which of the following interventions would be least helpful in stabilizing her condition until an open surgical correction can be performed?

   A. Antibiotics for endocarditis prophylaxis
   B. Supplemental iron
   C. Supplemental oxygen
   D. Beta-blockers
   E. Hydralazine

HPI: MW is a 15-year-old girl who presents with 2 years of increasing dyspnea and fatigue with exercise. Over the past 2 months, she has also noted increasing cyanosis and peripheral edema. Your colleague documented a "continuous machinery-like" murmur 6 months ago but she was lost to follow-up. Past Medical History (PMH): Other than premature birth at 34 weeks, patient is healthy.

PE: **Vitals:** T 37.0°C, HR 110 beats/min, BP 130/60 mm Hg, RR 22 breaths/min. **H/N:** JVP elevated at 9 cm. **Chest:** Basilar crackles. **Cardiac:** Tachycardic, RV lift, accentuated P_2, enlarged PMI, no significant murmur. **Extremities:** Cyanosis and clubbing present, mild peripheral edema. **ECG:** Sinus tachycardia with LV and RV hypertrophy. **CXR:** Enlarged cardiac silhouette, mild heart failure, and dilated pulmonary arteries.

Thought Questions

- How is the fetal circulation different from the adult circulation?

- What changes to the fetal circulation occur after birth?

- What is the classic murmur associated with patent ductus arteriosus (PDA)?

- What are the major chronologic milestones of cardiovascular embryologic development?

Basic Science Review and Discussion

Congenital heart disease is defined as a cardiac abnormality in structure and/or function present at birth. About 0.8% of live births are complicated by a congenital heart abnormality. Normal cardiovascular embryologic development will be reviewed in the Thumbnail section since congenital abnormalities are usually the result of altered embryonic development of a cardiac structure.

Fetal Circulation

1. Oxygenated blood leaving the placenta via the umbilical vein flows into either the ductus venosus or portal vein.

2. Blood routed to the ductus venosus bypasses the liver and is routed to the inferior vena cava (IVC).

3. Blood routed to the portal vein enters the liver and returns to the IVC via the hepatic vein; this hepatic blood pool has lower oxygen content than the ductus venosus blood pool.

4. Hepatic (less oxygenated) and ductus venosus (more oxygenated) blood pools remain separated in the IVC and enter the left atrium.

5. When the IVC enters the RA, the majority of the more oxygenated blood (from the ductus venosus pool) is shunted via the foramen ovale into the LA. This blood then flows into the LV and is pumped into the aorta to preferentially supply the heart, brain, and body with the most oxygen-enriched blood. The fetal LV accounts for only 34% of the total cardiac output.

6. The remainder of the less oxygenated blood from the hepatic blood pool enters the RA and RV. The minority of blood (12%) is pumped into the pulmonary arteries since there is a high resistance to pulmonary blood flow across the fluid-filled lungs (which are also incapable of oxygenating the blood). The RV pumps most of this blood (88%) into the descending aorta via the ductus arteriosus to be reoxygenated by the placenta (Figure 14-1).

Transitional Circulation   At birth, the systemic vascular resistance increases since the low-resistance placental circulation is removed. The pulmonary vascular resistance

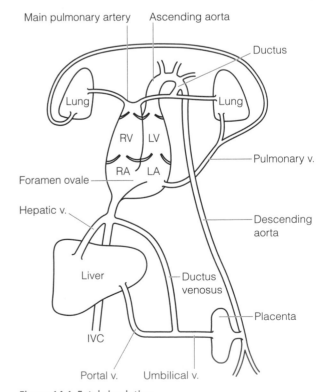

Figure 14-1 Fetal circulation.

decreases with the expansion of the lungs and vaso-dilatation of the pulmonary vessels. As a result, the RV preferentially pumps deoxygenated blood into the pulmonary circulation instead of shunting the blood through the ductus arteriosus into the aorta. Since the ductus is no longer needed, prostaglandin E$_2$ (PGE$_2$) levels decline, with resultant constriction and closure of the ductus.

At birth, the RA pressure declines due to decreased blood flow from the now ligated umbilical vein, and the LA pressure increases secondary to the increased venous return from the lungs via the pulmonary veins. With the LA pressure greater than the RA pressure, the septum primum is pushed rightward against the septum secundum, and the previously open foramen ovale is closed

Patent Ductus Arteriosus

Anatomy and pathology   The ductus arteriosus (DA) in fetal circulation permits oxygenated blood to bypass the immature lungs by serving as a conduit between the pulmonary artery/RV and the descending aorta (right-to-left shunt).

Pathophysiology   In utero, over 90% of the RV cardiac output bypasses the immature lungs and is directed via the DA into the systemic flow of descending aorta. After birth, a decrease in circulating prostaglandins and increased oxygen tension causes the DA to close spontaneously. If the DA remains patent postnatally, blood is shunted left to right, from the high-pressure systemic circulation (descending aorta) into the low-pressure pulmonic circulation (pulmonary artery). A large PDA can result in LV volume overload and subsequent CHF. In addition, the increased blood flow across the pulmonary vasculature as a result of the left-to-right shunt can increase pulmonary vascular resistance and cause pulmonary HTN. When the pulmonic pressure equals the systemic pressures, the shunt reverses in a right-to-left direction (reverse PDA).

Clinical presentation   Most patients are asymptomatic but some patients present with decreased exercise tolerance or CHF symptoms. The pathognomonic PDA murmur is a continuous "machine-like" murmur localized in the third intercostal space radiating to the supraclavicular region. With the onset of pulmonary HTN and reverse PDA flow (right-to-left), the murmur may disappear and cyanosis may become apparent. The diagnosis of a PDA is usually confirmed with cardiac echocardiography or cardiac catheterization.

Management   In premature infants, prostaglandin inhibition with indomethacin may accelerate closure. PDA patients should all receive antibiotic prophylaxis to prevent bacterial endarteritis. The final treatment is physical closure of the PDA either by surgical ligation or percutaneous device occlusion.

Case Conclusion   MW presents with a PDA secondary to incomplete closure at birth. Preterm birth is a risk factor for PDA. Six months ago, she presented with the typical "machinery-like" PDA murmur and left-to-right shunting. However, she has developed pulmonary HTN secondary to Eisenmenger's syndrome and now presents with "reversed ductus arteriosus" and right-to-left shunting. Her RV lift, accentuated P$_2$, and dilated pulmonary arteries on CXR are consistent with pulmonary HTN. Her elevated JVP and peripheral edema are secondary to right heart failure. Her pulmonary congestion and fatigue are secondary to LV dysfunction from chronic volume overload. Her "typical" PDA murmur has disappeared since the shunt flow is now reversed.

Thumbnail: Synopsis of Human Cardiovascular Embryologic Development

Embryo Day	Event	Diagram
Day 18	Cardiovascular system first appears as angiogenic clusters in mesoderm to form two heart tubes	

Day 21	Two heart tubes fuse to form single heart tube; outflow (cephalad) becomes aortic arches; inflow (caudal) becomes embryonic venous system	

A: Angiogenic cell clustering and fusion of the heart tube.

Day 22	Constrictions (sulci) divide single heart tube into five separate chambers; heart begins to beat; heart divided into three layers → endocardium, myocardium, and epicardium	

B: Five chambers of the heart tube and sulci.

Day 23	Folding of the heart tube positions the bulbus cordis (which becomes the RV) anteriorly and to the right and shifts the primitive ventricle and primitive atrium posteriorly and superiorly	

C: Folding of the heart tube.

Day 28	Septation of the atria and division of the common AV canal into right and left canals in order to separate the systemic and pulmonary circulations. Two embryonic partial septa, the septum primum and septum secundum, fuse to form the mature interatrial septum. The foramen ovale is the interatrial conduit formed by the opening of the septum secundum and lower septum primum; it allows blood to flow from the right to left atrium in the fetal circulation. Ventricular septal formation also begins on day 28 and is completed by the 8th week.	

D: Atrial septal formation.

Continued

5th week	Four endocardial cushions proliferate to form the AV canals and the conal septum (which divides the truncus arteriosus into the ascending aorta and the pulmonary trunk).

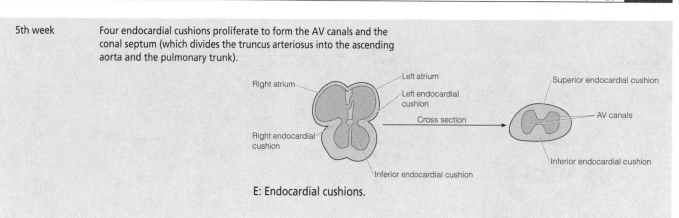

E: Endocardial cushions.

Key Points

▶ Fetal circulation: The LA/LV preferentially pump oxygenated blood shunted across the foramen ovale to the heart and brain; the RA/RV pump less oxygenated blood to the placenta to be reoxygenated.

▶ Transitional circulation: At birth, the DA and foramen ovale are physiologically closed. Cyanosis is the result of right-to-left shunting, not left-to-right shunting.

▶ PDA: Pathognomonic murmur is a continuous (during both systole and diastole), "machine-like" murmur.

Questions

1. A 45-year-old man undergoes right heart catheterization in which a catheter is advanced from the right femoral vein into the IVC, through the RA, RV, and into the distal left pulmonary artery. Blood samples are taken at each site. What would be the expected oxygenation values if the patient had a PDA (normal venous blood saturation is 70%)?

	IVC	RA	RV	Left pulmonary artery
A.	70%	70%	71%	71%
B.	70%	70%	70%	90%
C.	70%	84%	79%	79%
D.	70%	70%	92%	88%
E.	80%	80%	80%	80%

2. A newborn infant is diagnosed with a very large PDA and is scheduled for open surgical repair. In the interim period, which of the following treatments could potentially worsen the clinical situation?

A. Supplemental oxygenation
B. Indomethacin
C. Aspirin
D. Inhaled nitric oxide
E. Low-dose phenylephrine infusion into pulmonary artery

Answer Key—Part I: Cardiovascular

Case 1

1. C
2. D

Case 2

1. B
2. E

Case 3

1. C
2. D

Case 4

1. C
2. D

Case 5

1. C
2. D

Case 6

1. B
2. E

Case 7

1. C
2. C

Case 8

1. B
2. A
3. C

Case 9

1. E
2. D

Case 10

1. E
2. C

Case 11

1. D
2. E

Case 12

1. E
2. D

Case 13

1. D
2. E

Case 14

1. B
2. D

Part II

Endocrine

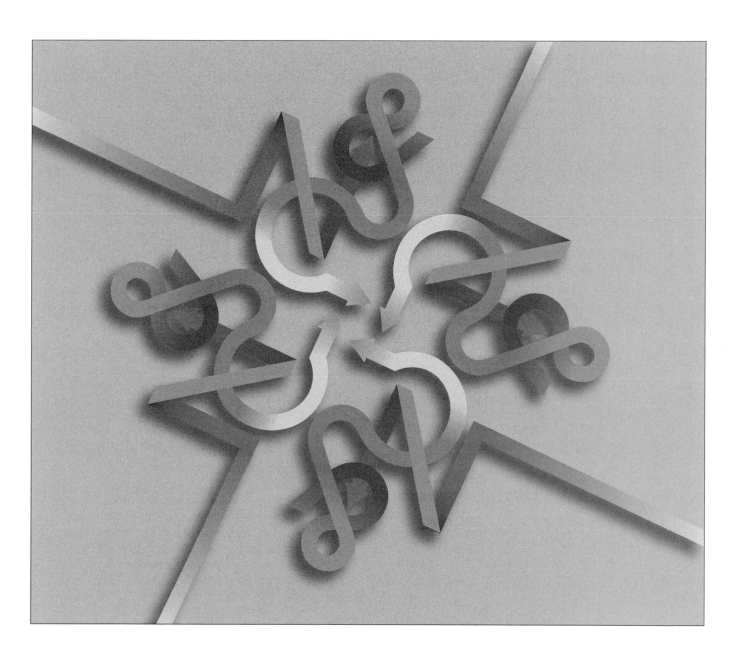

HPI: PY is a 19-year-old white man who presents to the emergency department (ED) with complaints of abdominal pain, nausea, and vomiting for 3 days. The patient states that he had a mild fever with chills for 1 day last week, but attributed his symptoms to "the flu." He has also noted increased thirst and urination for the past month. Patient denies diarrhea, constipation, dysuria, hematuria, headache, or flank pain, and he has not vomited any blood. He has complained of blurry vision recently, but has otherwise been free of known medical problems and is not on any medications. Systems review is significant for a 15-pound weight loss over the past 2 months and generalized fatigue for the same period.

PE: On physical exam, PY is a drowsy, thin man with an unusual fruity odor to his breath. He appears to be dehydrated, with poor skin turgor and dry mucous membranes in his mouth. The patient breathes both rapidly and heavily. He is tachycardic with normal heart sounds. He also exhibits mild epigastric tenderness, but no masses and normal bowel sounds.

Labs: Urinalysis reveals 4+ glucose and large ketones. Other significant labs include a serum glucose level of 645 mg/dL, positive ketones in serum, altered serum electrolytes, and an elevated BUN/creatinine level. Arterial blood Gas (ABG) reveals an elevated anion gap metabolic acidosis, with pH 7.05, P_{CO_2} 15 mm Hg, P_{O_2} = 106 mm Hg, and HCO_3^- 6 mEq/L.

Thought Questions

- This is an acute presentation of what chronic disease process?

- How do insulin and glucagon function to regulate glucose metabolism?

- What is the pathogenesis behind this condition?

Basic Science Review and Discussion

PY presents to the emergency room in acute **diabetic ketoacidosis** (DKA). DKA is a metabolic complication of type 1 diabetes mellitus, characterized by hyperglycemia, excess serum ketones, and metabolic acidosis. Although DKA can evolve rapidly, it is actually an acute manifestation of the chronic disease process of **type 1 diabetes.** Patients with type 1 diabetes often have a sudden onset of symptoms, commonly preceded by a viral-like syndrome. These symptoms can include polyuria, polydipsia, and polyphagia, as well as weight loss and blurry vision. In this instance, although PY attributed his condition to "the flu," laboratory studies and diagnostic signs help confirm that there is a serious underlying condition at hand.

Type 1 diabetes accounts for about 10% of all cases of diabetes. It is common in children, young adults, and people of European (especially Scandinavian) descent. The primary defect behind type 1 diabetes is a complete lack of endogenous insulin. Most commonly, this lack of insulin is caused by **autoantibodies directed against pancreatic beta cell antigens**. These autoantibodies start a destructive cascade within the pancreatic islet (Figure 15-1). It has been hypothesized that a precipitating event, such as a viral illness can initiate this cascade within genetically susceptible persons. Although insulin secretion is only impaired at first, continued destruction and loss of **beta cells** eventually eliminates insulin secretion completely. This process can take years to complete, and patients can remain asymptomatic until late in the disease process. After loss of about 70% of their beta cells, however, patients become symptomatic and may develop DKA rapidly. They are *dependent on exogenous*

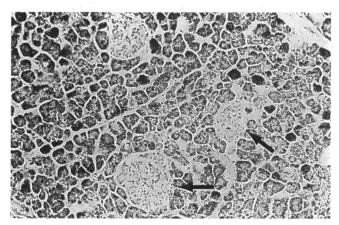

Figure 15-1 The endocrine functions of the pancreas arise from the islets of Langerhans. These islets contain numerous cell types, including beta cells, which secrete insulin, alpha cells, which synthesize glucagon, and delta cells, which produce somatostatin. The beta cells comprise about 75% of the cells in the islet and are the cells that are affected in type 1 diabetes mellitus. (Image courtesy of Joel Schechter, PhD, Keck School of Medicine at the University of Southern California.)

insulin secretion for day-to-day survival. Rarely, type 1 diabetes can occur in patients with severe insulin deficiency and no evidence of autoimmunity.

Glucose is the primary fuel source for all cells of the body. Plasma glucose levels are normally regulated by the balance of insulin and glucagon. Insulin is an anabolic hormone produced by the beta cells of the pancreas. The precursor molecule of insulin consists of a C-peptide, an α chain, and a β chain, connected by two disulfide bonds. The C-peptide portion must be cleaved off the proinsulin molecule before it becomes activated as insulin. Once activated, it promotes the burning of carbohydrate, the storage of fat, and a reduction in circulating levels of glucose, amino acids, and fatty acids.

Insulin and Glucagon   The primary stimuli for insulin secretion are an *increase in circulating glucose and amino acids.* Insulin lowers blood glucose by promoting glucose uptake and utilization by tissues that express GLUT-4 glucose transporters, namely skeletal muscle, cardiac muscle, and adipose tissue. In contrast, brain, liver, and RBCs take up glucose independent of insulin. Insulin also *suppresses hepatic glucose production* (glycogenolysis and gluconeogenesis) and *inhibits glucagon release* by the islet cells of the pancreas. Glucagon is a catabolic hormone that opposes the action of insulin on liver and fat, and acts to raise blood glucose. It does this by promoting the release of fatty acids from adipose tissue and promoting glycogenolysis and glucose release from the liver. A fall in plasma glucose is the main stimulus for the release of glucagon. Together, the actions of insulin and glucagon work to maintain normal glucose homeostasis. When there is an absolute or relative lack of insulin, however, diabetes mellitus can occur and manifests as the signs and symptoms of hyperglycemia.

Diabetic Ketoacidosis   DKA is an acutely dangerous complication of type 1 diabetes that results in a rapid spiraling sequence of events that can lead to coma and death. The diagnostic features of DKA are **hyperglycemia, excess ketones** (acetoacetate and β-hydroxybutyrate) in serum, and **high anion gap metabolic acidosis.** Other associated features include dehydration, electrolyte abnormalities, and severe metabolic "stress" such as infection, MI, or trauma. Because type 1 diabetics have an absolute lack of insulin, they are unable to use glucose as a source of energy. Paradoxically, this reduced glucose utilization by muscle and fat stimulates increased glucose production by the liver. Stress hormones such as epinephrine further stimulate glucose production and limit utilization, contributing to the hyperglycemia. As an alternate fuel source, increased free fatty acids are released for conversion into ketones for energy. The build-up of excess ketones in the blood results in an increased anion gap metabolic acidosis. Acidemia stimulates increased ventilation as a compensatory mechanism and thus lowers the P_{CO_2} of blood. Glucose excretion into the urine results in the loss of water from the body and creates an extremely dehydrated state. Correction of the hyperglycemia requires both hydration and insulin to reverse ketone production and ketoacidosis.

Case Conclusion   Taking note of PY's rapidly deteriorating state, physicians in the ED immediately begin rehydrating PY with IV fluids and administer insulin therapy. As hydration is corrected and ketone overproduction is shut off by insulin, PY's anion gap slowly begins to normalize. He remains in the ED until stabilized and is transferred to the diabetes unit for further monitoring.

Thumbnail: Type 1 Diabetes Mellitus

Primary defect
Absolute insulin deficiency

Pathogenesis
Autoimmune attack against pancreatic beta cells

Frequency
~10% of diabetes cases

Age of onset
Usually prior to age 20

Clinical onset
Acute symptoms

HLA association
DR3/DR4

Identical twin concordance
20%–30%

Islet antibodies
> 90%

Islet histology
Beta cell destruction

Insulin resistance
No

Blood insulin/C-peptide levels
Low or absent

High-risk groups
European, especially Scandinavian

Primary treatment options
Exogenous insulin therapy

Key Points

▶ Autoimmune etiology: antibodies are directed against pancreatic beta cells.

▶ Eventually results in absolute insulin deficiency.

▶ **Insulin is required for treatment.** Insulin secretagogues that stimulate insulin secretion (glyburide, glipizide, tolbutamide) become ineffective when all the beta cells are destroyed.

▶ Young age of onset, usually no family history of diabetes.

Questions

1. DKA is associated with several metabolic abnormalities. These abnormalities include dehydration, hyperglycemia, and an accelerated state of lipolysis and ketone production. These metabolic imbalances are reflected in irregular laboratory values, including an altered anion gap. Using the laboratory values Na$^+$ 140 mEq/L, K$^+$ 4.0 mEq/L, Cl$^-$ 103 mEq/L, and HCO$_3^+$ 6 mEq/L, PY's calculated anion gap is:

   A. 12 mmol/L
   B. 20 mmol/L
   C. 31 mmol/L
   D. 35 mmol/L
   E. 44 mmol/L

2. A 26-year-old bulimic woman is found weak and lethargic in her apartment by a neighbor. Mucous membranes are dry and she is minimally responsive. The neighbor dials 911 and the woman is rushed to the nearest hospital where laboratory tests reveal blood glucose levels of 800, serum pH 7.1, Pco$_2$ 18 mmHg, Po$_2$ 98 mmHg, and HCO$_3^-$ 10 meq/L. The patient is rapidly rehydrated with IV fluids and given an injection of exogenous insulin. When using exogenous insulin therapy, serum C-peptide levels are:

   A. Increased
   B. Decreased
   C. Normal
   D. Indicative of long-term glycemic control
   E. Necessary for acute therapeutic monitoring

HPI: CJ is a 63-year-old African-American woman who presents to her primary care physician complaining of nocturia twice nightly for the past 6 months. She states that she was reluctant to go to the doctor because she didn't think there was anything wrong, but the nocturia was beginning to interfere with her sleep. CJ states that she has felt otherwise well, but admits to being "thirsty all the time." Upon further questioning, the patient revealed that while pregnant with her daughter many years ago, she vaguely remembered her doctor mentioning that her blood sugar was "a little high." She received no medications at that time and recalls that the problem resolved shortly after delivering the baby. The patient is a pleasant and cooperative, mildly obese female. She admits to putting on "a few pounds" over the past 5 years, especially after the death of her husband. She says that the two of them used to take walks in the park together on a regular basis, but now she has no one to walk with. Patient denies any headache, visual loss, or numbness/tingling in her extremities.

PE: On physical exam, CJ appears to have scattered dot/blot hemorrhages and hard exudates in the periphery of her left eye; macula are intact bilaterally. She also exhibits reduced sensation to touch and vibration in both feet and ankles. The remainder of the exam is normal.

Labs: Blood tests reveal plasma glucose levels to be elevated at 232 mg/dL. Both BUN and creatinine are also slightly increased above normal. Urinalysis shows 3+ glucose and 2+ protein in her urine.
Upon receiving these results, the physician asks CJ to return the next morning for a fasting glucose level. Fasting results are also elevated at 170 mg/dL. The physician diagnoses CJ with type 2 diabetes mellitus (DM) and asks her to make an appointment to discuss her diagnosis and treatment options.

Thought Questions

■ What is the primary defect behind type 2 DM?

■ What risk factors does CJ have for developing diabetes?

■ What are the complications of this disease process?

Basic Science Review and Discussion

CJ has been diagnosed with type 2 DM. Although the symptoms of **polyuria, polydipsia,** and **hyperglycemia** are common to both type 1 and type 2 diabetes, the gradual onset, increased age of the patient, and obese body habitus suggest that type 2 DM is more likely. Type 2 DM results from a decreased sensitivity to insulin resulting in a "relative" insulin deficiency. Although patients can produce insulin in their pancreas, they cannot make enough to compensate for their increased needs. This insulin resistance is in part genetic; **central obesity, high carbohydrate diet,** and **reduced physical activity** are the most common environmental contributing factors. Also, the condition is most common in people of Latino, African, Native American, and Asian origin. Women with a history of gestational diabetes are at increased risk for getting type 2 DM later in life.

Pathophysiology Physiologically, the primary defect in type 2 DM is peripheral **insulin resistance.** This resistance disturbs the delicate balance between the glucose-regulating actions of insulin and glucagon. Namely, insulin is deficient and glucagon is excessive. This imbalance results in **impaired**

glucose uptake and utilization by cells (particularly skeletal muscle and fat cells), **increased protein catabolism,** and **increased lipolysis.** These changes are evident in patients as hyperglycemia and glucosuria, nitrogen loss in urine from protein breakdown, and ketonemia/ketonuria from increased fat metabolism. As the body senses decreased glucose uptake, it stimulates the pancreatic beta cells to compensate and make more insulin. However, the beta cells eventually become overworked and fail to maintain blood glucose at normal levels. Hepatic glucose overproduction occurs secondary to the perceived lack of glucose availability, further contributing to the hyperglycemia.

Acute Complications Because type 2 diabetics make some insulin, they can suppress lipolysis and do not develop the acute, life-threatening complication of DKA that is seen in type 1 diabetics. Instead, type 2 patients are susceptible to a **nonketotic hyperosmolar state** that can occur with infection or other metabolic stress. Although there is no ketoacidosis, these states are characterized by **hyperglycemia, dehydration,** and **altered mental status.** With blood glucose values of greater than 600 to 800 mg/dL, a hyperosmolar coma may ensue. Electrolyte abnormalities are also common. Treatment is slow fluid rehydration to correct the hyperosmolar state.

Chronic Complications Chronic complications of diabetes include **nephropathy, retinopathy,** and **neuropathy.** In addition, **atherosclerosis** is often present prior to the onset of symptomatic hyperglycemia, and its course is hastened and aggravated by DM. Complications are not usually present at the onset of diabetes, but develop after years of hyperglycemia. Abnormal microvascular hemodynamics and glycosolation of proteins are possible mechanisms contributing to the atherosclerosis, retinopathy, and nephropathy. In addition, individuals differ in their susceptibility to the effects of diabetes on their renal, retinal, and neural tissues.

CJ already shows signs of chronic hyperglycemia, as she has evidence of background retinopathy in her left eye (dot/blot hemorrhages from microvascular changes), though the initial changes have not yet impinged on her vision (macula are intact). Also, she may have some early symmetric polyneuropathy, as shown by the bilateral loss of touch and vibration sensation in her feet and ankles. Cells that are freely permeable to glucose, such as peripheral nerves, experience a large influx of glucose during periods of hyperglycemia. This excess glucose is converted to sorbitol within the cells. Diabetic neuropathy may be caused by **sorbitol accumulation** and **myoinositol depletion** within peripheral nerves, resulting in decreased Na^+-K^+ ATPase activity and impaired nerve conduction. CJ's renal function has also been affected, as shown by the elevated BUN and creatinine. Low glomerular filtration rate (GFR), proteinuria, and HTN may be indicative of impending renal failure. Obesity is a risk factor for the development of type 2 DM, but it is not a result of long-term DM. More than 80% of all patients with type 2 DM are obese, because obesity is associated with resistance to the glucose-lowering effects of insulin. Weight loss often lowers elevated blood glucose in patients with type 2 DM.

Clinical Management Because of the acute and particularly the chronic complications of type 2 DM, it is imperative that patients are followed closely and their disease carefully managed. Aggressive management can involve patients checking their blood glucose values four times per day, although this can decrease once a stable management regimen is achieved. A hemoglobin A_{1c} (**HbA$_{1c}$**), or **glycosylated hemoglobin,** can be sent to assess the average glucose values over the past 3 months, since the average life span of a red blood cell is 120 days. In patients who achieve tight control of their sugar levels, keeping HbA$_{1c}$ below 7%, it has been shown that they are less likely to suffer the chronic microvascular complications of diabetes.

Diet and exercise are mainstays of treatment, and patients who are actually able to maintain a low-carbohydrate diet and lose weight have been known to decrease or discontinue medications. Oral medications are commonly used, including the **sulfonylureas** (e.g., glyburide, glipizide), **biguanides** (metformin), **thiazolidinediones** (rosiglitazone, pioglitazone), and the **meglitinides** (repaglinide). The most common of these medications, the sulfonylureas, act to increase insulin release from the beta cell of the pancreas. Another common medication, metformin, a biguanide, acts to decrease postprandial glucose levels, although the exact mechanism is unclear. Because these two medications operate in different ways, they can be used together to keep patients from requiring insulin. In patients who fail oral agents, insulin therapy is used. It can be used similarly to that in type 1 patients, although the risk of hypoglycemia is lower.

Case Conclusion CJ returns to her physician and is encouraged to find a new walking partner, as well as maintain a low-fat, low-simple sugar, and high-fiber diet. She is also started on a regimen of glyburide to help stimulate insulin secretion by the pancreas and increase tissue sensitivity to insulin. This approach brings her glucose levels back to normal and gives CJ a chance to get more rest.

Key Points

▶ Type 2 DM results from a combination of **insulin resistance** and a **pancreatic beta cell defect** leading to abnormal glucose homeostasis.

▶ Common signs and symptoms include polyuria, polyphagia, increased thirst, weight loss, sexual dysfunction, and poor wound healing.

▶ Complications include accelerated atherosclerosis, diabetic nephropathy, diabetic retinopathy, and peripheral neuropathy.

Thumbnail: Type 2 Diabetes Mellitus

Primary defect
Peripheral insulin resistance

Pathogenesis
Genetic/environmental influences

Frequency
~90% of cases

Age of onset
> 40 years old

Clinical onset
Gradual symptoms

HLA association
None

Identical twin concordance
60%–90%

Islet antibodies
Rare

Islet histology
Beta cells present/reduced

Insulin resistance
Yes

Blood insulin/C-peptide levels
Low for insulin resistance

High-risk groups
Native American, Asian, African American, Hispanic

Primary treatment options
Weight loss, diet/exercise, insulin sensitizers/secretion enhancers, with or without exogenous insulin

Questions

1. A 72-year-old man with a long history of type 2 diabetes treated with insulin visits his family physician for a routine check-up. He states that he administers his insulin just as the doctor ordered, but continues to present with random blood sugar levels well above 200 mg/dL. The doctor suspects the patient has not been using his insulin appropriately for some time now. What is the best way to measure long-term diabetic control of blood glucose?

   A. Glucose tolerance test
   B. Fasting serum glucose
   C. HbA_{1c}
   D. Urinalysis
   E. CBC

2. A 42-year-old woman is diagnosed with type 2 diabetes after two pregnancies complicated by gestational diabetes. She has never been on medications for diabetes before. Which of the following is not a first-line treatment option for type 2 DM?

   A. Metformin
   B. Insulin
   C. Glyburide
   D. Acarbose
   E. Pioglitazone

3. A 38-year-old Latina woman with borderline high-glucose levels is referred to the diabetes clinic by her gynecologist. She is currently not on any diabetes medications. She is moderately overweight, eats mostly fast food, does not exercise, and smokes half a pack of cigarettes daily. The physician suggests a diabetes educational class to help her learn more about her condition and how she can take better care of herself. Her risk factors for developing overt type 2 diabetes do not include:

   A. Obesity
   B. Ethnicity
   C. Poor diet
   D. Smoking
   E. Lack of exercise

HPI: LG is a 35-year-old white woman who presents with a history of anxiety, nervousness, and difficulty sleeping for the past 3 months. She complains of feeling hot and sweaty, even in air-conditioned rooms, and has noticed her heart beating irregularly at times during the day. LG had attributed her anxiety and symptoms to increasing stress at work, but became concerned after friends and family kept commenting on her recent weight loss. She failed to notice it at first, but after stepping on the scale at the gym, LG realized she had lost some 20 lbs over the past 3 months—despite having a voracious appetite. She also complains of having puffy eyes, but thinks it is mostly due to lack of sleep. She would like a prescription for something to help calm her anxiety so she can get some rest and finally get rid of the "bags under her eyes." LG's family history is significant for her mother having a history of thyroid disease.

PE: **Vitals:** Thin, mildly tachypneic female in no acute distress. Skin appears warm and moist. **Head, Eyes, Ears, Nose, and Throat (HEENT):** Prominent eyes with lid lag, stare, and infrequent blinking. Moderate degree of periorbital edema. Patient has difficulty looking up and out but no limitation of downward gaze. **Neck:** Thyroid gland appears diffusely and symmetrically enlarged, soft, and nontender. **Cardiac:** Precordium and carotid pulses hyperdynamic to palpation. No murmurs detected. **Extremities:** Nontender, erythematous nodule on anterior aspect of left lower extremity. Brisk deep tendon reflexes.

Thought Questions

- What is the likely cause of LG's symptoms and what clues lead you to this conclusion?

- What diagnostic tests would you order to confirm her diagnosis? What would these tests show?

- What is the pathophysiology of this condition?

Basic Science Review and Discussion

LG appears to have many of the classic signs and symptoms of hyperthyroidism. These include heat intolerance, weight loss, tachycardia, arrhythmias, chest pain, palpitations, anxiety, sweating, diarrhea, hyperreflexia, fine hair, and sleep disturbances. Hyperthyroidism can have multiple causes, but the most likely cause in this case is Graves' disease. The combination of ophthalmopathy (proptosis, extraocular muscle swelling), pretibial myxedema, and diffuse goiter all point to the clinical diagnosis of Graves' disease as the cause of LG's hyperthyroidism.

Graves' Disease Graves' disease is an **autoimmune hyperthyroidism** caused by **antibodies to the thyroid stimulating hormone (TSH) receptor** in the thyroid gland. It has a female predilection of 5:1 and occurs in about 0.5% of the adult population. Autoantibodies (also known as thyroid-stimulating immunoglobulin) bind to and stimulate the TSH receptor, producing glandular growth and excess secretion of thyroid hormone [preferential tri-iodothyronine (T_3) secretion]. On physical exam, the glandular growth is present as a diffuse goiter and the preferential secretion of the **active form of thyroid hormone (T_3)** produces moderate to severe thyrotoxicosis. In addition, **infiltrative ophthalmopathy** is present in about 5% of the patients with Graves' disease. Though LG attributes her puffy eyes to lack of sleep, the swelling and "bags under her eyes" are actually due to antibodies directed against her extraocular eye muscles. These antibodies cause a local immune response and result in inflammation of the muscles and deposition of glycosaminoglycans by orbital fibroblasts. Patients may complain of pain or double vision with reading, burning or tearing of the eyes, and may lose the ability to look up and out. Another rare complication of Graves' disease is **pretibial myxedema,** which occurs in about 1% of all cases. The nontender erythematous nodule on the anterior aspect of LG's left leg is an example of pretibial myxedema, which is caused by mucopolysaccharide infiltrate in the skin of the pretibial area.

Laboratory studies can confirm the clinical diagnosis of Graves' disease. Important thyroid function tests include TSH, free thyroxine (T_4), T_3, and antithyroid peroxidase antibodies (anti-TPO, also known as antimicrosomal antibodies). TSH from the anterior pituitary is the best thyroid function test, as it will reveal abnormalities well before T_3 or T_4. In Graves' disease, TSH levels will be markedly suppressed, while T_4 and T_3 values will be markedly elevated ($T_3/T_4 > 20:1$). Anti-TPO antibody will be positive and serves as a marker for autoimmune thyroid disease. In addition, because the gland is actively taking up iodine for thyroid hormone synthesis, administration of radioactive iodine will show elevated and diffuse uptake, indicating a general increase in thyroid gland activity.

Case Continued LG is diagnosed with Graves' disease and treated successfully with radioactive iodine. She remains euthyroid and symptom free for the next 5 years, but slowly starts to notice increasing fatigue, muscle cramps, and weight gain. She returns to her primary care physician, hoping he may be able to help her once again.

Thought Questions

- What is the most likely cause of LG's symptoms now? What are the associated symptoms of this condition?

- What would LG's lab results show?

Basic Science Review and Discussion

Radioactive iodine (RAI) is the most commonly prescribed treatment for Graves' disease. Iodine 131 (^{131}I) is selectively absorbed by thyroid tissue, where it destroys some or all of the hyperfunctioning thyroid follicles by emitting beta particles. Unfortunately, 50% to 90% of patients with Graves' disease treated this way eventually become hypothyroid. This is the most likely cause of LG's current symptoms. Other signs and symptoms associated with hypothyroidism include cold intolerance, reduced heart rate, hypoactivity, decreased appetite, decreased reflexes, constipation, cool/dry skin, myxedema (facial/periorbital), and coarse, brittle hair. Hypothyroidism can also be caused by a variety of conditions, the most common of which are RAI therapy for hyperthyroidism and Hashimoto's thyroiditis. **Hashimoto's thyroiditis** is a cell-mediated autoimmune destruction of the thyroid gland. It occurs in 1% to 2% of the population, with a female predilection of 5:1. The condition begins in adolescence, but is usually not evident until after 50 years of age. The result is an atrophic, fibrotic thyroid gland in a patient with the signs and symptoms of hypothyroidism. Laboratory studies for hypothyroidism will reveal an increased TSH and low T_3, free T_4 levels. Since Hashimoto's thyroiditis is an autoimmune condition, anti-TPO antibody levels will be positive. All permanent forms of hypothyroidism are treated with life-long thyroid hormone replacement.

Case Conclusion LG was started on levothyroxine 100 μg/day for treatment of her subsequent hypothyroidism. TSH levels were monitored periodically to ensure a euthyroid state.

Thumbnail: Hyper- versus Hypothyroidism

	Hypothyroid	Hyperthyroid
Etiology	Hashimoto's thyroiditis RAI therapy Idiopathic or atrophic thyroiditis Pituitary or hypothalamic disease Thyroid aplasia Inborn defects in hormone synthesis or action	Graves' disease Toxic multinodular goiter Iodide-induced thyrotoxicosis Autonomous hyperfunctioning nodule Subacute thyroiditis Postpartum thyroiditis Factitious thyrotoxicosis
Symptoms	Decreased metabolic rate Cold intolerance Decreased heart rate Weight gain Fatigue, lethargy Myxedema Cool, dry skin Coarse, brittle hair Constipation Hyporeflexia	Increased metabolic rate Heat intolerance Palpitations, irregular heart rate Weight loss Hyperactivity Pretibial myxedema (Graves') Warm, moist skin Fine hair Diarrhea Hyperreflexia
Labs	↑ TSH ↓ total T_4 ↓ free T_4 ↓ T_3 uptake	↓ TSH ↑ total T_4 ↑ free T_4 ↑ T_3 uptake

Key Points

- The etiology of hyperthyroidism is usually autoimmune, caused by antibodies to the TSH receptor.
- Signs and symptoms include increased metabolism, heat intolerance, weight loss, arrhythmias, and diarrhea.
- TSH measurement is the best thyroid function test; TSH levels are markedly decreased in hyperthyroid states.
- Treatment: radioactive iodine ablation of the overactive thyroid gland.

Questions

1. A 33-year-old woman presents with signs and symptoms of hyperthyroidism. She complains of anxiety, tremor, nervousness, weight loss, and inability to sleep at night. Laboratory evaluation confirms hyperthyroidism with a free T_4 of 25 mg/dL and undetectable levels of TSH. Which of the following is not an appropriate option for treatment of her hyperthyroidism?

   A. Propylthiouracil (PTU)
   B. Radioactive iodine
   C. Levothyroxine (Synthroid)
   D. Propranolol
   E. Surgery

2. A 22-year-old woman presents to her obstetrician/gynecologist for follow-up 8 weeks after the delivery of her baby. There were no complications during her pregnancy or during delivery. On this visit, her thyroid gland is diffusely, but minimally enlarged and nontender to palpation. The doctor decides to obtain a thyroid function panel to aid her diagnostic evaluation. In this thyroid function panel, the most sensitive indicator of thyroid function is:

   A. T_3 uptake
   B. Free T_4
   C. Total T_4
   D. T_3/T_4 ratio
   E. TSH

> **HPI:** KM is a 51-year-old Hispanic woman who complains of increasing fatigue and lethargy over the past 6 months. She states that her husband has been pushing her to go see her doctor because she hasn't been her usual active self recently. In addition to the weakness and fatigue, KM admits to having some difficulty concentrating and focusing on simple tasks. Even putting together her weekly grocery list has become increasingly more difficult. She thought her symptoms may have something to do with the onset of menopause, but instead of the typical "hot flashes" one would expect, KM found herself extremely sensitive to cold. In addition, she describes a 25-pound weight gain over the past few months despite a markedly reduced appetite.
>
> **PE:** On physical exam, KM is a mildly obese female in no acute distress. Pulse is 60 beats/min and BP is elevated at 160/100 mm Hg. Her skin is cool and dry; her hair appears coarse and brittle. Thyroid gland is nontender and not palpable. Heart, lung, and abdomen exams are all within normal limits, but neurologic exam reveals decreased muscle strength and hypoactive reflexes.
>
> **Labs:** Laboratory studies include a thyroid function panel that demonstrates decreased T_4 levels and increased TSH.

Thought Questions

- What is KM's diagnosis and what laboratory results confirm this?

- What is the function of thyroid hormone and how does this explain KM's signs and symptoms?

- How would you treat this patient?

Basic Science Review and Discussion

Thyroid hormones (T_3 & T_4) function to control the body's metabolic rate. Thyroid hormone production is regulated by thyroid-releasing hormone (TRH) from the hypothalamus and TSH from the pituitary. TSH promotes the synthesis of both T_3 and T_4 from thyroglobulin in the thyroid follicles. T_3 is the more active form of the hormone; however, greater amounts of T_4 are released from the gland than T_3. T_4 is subsequently deiodinated to T_3 in the periphery. Production is further regulated by negative feedback by T_3 on the anterior pituitary, which decreases sensitivity to TRH.

Hypothyroidism KM presents with many of the classic signs and symptoms of hypothyroidism. Insufficient thyroid hormone production causes a decrease in the body's basal metabolic rate. Nonspecific symptoms include **fatigue, lethargy,** and **weight gain.** Patients may also complain of **constipation** and **decreased appetite. Cold intolerance** is a clinical manifestation of the body's reduced heat production secondary to decreased metabolism. Clinical signs of hypothyroidism also result from altered rates of metabolism. These signs include **slow mentation, muscle weakness, dry/coarse skin, brittle hair,** and **decreased reflexes.** Because the physiologic response to hypothyroidism is to conserve heat, patients may present with HTN secondary to

vasoconstriction and a reduced HR. CXR may reveal cardiomegaly in response to the systemic vasoconstriction and reduced blood volume. In general, there is a decrease in β-adrenergic responsiveness (α-adrenergic receptors are not affected) and a decrease in systemic oxygen consumption.

Hashimoto's Thyroiditis The most common cause of hypothyroidism is chronic lymphocytic thyroiditis, also known as **Hashimoto's thyroiditis.** It is a chronic disease process that begins subclinically in adolescence and progresses throughout one's lifetime, becoming clinically apparent in middle-age. The disease primarily affects women and is characterized by circulating **thyroid antibodies** (α-microsomal Ab, α-thyroglobulin Ab, and α-TSH Ab). An autoimmune disease process is thus suspected, but the exact cause of the disease is unknown. Pathologically, there is a slow **lymphoid replacement of thyroid tissue accompanied by fibrosis.** Eventually, the entire gland becomes atrophic and fibrotic. CBC will reveal lymphocytosis, with an excess of CD8+ lymphocytes; patients with Hashimoto's thyroiditis are thus predisposed to B-cell lymphomas (Figure 18-1).

Patient symptoms at the time of presentation will depend on the stage of their disease process. During the early stage (adolescence), patients are asymptomatic and clinically euthyroid because there is sufficient thyroid tissue to produce adequate amounts of hormone. The gland may feel rubbery and diffusely enlarged, but nontender. As functioning thyroid tissue is progressively obliterated by lymphocytes and fibrosis, destruction of the gland releases existing thyroid hormone into the circulation. At this stage, patients may actually present as hyperthyroid due to the release of excess hormone secondary to destruction of the gland. Late-stage disease usually presents after age 50 with a completely atrophic and fibrotic thyroid gland and the

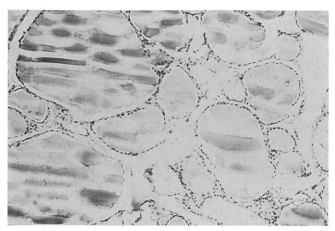

Figure 18-1 Hematoxylin and eosin stain of the thyroid gland showing numerous follicles filled with colloid, the storage form of thyroglobulin. Thyroglobulin is the precursor molecule to thyroid hormone. In Hashimoto's thyroiditis, these follicles become atrophic and fibrotic as the gland is replaced by lymphocytes. (Image courtesy of Joel Schechter, PhD, Keck School of Medicine at the University of Southern California.)

clinical signs and symptoms of hypothyroidism. Hashimoto's thyroiditis is the cause of most, if not all, spontaneous hypothyroidism in adults.

Laboratory evaluation of a patient with late-stage Hashimoto's thyroiditis will demonstrate **low free and total T_4 levels.** Increased TSH in a clinically euthyroid patient may signal early gland failure. TSH will be markedly elevated in a patient with end-stage lymphocytic thyroiditis. The presence of circulating anti-TPO antibodies in a patient with hypothyroidism will point to the diagnosis of Hashimoto's thyroiditis. This condition is often associated with other autoimmune disorders occurring in the same patient.

Other Causes of Hypothyroidism   Hypothyroidism can also result from a variety of other known causes. These include both exogenous and endogenous etiologies. Exogenous causes are usually iatrogenic; patients may have undergone thyroidectomy, received radioactive iodine therapy, external beam radiation, or taken drugs that cause hypothyroidism [lithium, propylthiouracil (PTU), methimazole, amiodarone]. Endogenous causes may be due to defects within the thyroid gland itself (**primary hypothyroidism**) or farther up in the pituitary or hypothalamus (**secondary hypothyroidism**). In secondary hypothyroidism, TSH and/or TRH levels will remain low or normal, despite low T_4 levels.

Sporadic hypothyroidism in children results from ineffective thyroid gland development or T_4 biosynthesis/action. This condition is known as **cretinism;** affected children characteristically exhibit mental retardation, facial/periorbital edema, and are of short stature with a protuberant tummy and tongue. These findings occur due to the lack of thyroid hormone necessary for proper development, specifically bone growth and CNS maturation.

In adults, severe hypothyroidism over a long period of time can lead to a condition known as **myxedema** (also known as idiopathic hypothyroidism, primary atrophy of the thyroid). The thyroid gland is completely shrunken and fibrotic, with only a few scattered lymphocytes present. Patients will exhibit changes consistent with chronic hypothyroidism and with the **deposition of mucopolysaccharides** throughout the body. Deposition of mucopolysaccharides occurs most notably in the skin, larynx, and heart, leading to edema of the face and eyelids, thick tongue, slow speech, lethargy, and dry skin. Increased deposition in the heart can even lead to cardiac arrest. Idiopathic myxedema appears to be the end result of chronic Hashimoto's disease, in which the early phase of thyroid enlargement was not apparent clinically.

Case Conclusion   Further laboratory evaluation confirms the presence of lymphocytosis, accompanied by high circulating levels of anti-TPO antibody. KM is diagnosed with chronic lymphocytic thyroiditis and is advised that because her thyroid gland is no longer functional, she will need to be treated with lifelong thyroid hormone replacement; she will also need to be followed regularly to make sure her TSH value remains within normal limits with hormone replacement. She is immediately started on 100 µg of daily oral thyroxine. KM returns to the clinic in 3 months to measure T_3, T_4, and TSH levels. At that time, serum hormone concentrations appear normal and her symptoms have all but disappeared.

Thumbnail: Hypothyroidism

Etiology
Chronic lymphocytic (Hashimoto's) thyroiditis
Idiopathic or atrophic thyroiditis
Iatrogenic: thyroidectomy, ^{131}I therapy, external beam radiation, drugs
Pituitary or hypothalamic disease (secondary)
Thyroid aplasia
Inborn defects in hormonal biosynthesis or action

Symptoms and signs

Lethargy	Cool, dry skin
Weight gain	Coarse, brittle hair
Fatigue	Slow mentation
Constipation	Slow speech
Decreased appetite	Thick tongue
Cold intolerance	Facial/periorbital myxedema
Weakness	Irregular menstrual cycles
Decreased reflexes	Decreased muscle strength
Normocytic anemia	

Primary hypothyroidism
↓ free T_4
↓ total T_4
↓ T_3
↑ TSH

Secondary hypothyroidism
↓ free T_4
↓ total T_4
↓ T_3
↓ or normal TSH

Hyperthyroidism vs. Hypothyroidism Laboratory Values

Laboratory measurements	Hyperthyroidism	Primary Hypothyroidism	Secondary Hypothyroidism
TSH	↑	↑	↓
Free T_4	↑	↓	↓
Total T_4	↑	↓	↓
T_3 uptake	↑	↓	↓

Key Points

- Primary hypothyroidism = problem in thyroid gland itself.

- Secondary hypothyroidism = problem in pituitary or hypothalamus.

- Most common primary etiology is Hashimoto's thyroiditis.

- Symptoms and signs of decreased metabolism, fatigue, lethargy, weight gain, constipation, cold intolerance.

- TSH levels are markedly elevated in primary hypothyroidism, normal or low in secondary hypothyroidism.

- Treatment: exogenous thyroid hormone replacement.

Questions

1. A 24-year-old woman presents to her primary care physician with symptoms of hypothyroidism 8 weeks following resolution of a viral upper respiratory tract infection. Her thyroid gland is diffusely enlarged and tender to palpation; her ears are bilaterally tender as well. What can she be told about the nature and clinical course of her condition?

   A. She most likely has Hashimoto's thyroiditis and will need to be treated with exogenous thyroid hormone indefinitely.

   B. She most likely has subacute thyroiditis and her symptoms will resolve spontaneously within 6 months.

   C. Her symptoms are due to insufficient iodine intake and will improve if she changes her diet.

   D. She most likely has a thyroid neoplasm that will need to be further evaluated with fine-needle aspiration.

   E. She most likely has a pituitary adenoma that will need to be excised immediately.

2. A 72-year-old man complains of increasing fatigue and weakness over the past 2 to 3 years. Physical exam reveals scant beard growth and axillary hair. Laboratory blood tests reveal hemoglobin/HCT of 11.8 mg/34%; cells are normochromic, normocytic. Serum free T_4 index is decreased at 2.6 (normal 5–12). Which of the following is the best test to determine the etiology of his symptoms?

   A. Serum free T_3 index

   B. Visual field testing

   C. Serum TRH level

   D. Serum TSH level

   E. Serum testosterone

HPI: LS is a 31-year-old Filipino-American woman who initially presented to her gynecologist because of irregular and prolonged menses and inability to become pregnant after discontinuing birth control pills. Over the past year she has noticed increasing acne on her face and prominence of facial hair. LS complains that she can barely recognize herself in the mirror anymore—not only has her face been getting rounder, but she appears to be putting on weight in peculiar places like the back of her neck and around her abdomen. She denies any history of increased bruising or poor wound healing, but does notice that her skin appears darker and she has prominent stretch marks around her ever-enlarging abdomen.

PE: The patient is mildly hypertensive, with BP 140/90 mm Hg. Physical exam reveals an anxious but cooperative female with a full, rounded face. She has acne and excess hair over the neck. There is also excess fat over the dorsal cervical and supraclavicular areas. Skin around the waistline is significant for multiple purple striae. Musculoskeletal exam reveals slight muscle weakness.

Labs: Laboratory results demonstrate an elevated fasting glucose level, elevated 24-hour urinary free cortisol, and a slightly elevated adrenocortiotropic hormone (ACTH) level.

Thought Questions

■ Where is cortisol produced? What regulates its secretion?

■ What are the clinical manifestations of excess cortisol production?

■ What is the difference between Cushing's disease and Cushing's syndrome?

■ Why do patients with Cushing's disease/syndrome often have concurrent DM?

Basic Science Review and Discussion

The adrenal glands, located bilaterally above the kidneys in the retroperitoneal space, serve to produce glucocorticoids, mineralocorticoids, and androgens from the adrenal cortex. In addition, catecholamines are secreted from the medulla. The adrenal cortex itself is one of the most productive endocrine glands, responsible for much of the body's hormone production. This hormone production is regulated primarily by input from both the hypothalamus, in the form of corticotropin-releasing hormone (CRH) and the anterior pituitary, in the form of ACTH. CRH from the hypothalamus regulates ACTH release in response to decreased serum cortisol levels. In turn, cortisol inhibits both CRH and ACTH secretion. This negative feedback loop regulates daily glucocorticoid homeostasis. Glucocorticoid secretion normally oscillates with a 24-hour periodicity. This pattern of secretion is due to the fact that CRH and ACTH are secreted in a diurnal pattern with secretory bursts that are highest in the early morning hours. Therefore, cortisol levels are usually highest in the morning and lowest at night.

Adrenal Anatomy The adrenal cortex is divided into three functional and histologically distinct regions (Figure 19-1). These three regions are (1) the **zona glomerulosa,** the outermost layer; (2) **zona fasciculata,** the middle layer; and (3) **zona reticularis,** the inner layer. The zona glomerulosa produces aldosterone and is not dependent on the pituitary or the hypothalamus for its stimulus to secrete. Instead, aldosterone production is regulated by the renin-angiotensin system. In contrast, both the zona fasciculata and the zona reticularis are dependent on signals from the pituitary and hypothalamus. The zona fasciculata synthesizes mostly glucocorticoids (cortisol), while the zona reticularis produces

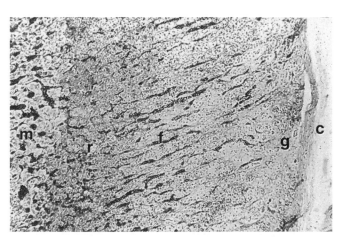

Figure 19-1 H&E stain of the adrenal gland, showing the adrenal cortex, medulla, and vasculature. From left to right: the adrenal medulla (m), zona reticularis (r), zona fasciculata (f), zona glomerulosa (g), and adrenal capsule (c). The adrenal medulla is responsible for synthesis of the catecholamines norepinephrine and epinephrine. (Image courtesy of Joel Schechter, PhD, Keck School of Medicine at the University of Southern California.)

mostly androgens (dehydroepiandrosterone [DHEA] and androstenedione).

Glucocorticoids Glucocorticoids are important for the physiologic response to stress. They initiate a variety of biological processes that relate to stress, including stimulation of gluconeogenesis, anti-inflammatory reactions, and suppression of the immune response. In addition, glucocorticoids function to maintain the vascular responsiveness to catecholamines; this action is especially critical during the sympathetic "fight or flight" response. Cortisol increases gluconeogenesis by a number of mechanisms. There is an increase in protein breakdown and a decrease in protein synthesis; this provides more amino acids to the liver for gluconeogenesis. In addition, there is a decrease in glucose utilization and insulin sensitivity, primarily in adipose tissue. Furthermore, an increase in lipolysis provides additional glycerol to the liver for gluconeogenesis. The anti-inflammatory actions of cortisol result from its inhibitory effects on prostaglandin formation. Suppression of the immune response occurs through the inhibition of interleukin-2 (IL-2) production and reduction of T-lymphocytes critical for the cell-mediated immune response.

Cushing's Disease This patient's most likely diagnosis is Cushing's disease. Cushing's disease is an excess of adrenocortical hormones due to a **pituitary corticotroph adenoma** producing large amounts of ACTH. The disease is named after Harvey Cushing, the neurosurgeon who delineated its features in 1932. Because ACTH stimulates both the zona fasciculata and the zona reticularis, the symptoms seen in Cushing's disease are due to **overproduction of both cortisol and androgens.** Clinically, patients with glucocorticoid excess present with a typical "cushingoid" appearance. There is a redistribution of adipose tissue to specific areas of the body, namely the face, abdomen, posterior neck, and supraclavicular areas. Patients are usually described as centrally obese with "moon facies" and a "buffalo hump." These patients also exhibit muscle wasting and weakness due to the increased protein catabolism. Associated DM is often present because the increase in gluconeogenesis and insulin resistance raises serum glucose levels. The excess cortisol also induces atrophic skin changes such as thinning; this thinning is evident as prominent purple striae in affected areas. A history of poor wound healing and easy bruising would be consistent with the immunosuppressive

effects of glucocorticoids. The increase in circulating androgens is manifested as hirsutism, acne, and virilization with menstrual irregularities. Because anterior pituitary corticotrophs are also responsible for the synthesis of melanocyte-stimulating hormone (MSH), many patients with Cushing's disease also complain of skin darkening. This increased pigmentation is due to an increase in MSH production from the adenoma. It is particularly prominent in areas of friction (e.g., under the bra straps). Because glucocorticoids also have weak mineralocorticoid activity, excess cortisol can cause mild sodium retention and contribute to elevated blood pressures.

Cushing's Syndrome In contrast to Cushing's disease, which is glucocorticoid excess specifically due to a pituitary adenoma secreting ACTH, Cushing's syndrome refers to any condition in which there is an excess of glucocorticoids. This excess may be ACTH dependent or ACTH independent. ACTH dependent glucocorticoid excess occurs with a pituitary adenoma or with paraneoplastic syndromes, in which a neoplasm (most commonly small cell lung carcinoma) produces ectopic ACTH that stimulates the adrenals. Ectopic ACTH syndrome affects men three times more frequently than women. Laboratory evaluation of ACTH dependent conditions will demonstrate an increase in both ACTH and 24-hour urinary free cortisol. Ectopic ACTH conditions tend to have very high ACTH levels. Glucocorticoid excess due to ACTH independent conditions results from primary adrenal neoplasms or exogenous glucocorticoid administration. In these instances, urine cortisol will be increased despite low or undetectable levels of ACTH.

Treatment for glucocorticoid excess depends on the etiology of the condition. Possibilities include surgery, radiation, chemotherapy, or the use of cortisol-inhibiting drugs. If the cause is long-term use of glucocorticoid hormones to treat another disorder, it is best to gradually taper the dosage to the lowest dose adequate for control of that disorder. Surgical resection is the mainstay of treatment for pituitary adenomas; the procedure is called a trans-sphenoidal adenomectomy. If surgery is not possible in such patients, pituitary irradiation is an effective alternative. Adrenal tumors and ectopic ACTH-secreting tumors can be treated with surgery, radiotherapy, or chemotherapy. Medications such as ketoconazole, which inhibits steroid synthesis, can also be used in the treatment of Cushing's.

Case Conclusion The endocrinologist orders an MRI of the head which is read as "enlarged pituitary fossa with irregular pituitary mass." LS is immediately scheduled for surgical excision of the mass. Pathology report confirms the presence of a pituitary corticotroph adenoma.

Thumbnail: Adrenal Gland

CRH (hypothalamus)

↓

ACTH (pituitary) → Androgens (zona reticularis)

↓

Cortisol (zona fasciculata)

Causes of glucocorticoid excess

ACTH dependent

Cushing's disease (pituitary ACTH adenoma)

Ectopic ACTH production (paraneoplastic)

ACTH independent

Exogenous glucocorticoid administration

Adrenal neoplasm (benign or malignant)

Symptoms and signs of glucocorticoid excess

Catabolic effects on skin and muscle (striae, skin atrophy)

Classical facies and body habitus

Increased brown fat

Poor wound healing

HTN (50%)

Hypokalemia (20%)

Amenorrhea or decreased libido

Psychological disturbances

Osteoporosis

Impaired glucose tolerance

Increased pigmentation

Key Points

▶ Cushing's disease = pituitary adenoma producing excess ACTH.

▶ Cushing's syndrome = nonpituitary source of excess cortisol.

▶ Symptoms and signs include body fat redistribution (moon facies, buffalo hump), skin atrophy, poor wound healing, glucose intolerance.

▶ Initial screen for suspected glucocorticoid excess is 24-hour urinary free cortisol measurement.

▶ Cushing's disease is treated with pituitary surgery or radiation.

Questions

1. A 26-year-old man presents to his primary care physician complaining of multiple episodes of easy bruising after playing basketball. He recently started playing ball again after he noticed that he was growing a "beer belly" even though he hardly drank any alcohol. He also complains of little to no libido. Among other findings, the physician notes a plethoric, round face and skin atrophy, particularly over the pretibial areas. The most useful screening test for Cushing's in this case is:

   A. Measure plasma cortisol.
   B. Measure 24-hour urinary cortisol production.
   C. Perform a low- and high-dose dexamethasone suppression test.
   D. Perform pituitary MRI.
   E. Perform an abdominal computed axial tomography scan.

2. An 11-year-old girl is prescribed oral prednisone to help control her severe persistent asthma. Which of the following actions of cortisol is most beneficial in helping her achieve long-term control of her asthma?

   A. Increased glucose formation and release
   B. Sodium retention
   C. Increases "stress response"
   D. Inhibits T-lymphocyte proliferation
   E. Inhibits prostaglandin formation

HPI: JV is a 44-year-old Scandinavian man who presents to his family doctor with a 1-year history of fatigue, weakness, and weight loss. He states that he doesn't eat very much now, and when he does, it is usually accompanied by nausea and vomiting. His two school-aged children have been complaining that "Daddy doesn't play with us much anymore." JV's response is that he simply doesn't have the energy he did in the past. Even standing up from a reclining position makes him feel dizzy and faint.

PE: On physical exam, JV is tachycardic, with blood pressures of 110/64 mm Hg supine and 92/50 mm Hg while standing. He is a thin man who appears older than his stated age. His skin exhibits peculiar areas of hyperpigmentation, most notably around his palmar creases and buccal mucosa. His eyes appear sunken, and mucous membranes are pale and dry. His verbal responses and mentation appear delayed, but the rest of his physical exam is within normal limits.

Labs: Subsequent laboratory tests are significant for hyponatremia, hyperkalemia, lymphocytosis, and marked eosinophilia.

Thought Questions

- What endocrine disorder could be responsible for JV's relatively nonspecific signs and symptoms? What physical sign is most specific for this diagnosis?

- What laboratory tests would confirm your hypothesis? What would these labs show?

- What is the difference between primary and secondary adrenal insufficiency?

- How should this patient be treated for his condition?

Basic Science Review and Discussion

JV presents with many nonspecific signs and symptoms. These include a chronic history of fatigue, weakness, weight loss, anorexia, nausea, and vomiting. When taken into consideration with his significant dehydration, hypotension, and hyperpigmentation, however, one must consider the diagnosis of Addison's disease. Addison's disease is also known as primary adrenal insufficiency. **Primary adrenal insufficiency** is distinguished from **secondary adrenal insufficiency** in that the defect in primary disease is end-organ failure of the adrenal gland itself, while secondary disease is caused by defects in the hypothalamus or pituitary resulting in decreased production of CRH or ACTH. The signs and symptoms of both conditions are caused by the loss of mineralocorticoid and glucocorticoid production.

Adrenal Gland The adrenal gland is made up of two anatomically distinct regions: the outer cortex and the inner medulla. The cortex is further divided into three different hormone-synthesizing areas: the **zona glomerulosa, zona fasciculata,** and **zona reticularis.** These zones are responsible for the synthesis of mineralocorticoids (primarily aldosterone), glucocorticoids (primarily cortisol), and androgens,

respectively. The fasciculata and reticularis zones of the adrenal gland are under regulatory control of the hypothalamic-pituitary axis. The hypothalamus secretes CRH, which acts on the anterior pituitary gland to produce ACTH. The action of ACTH on the adrenal gland is to stimulate the production of cortisol from the zona fasciculata. In addition, ACTH stimulates the zona reticularis to produce androgens. The zona glomerulosa is unique in that its producing capacity is regulated by the **renin-angiotensin system.** A decrease in blood pressure sensed by decreased sodium or chloride transport to the macula densa in the kidney stimulates the juxtaglomerular cells to secrete renin. Renin catalyzes the conversion of angiotensinogen to angiotensin I, which is subsequently converted to angiotensin II in the lungs. Angiotensin II then stimulates the zona glomerulosa to secrete aldosterone. Aldosterone causes an increase in BP through sodium (and water) retention.

Primary Adrenal Insufficiency The etiologic defect in Addison's disease occurs in the adrenal gland. There are numerous causes, but an autoimmune mediated destruction of the adrenal gland is the most common cause in the United States. Other causes include tuberculosis and other granulomatous diseases, acquired immunodeficiency syndrome (AIDS), sarcoidosis, bacterial infections, adrenal hemorrhage, and coagulation disorders. The disease process is characterized by **atrophy of all three cortical divisions,** resulting in the complete absence of hormone production.

Secondary Adrenal Insufficiency In contrast, secondary adrenal insufficiency occurs as a result of decreased production of CRH from the hypothalamus or ACTH from the pituitary. Atrophy of the adrenal cortex occurs as a result of **insufficient stimulation from higher regulatory centers.** The most common cause of isolated secondary insufficiency is long-term exogenous glucocorticoid therapy. Administration of exogenous cortisol decreases production of both

CRH and ACTH through negative feedback regulation. Less common causes of secondary insufficiency include craniopharyngioma, empty sella syndrome, sarcoidosis, histiocytosis X, hypothalamic tumors, head trauma, and Sheehan's syndrome.

Primary versus Secondary Adrenal Insufficiency Many of the signs and symptoms of primary adrenal insufficiency are the same as those of secondary insufficiency. These common findings are caused by a lack of both aldosterone and cortisol activity. The symptoms are generally nonspecific and include tiredness, weakness, confusion, weight loss, nausea, vomiting, and occasionally hypoglycemia. Hyponatremia and hyperkalemia is characteristic of primary disease, because the absence of aldosterone causes sodium to be lost in the urine and potassium to be retained in the body. Hypotension and volume depletion are due to the inability to retain sodium, and thus water, since water follows sodium. Because the zona glomerulosa is not dependent on ACTH for stimulation, aldosterone levels are normal in secondary failure and hypotension is not a primary feature of the disease. In addition, skin pigmentation is only seen in primary adrenal failure. The hyperpigmentation occurs all over the skin, but characteristically in the palmar creases and buccal mucosa. Because ACTH and MSH are formed by the same precursor, the hyperpigmentation is caused by an increase in MSH secondary to the increase in ACTH seen in primary failure. If the cause of primary failure is due to an autoimmune mechanism, patients may also present with other autoimmune conditions such as thyroid disorders or vitiligo. Secondary failure is usually associated with the loss of gonadotropins, TSH, and/or growth hormone (GH). These deficiencies manifest as scanty secondary sex characteristics (axillary hair, pubic hair), amenorrhea in women, decreased libido/potency, delayed puberty, or hypothyroidism. Pituitary tumors may also present with headache or visual changes, while hypothalamus defects can also present with diabetes insipidus.

Diagnosis Diagnosis of adrenal insufficiency is made based on the constellation of clinical signs and symptoms in

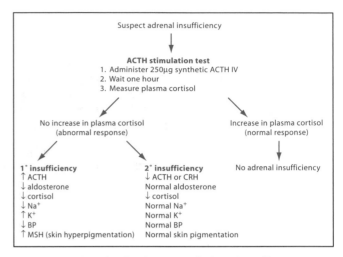

Figure 20-1 Algorithm for diagnosis of adrenal insufficiency.

combination with laboratory evaluation (Figure 20-1). Laboratory workup for a patient with suspected adrenal insufficiency should include a measurement of morning cortisol level and plasma ACTH. Primary adrenal insufficiency will reveal low morning plasma cortisol levels. Cortisol levels are usually highest around 8 to 9 a.m. because CRH and ACTH are secreted in a diurnal pattern with secretory bursts that are highest in the early morning hours. ACTH from the pituitary will be increased in primary insufficiency secondary to the low circulating cortisol. On the other hand, both ACTH and cortisol levels will be decreased in secondary adrenal insufficiency because the defect occurs in the pituitary or hypothalamus. An ACTH stimulation test with 250 μg of synthetic ACTH can also be used to confirm adrenal insufficiency. Administration of ACTH should increase plasma cortisol to a level > 17 μg/mL within 1 hour of IV dose. Inadequate response indicates adrenal insufficiency but does not distinguish primary from secondary failure. Head CT or MRI scan may be necessary if a secondary cause of adrenal insufficiency is suspected.

Case Conclusion JV's family physician refers him to an endocrinologist who diagnoses Addison's disease based on physical evidence of hyperpigmentation, low morning plasma cortisol, and elevated ACTH. He is started on glucocorticoid and mineralocorticoid replacement therapy with rapid improvement of symptoms. JV's children are much happier now that their daddy is back to his usual playful and energetic self again.

Thumbnail: Adrenal Insufficiency

Primary (Addison's disease)	Secondary
End-organ failure	Decreased production of CRH or ACTH
Most common cause is autoimmune adrenalitis	Most common cause is exogenous glucocorticoid administration
Low plasma cortisol, low aldosterone, high ACTH	Low plasma cortisol
Presents with hyponatremia, hyperkalemia, hypotension, and hyperpigmentation	Normal aldosterone
Hyperpigmentation is most specific sign of primary disease	Normal blood pressure, sodium, and potassium
	No hyperpigmentation, but may have signs and symptoms related to loss of gonadotropins, TSH, or GH

Key Points

▶ Can be primary (adrenal gland failure) or secondary (pituitary or hypothalamic defect).

▶ Nonspecific symptoms and signs of fatigue, weakness, weight loss, confusion, nausea, and vomiting from lack of cortisol.

▶ Skin pigmentation, hypotension, and hyperkalemia only present in primary disease.

▶ Initial screen for suspected adrenal insufficiency is measurement of morning cortisol level and plasma ACTH.

▶ Treatment with exogenous glucocorticoid and mineralocorticoid replacement.

Questions

1. A 16-year-old girl is brought to see her pediatrician because her mother is concerned that she has not started her monthly periods. On physical exam, the girl is mildly obese, of short stature, and without secondary sex characteristics. Further workup includes serum hormone levels and a CT scan of the head, which reveals a craniopharyngeoma. Adrenocortical function in this patient is most likely:

A. Absent
B. Decreased
C. Normal
D. Increased
E. Unassessable

2. A 36-year-old woman with a history of Graves' disease complains of lethargy, weight loss, and feeling faint often. Her Graves' disease was treated successfully with total thyroidectomy secondary to inadequate response to antithyroid medications and radioactive iodine. Physical exam reveals multiple patches of skin depigmentation and orthostatic hypotension. The physician suspects adrenal insufficiency and confirms her diagnosis with an morning cortisol level and plasma ACTH. What is the most likely cause of her adrenal insufficiency?

A. Autoimmune adrenalitis
B. Long-term exogenous levothyroxine therapy
C. Undiagnosed coagulation disorder
D. Long-term exogenous glucocorticoid therapy
E. Tuberculosis reactivation

HPI: MC is a 57-year-old woman who presents to the ED with an acute onset of severe left flank pain. She describes the pain as 10/10, radiating down the same side to her groin. During the interview, MC is writhing uncomfortably, unable to sit still. She states that she has never experienced pain like this before. She took ibuprofen at home, but the medication did nothing for her pain. She also complains of two episodes of vomiting before arriving in the ED.

PE: On physical exam, MC is pale and sweating profusely. She has significant left costovertebral angle tenderness, but the rest of the physical exam is within normal limits. A urine dipstick reveals a small quantity of blood in her urine. Suspecting renal colic secondary to nephrolithiasis, the ED physician orders a urinalysis, an abdominal x-ray of the kidneys, ureters, and bladder (KUB), and blood tests, including a serum Ca^{2+} and serum parathyroid hormone (PTH). KUB radiography confirms the presence of a stone obstructing the left ureter, while blood tests are significant for hypercalcemia with a normal PTH level. She is immediately started on IV morphine sulfate for relief of her pain.

Thought Questions

- Why would primary hyperparathyroidism cause kidney stones? What are the other signs and symptoms of a patient with primary hyperparathyroidism?

- What are the functions of PTH?

- How is PTH secretion regulated?

- What is the differential diagnosis for hypercalcemia?

Basic Science Review and Discussion

The **parathyroid gland** is a paired hormone-secreting organ situated on the posterior surface of the thyroid gland. There are four glands in all, two on each side. The chief cells of the parathyroid gland secrete **PTH,** which is critical for calcium homeostasis. PTH functions to increase serum calcium via three main mechanisms: (1) increasing bone resorption, (2) increasing tubular reabsorption of calcium, and (3) stimulating conversion of 25-hydroxy-cholecalciferol (25OH-vitamin D) to 1,25-dihydroxycholecalciferol [1,25(OH)$_2$-vitamin D] in the kidney. In turn, vitamin D and its metabolites increase both bone and intestinal calcium and phosphate reabsorption. PTH also decreases serum phosphate by decreasing kidney reabsorption of phosphate. The stimulus for PTH secretion from the parathyroid glands is low free serum calcium.

The biologic action of PTH is partially mediated through cyclic AMP. PTH stimulates calcium release from bone through an indirect effect on osteoclasts, the cells involved in bone reabsorption. PTH receptors are actually present on bone-forming osteoblasts. When PTH binds to these receptors, osteoblasts move out of the way. This allows osteoclasts to enter the matrix and reabsorb bone, thereby releasing calcium into the circulation. The increase in serum calcium negatively feeds back on the parathyroid gland to decrease PTH release. When serum calcium becomes low again, more PTH is secreted.

Primary Hyperparathyroidism Primary hyperparathyroidism refers to multiple disorders of the parathyroid gland characterized by excessive and inappropriate secretion of PTH, resulting in hypercalcemia. The most common cause of primary hyperparathyroidism is a single adenoma in one gland secreting excessive amounts of PTH. Multiple adenomas have been reported in 2% to 4% of patients undergoing surgical excision. Approximately 15% of patients have diffuse hyperplasia of all four parathyroid glands, which frequently occurs as a hereditary trait. The familial pattern is also found associated with multiple endocrine neoplasia type I (MEN I: primary hyperparathyroidism, pituitary adenomas, and pancreatic islet cell tumors) and type IIa (MEN IIa: primary hyperparathyroidism, thyroid medullary carcinoma, and pheochromocytoma). Parathyroid carcinoma is the least common cause of primary hyperparathyroidism, accounting for less than 1% of all cases.

Patients with primary hyperparathyroidism exhibit the signs and symptoms associated with **hypercalcemia.** None of these symptoms, however, are specific to hypercalcemia or primary hyperparathyroidism itself. Because the rise in serum calcium is usually chronic and of slow onset, patients are usually asymptomatic and the diagnosis is an incidental finding based on serum laboratory tests. The gastrointestinal symptoms include dry mouth, thirst, and polydipsia. Constipation is also common. Genitourinary complaints may include polyuria and nocturia. As in this patient, renal stones and nephrocalcinosis are potential serious complications. Metastatic calcification can occur in the cornea, conjunctiva, or throughout the vascular system. Musculoskeletal symptoms range from muscle weakness and decreased deep tendon reflexes to bone and joint pain secondary to cystic changes within bone and calcium deposition in the joints. In general, patients can feel drowsy and fatigued or experience speech deficits or blurry vision.

Hypercalcemia There are numerous causes of hypercalcemia besides hyperparathyroidism. Hypercalcemia can be secondary to drugs (vitamin D or vitamin A intoxication, chlorothiazide diuretics, lithium), granulomatous disorders (sarcoidosis, tuberculosis, coccidioidomycosis), renal failure, endocrine disorders (hyperthyroidism, acromegaly, addisonian crisis), or prolonged bed rest. In hospitalized patients, however, the most common cause of hypercalcemia is malignancy. Together, primary hyperparathyroidism and malignancy account for over 90% of hypercalcemia cases. Malignancies can cause hypercalcemia through various mechanisms. When no skeletal metastases are present, hypercalcemia occurs through **PTH-related protein (PTHrP),** a factor known to be produced by some tumors that will bind to the PTH receptor in the bone and kidney and thereby cause hypercalcemia. Lung and breast cancers are the two most common malignancies to produce PTHrP. Cancers can also cause hypercalcemia through bone invasion and the release of calcium-stimulating factors such as PGE_2, TGF-α, or PDGF. In contrast to hyperparathyroidism, patients with an underlying malignancy tend to have a more rapid rise in serum calcium concentration. This rapid rise is associated with the acute signs and symptoms of nausea/vomiting and altered mental status not seen in chronic disease. In these instances, altered mental status can range from confusion to coma.

Diagnosis Because most patients are asymptomatic, the diagnosis of hyperparathyroidism is based on laboratory examination. A direct measurement of the simultaneous concentrations of calcium and PTH in the serum are critical for diagnosis. Serum calcium should always be assessed with concomitant serum protein level, because changes in protein level can alter serum calcium assessment. Forty percent of the total serum calcium is bound to plasma proteins (primarily albumin), 10% is complexed to anions, and only 50% is available for action as free ionized calcium. Multiple determinations of calcium of greater than 10.2 mg/dL is consistent with hypercalcemia (normal range 8.4–10.2 mg/dL). To assess parathyroid function, serum PTH is the best test. Because PTH secretion is regulated by serum calcium levels, the PTH level should be low or undetectable with hypercalcemia. With primary hyperparathyroidism, however, the PTH level can be normal or elevated. A normal serum PTH in the presence of hypercalcemia is inappropriately normal relative to serum calcium and indicates hyperparathyroidism. Other laboratory findings that are consistent with primary hyperparathyroidism include elevated serum 1,25(OH)$_2$-vitamin D levels, decreased serum phosphate, increased alkaline phosphatase from bone reabsorption, and elevated urinary cyclic AMP. In addition, because PTH acts to lower the renal tubular maximum for bicarbonate, there is a tendency to develop mild hyperchloremic metabolic acidosis with primary hyperparathyroidism.

Case Conclusion   MC passes her stone successfully and returns home the next day. She is followed up by her primary doctor who explains to her the diagnosis of primary hyperparathyroidism and the need for neck exploration and resection of the abnormal parathyroid tissue. At the time of surgery, a single adenoma is found in one of her parathyroid glands. The remaining three glands, however, appear to be shrunken and atrophic. The affected gland is removed in its entirety while the other glands are left intact. When MC returns for postsurgical follow-up, a serum calcium of 3.4 mg/dL is documented. PTH levels at that time are undetectable.

Thought Questions

- What is the cause of MC's subsequent hypocalcemia?
- What are the signs and symptoms of hypocalcemia?

Discussion Continued

MC now presents with postsurgical **hypoparathyroidism,** the most common cause of hypoparathyroidism. This surgical complication occurs frequently during thyroid surgery because the close proximity of the parathyroid glands in relation to the thyroid makes them particularly vulnerable to damage. Postsurgical hypoparathyroidism can be transient or permanent, and is usually caused by ischemia to the glands secondary to ligation of the thyroid artery. In this case, the hypoparathyroidism is probably transient and caused by suppression of the unaffected glands by the adenoma. Hypoparathyroidism is characterized by **hypocalcemia** and low/undetectable PTH levels. Other causes of hypoparathyroidism are parathyroid agenesis or polyglandular failure, an autoimmune condition often associated with adrenal and ovarian failure. Rare causes are invasion by metastatic tumor and destruction of the gland due to radiation therapy.

Hypocalcemia Hypocalcemia in general also has multiple causes. These include magnesium deficiency, decreased serum albumin, and pseudohyperparathyroidism. **Pseudohyperparathyroidism** is a condition characterized by end-organ resistance to PTH. Patients with this condition exhibit hypocalcemia, but have increased levels of serum PTH. The condition is caused by a defect in adenylate cyclase resulting in an inability to generate cyclic AMP. Patients are short-statured secondary to early epiphyseal closure and have mild mental retardation. Interestingly, patients with pseudohypoparathyroidism often have a shortened fourth metacarpal on x-ray examination.

The signs and symptoms of hypocalcemia are neuromuscular, neurologic, dermatologic, and ophthalmologic. More specifically, patients complain of paresthesias (perioral numbness, numbness of extremities), have dry/scaly skin and brittle nails, and are hyperreflexic. Neurologically, patients can present with seizures, depression, anxiety, or irritability. Papilledema and cataracts may also be present. Trousseau's sign (tap the facial nerve →twitching of lip and cheek) and Chvostek's sign (inflation of blood pressure cuff on arm → carpal spasm) are both positive with hypocalcemia.

Treatment of hypocalcemia involves identifying the underlying cause and treating that cause appropriately. For hypoparathyroidism, the treatment consists of administering $1,25(OH)_2$-vitamin D (active form). The goal of treatment is to keep serum calcium at low-normal levels, around 8 mg/dL; this level will prevent the symptoms of hypocalcemia from developing while preventing kidney stone formation as well.

Thumbnail: Signs and Symptoms—Hypercalcemia versus Hypocalcemia

Organ system	Hypercalcemia	Hypocalcemia
Gastrointestinal	Dry mouth, thirst, polydipsia, anorexia, nausea, vomiting, constipation	No significant abnormalities
Genitourinary	Polyuria, nocturia, renal stones, nephrocalcinosis, uremia	No significant abnormalities
Musculoskeletal	Fatigue, muscle weakness, arthralgia, bone pain	Fasciculations, tetany
Neurologic	Drowsiness, lethargy, stupor, coma, confusion, speech deficits, blurry vision, decreased or absent deep tendon reflexes	Seizures, depression, anxiety, irritability, increased CSF pressure, hyperreflexia, positive Trousseau's and Chvostek's signs
Dermatologic		Dry/scaly skin, brittle nails
Ophthalmologic		Cataracts, papilledema

Key Points

Primary Hyperparathyroidism
▶ Causes: adenoma (most common), hyperplasia, carcinoma, familial, MEN I, MEN IIa.
▶ Eighty percent of patients are asymptomatic.
▶ Lab findings: elevated serum calcium, normal or elevated PTH.
▶ Treatment is surgical.

Hypoparathyroidism
▶ Causes: postsurgical (most common), autoimmune, congenital agenesis, metastatic tumor, radiation therapy.
▶ Symptoms and signs of hypocalcemia.
▶ Lab findings: low serum calcium, low/undetectable PTH.
▶ Treatment with $1,25(OH)_2$-vitamin D.

Questions

1. A 26-year-old Asian woman presents to her primary care physician for routine physical exam. She states that she likes to exercise often, but that her activities have been limited recently due to bone and joint pain in her lower extremities. One year ago, she fractured her tibia after lightly bumping her leg against a treadmill. A routine chemistry panel reveals a serum calcium of 11.5 mg/dL (normal 8.4–10.2 mg/dL) and an elevated PTH level. What could be the cause of her problems?

   A. Osteoporosis
   B. Osteoarthritis
   C. Rheumatoid arthritis
   D. Osteogenesis imperfecta
   E. Fibromyalgia

2. A 68-year-old man with a 40-pack per year history of smoking is diagnosed with squamous cell carcinoma of the lung. He has multiple skeletal metastases. His serum calcium is elevated at 14.3 mg/dL. What is the source of his hypercalcemia?

   A. PGE_2
   B. PTHrP
   C. TGF-α
   D. PDGF
   E. All of the above

HPI: TS is a 30-year-old white woman who presents to her new primary medical doctor for the first time. During the initial history and physical, TS reveals that her husband became alarmed recently while perusing through wedding photos from 2 years ago. He noticed that TS had changed significantly in appearance since their wedding day. According to her husband, TS now has a more prominent forehead and jaw line than she used to, and when he held her hands, they felt especially thick and rough. TS states that she had not noticed much change in her appearance until her husband forced her to look at her old pictures. She attributes her rough hands to working out in the garden frequently, but does admit that her feet feel bigger and coarser as well. She complains that her shoes have been feeling particularly tight, so she has been buying shoes a full size larger than she has in the past.

PE: Physical exam reveals a pleasant and cooperative woman with slightly slurred speech and a deep voice. Significant physical exam findings include a prominent brow bone, large tongue, and protuberant jaw. Her hands and feet are coarse and thickened. The doctor asks to see TS's driver's license photo for comparison; he suspects acromegaly and immediately orders the appropriate tests for workup.

Thought Questions

■ What is acromegaly?

■ What is the best test for the diagnosis of acromegaly?

■ What are the clinical signs and symptoms of acromegaly?

■ How is GH secreted and regulated?

Basic Science Review and Discussion

Growth hormone is secreted from acidophilic cells called somatotrophs in the anterior pituitary. Like all other pituitary hormones, secretion of GH is tightly regulated by the hypothalamic-pituitary axis. The hypothalamus secretes **growth hormone releasing hormone (GHRH),** which acts on the pituitary to stimulate GH secretion. The hypothalamus also secretes somatostatin, which inhibits the production and release of GH. Secretion of GH by the pituitary into the bloodstream stimulates the liver to produce **insulin-like growth factor 1 (IGF-1).** The actions of GH are mediated through IGF-1, which binds to the IGF receptor on tissues; the IGF receptor has tyrosine kinase activity. GH secretion is also regulated by a negative feedback mechanism. Namely, IGF-1 inhibits the secretion of GH by directly acting on the anterior pituitary as well as stimulating the release of somatostatin from the hypothalamus. GH also inhibits its own secretion by stimulating somatostatin release from the hypothalamus. GHRH, somatostatin, GH, and IGF-1 levels are all tightly regulated by each other and by sleep, exercise, stress, food intake, and blood sugar levels.

GH is critical during childhood for developing normal adult stature and proportions. GH has both direct and indirect effects mediated through IGF-1. The direct effects include decreased glucose uptake, increased lipolysis, and increased protein synthesis resulting in more lean body mass. Because GH also stimulates the production of IGF-1 from the liver, GH acts indirectly through IGF-1 to increase linear growth in long bones and increase organ size. A deficiency in GH prior to fusion of the epiphyseal growth plates in long bones results in **dwarfism.** Affected individuals are short statured, mildly obese, and have delayed onset of puberty. Because GH primarily affects long bones, the flat bones of the skull are not affected, resulting in abnormal skull-to-skeletal proportions.

An excess of GH can result in two different clinical presentations, depending on the time of the excess. Before puberty and closure of the epiphyseal growth plates, excess GH causes increased linear bone growth resulting in **gigantism.** After puberty, however, GH excess causes **acromegaly,** a condition characterized by periosteal bone growth, organomegaly, and changes in sugar and lipid metabolism associated with DM.

Acromegaly Over 90% of acromegaly cases are caused by a benign pituitary adenoma. The rest are caused by paraneoplastic production of GH or GHRH by tumors of the lung, pancreas, or adrenal glands. Most pituitary tumors arise spontaneously, without genetic predisposition. The adenoma produces excessive amounts of GH and as it expands, may compress surrounding brain and normal pituitary tissue. Patients can thus present with the headache and visual field abnormalities typical of pituitary tumors, or with additional endocrine defects associated with the compromised production of other pituitary hormones. The gonadotropins are often the first to be affected, leading to changes in menstruation in women or impotence in men. Both men and women can present with infertility as well. In certain cases, GH-secreting adenomas may simultaneously produce excess prolactin; patients with these tumors may also complain of galactorrhea.

The name *acromegaly* comes from the Greek words for "extremities" and "enlargement" and reflects one of its most common symptoms, the abnormal growth of the hands and feet (Figure 22-1). Soft tissue swelling of the hands and feet is an early feature, and patients may first notice a change in ring or shoe size. The hands and feet are usually thick and coarse, with significant edema. When tissue thickens, it may trap nerves, causing carpal tunnel syndrome characterized by weakness and tingling of the hands. Systemic edema can lead to HTN. Gradual bony changes will alter the patient's facial features: the brow and lower jaw protrude, the nasal bone enlarges, and the spacing of the teeth increases. GH-induced swelling in the tongue and vocal cords may cause speech to slur or the voice to deepen. In addition, there may be visceral enlargement of the liver, spleen, kidneys, and heart.

The most serious complications of acromegaly are HTN, DM, and increased risk for cardiovascular disease. Patients most often die from CHF as a result of the severe HTN and vascular disease. Patients with acromegaly are also at increased risk for growth of visceral tumors that are stimulated by GH. In particular, many patients have growth of colonic polyps that can subsequently develop into cancer.

Diagnosis GH is secreted in a rapid oscillating pattern that varies throughout the day. As a result, measurements of serum GH may not be an accurate indicator of GH excess. If acromegaly is suspected, **the most important diagnostic test is measurement of IGF-1** levels. Because IGF-1 levels are much more stable over the course of the day, they are a more practical and reliable measure than GH levels. Elevated IGF-1 is almost always consistent with acromegaly. Few exceptions include an elevated IGF-1 in pregnant women and decreased IGF-1 in elderly patients and patients with poorly controlled diabetes. Confirmation of a pituitary adenoma can be made with MRI of the head to visualize the tumor. Workup should also include measurements of prolactin, TSH with free T_4, luteinizing hormone (LH), follicle-stimulating hormone (FSH), and morning cortisol to rule out other endocrine abnormalities.

Treatment Acromegaly is primarily a surgical disease. Once the diagnosis is confirmed and the pituitary tumor identified, a trans-sphenoidal approach is used to remove the abnormal tissue. The physical changes secondary to edema and tissue thickening will often begin to resolve immediately following a successful surgery. Unfortunately, the bony defects will not improve following surgery. Other potential treatments include gamma knife surgery and medications such as somatostatin analogues (octreotide), which can decrease IGF-1 production in the liver. However, these other treatment modalities are not very effective and are associated with increased side effects; surgery thus remains the gold standard for treatment of acromegaly.

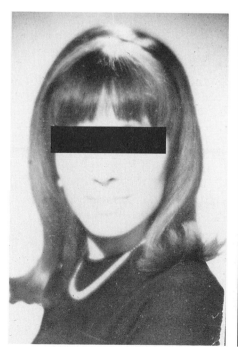 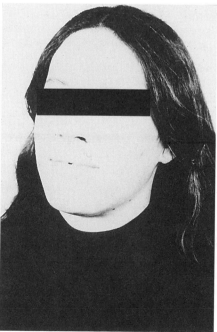 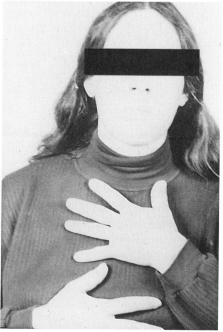

Figure 22-1 A 21-year-old female college student before and after the diagnosis of acromegaly. The student noticed a significant change in her physical appearance over a period of 1½ years. Notice the coarse facial features, prominent jawbone, and thickened hands caused by excess GH production after closure of the epiphyseal growth plates. (Images courtesy of Joel Schechter, PhD, Keck School of Medicine at the University of Southern California.)

Case Conclusion TS is diagnosed with acromegaly and undergoes trans-sphenoidal resection of her pituitary tumor.

Thumbnail: Acromegaly

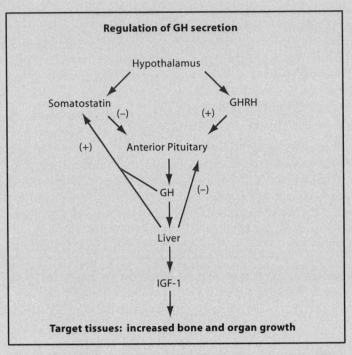

Regulation of GH secretion

Hypothalamus

Somatostatin   GHRH

(−)   (+)

(+)   Anterior Pituitary

GH   (−)

Liver

IGF-1

Target tissues: increased bone and organ growth

Functions of GH
- decreased glucose uptake
- increased lipolysis
- increased muscle mass
- increased bone growth
- increased organ size

GH abnormalities
Pre-puberty: Deficiency = dwarfism
               Excess = gigantism

Post-puberty: Excess = acromegaly

Key Points

▶ Excess growth hormone production after puberty due to pituitary adenoma.

▶ Symptoms and signs include bony and visceral organ enlargement, coarsening of facial features, and thickening of hands, feet, and tongue.

▶ Measure IGF-1 level for diagnosis—will be elevated in acromegaly.

▶ Definitive treatment is trans-sphenoidal excision of the pituitary tumor.

Questions

1. A 40-year-old man presents to your primary care clinic complaining of infertility. He and his wife have been trying unsuccessfully to have a child for the past 2 years. On physical exam, you notice that he is a peculiar looking man, with a protruding brow and lower jaw, a large nose, and wide spaces between his teeth. What is the most important diagnostic test you should order?

   A. MRI of the head
   B. Serum LH, FSH, and testosterone levels
   C. GH serology
   D. GHRH serology
   E. IGF-1 serology

2. A 36-year-old woman is diagnosed with acromegaly. She is not pregnant and her IGF-1 levels are 1020 mg/dL. Which of the following is not an important consequence of her new diagnosis?

   A. DM
   B. Colon cancer
   C. HTN
   D. Delayed puberty
   E. Arthritis

HPI: LW is a 47-year-old Asian-American woman who presents to her primary care doctor for follow-up of her HTN. She has a 2-year history of HTN, treated unsuccessfully with multiple trials of medications. On this visit, LW's BP is elevated at 180/120 mm Hg, despite combined treatment with a beta-blocker and a diuretic. LW also complains of persistent mild frontal headaches, nocturia, and generalized weakness of her extremities.

PE: Physical exam is significant for elevated systolic and diastolic BPs pressures, without evidence of retinopathy or abdominal bruits. LW also demonstrates normal tone, but 3/5 muscle strength in her upper and lower extremities. At this time, serum electrolyte evaluation reveals a K^+ of 2.5 mEq/L and a mild metabolic alkalosis with HCO_3^- of 32 mmol/L. LW's physician suggests that she discontinue her current medications and return in 3 weeks for further evaluation of her BP and electrolytes. On stopping her medications for 3 weeks, serum K^+ remained low at 3.0 mEq/L. Plasma renin was decreased at 0.1 ng/mL/h (normal 1–3 ng/mL/h), but plasma aldosterone was elevated at 22 ng/mL (normal 3–9 ng/mL).

Thought Questions

- What are the components of the renin-angiotensin system (RAS)?

- How does this system regulate BP?

- What are the features of primary hyperaldosteronism?

- What is the difference between primary and secondary hyperaldosteronism?

Basic Science Review and Discussion

Aldosterone is a mineralocorticoid hormone secreted by the zona glomerulosa cells of the adrenal cortex. Aldosterone acts on the distal tubule of the kidney to increase reabsorption of salt and facilitate excretion of potassium. Unlike the zona fasciculata and the zona reticularis, the zona glomerulosa is minimally regulated by ACTH from the hypothalamus. Instead, aldosterone secretion is primarily regulated via the RAS.

The Renin-Angiotensin System The **RAS** is responsible for long-term BP regulation in the body (Figure 23-1). The system is stimulated by a decrease in renal perfusion pressure to the kidney as sensed by the **juxtaglomerular apparatus (JGA).** The JGA consists of juxtaglomerular (JG) cells, specialized myoepithelial cells within the afferent arteriole that secrete renin, and the macula densa, cells in the distal convoluted tubule that can assess the amount of sodium that is delivered to the distal tubules per unit time. The JG cells respond to changes in stretch induced by changes in renal BP. When JG cells are stretched with increased renal BP, they respond by decreasing renin release. Conversely, a decrease in renal BP increases renal renin release.

Renin is a proteolytic enzyme that cleaves angiotensinogen to angiotensin I, an inactive intermediate in the plasma. Angiotensin I circulates to the lungs and other tissues, where it is converted to angiotensin II by ACE synthesized by pulmonary endothelial cells. Angiotensin II is the biologically active hormone that actually functions to increase BP. It does this via two primary mechanisms: (1) Angiotensin II causes vasoconstriction of arterioles; this vasoconstriction causes increased peripheral resistance and thus leads to an increased diastolic BP. (2) Angiotensin II also acts on the zona glomerulosa cells of the adrenal gland to release aldosterone; aldosterone then acts on the distal tubules of the kidney to increase sodium and water retention and promote potassium excretion. Increased salt and water reabsorption increases total blood volume and mean arterial pressure.

Primary Hyperaldosteronism This patient presents with the typical signs and symptoms of **primary hyperaldosteronism,** otherwise known as **Conn's syndrome.** Jerome Conn first described primary hyperaldosteronism in 1955. Primary hyperaldosteronism occurs in 1% of all people diagnosed with HTN, with the highest incidence between ages 30 and 50 and affecting men twice as often as women. The syndrome results from an abnormally large amount of aldosterone produced by the adrenal cortex. Most often, the excess aldosterone is due to an aldosterone-secreting adrenal adenoma in one of the adrenal glands. Less commonly, the excess can be due to idiopathic bilateral hyperplasia of the zona glomerulosa or adrenocortical carcinomas. The syndrome is characterized by HTN, hypokalemia, metabolic alkalosis, and low plasma renin levels. Plasma renin is low because the retained sodium feeds back to the JGA and decreases renal renin release. Low renin levels are key to distinguishing primary from secondary sources of hyperaldosteronism.

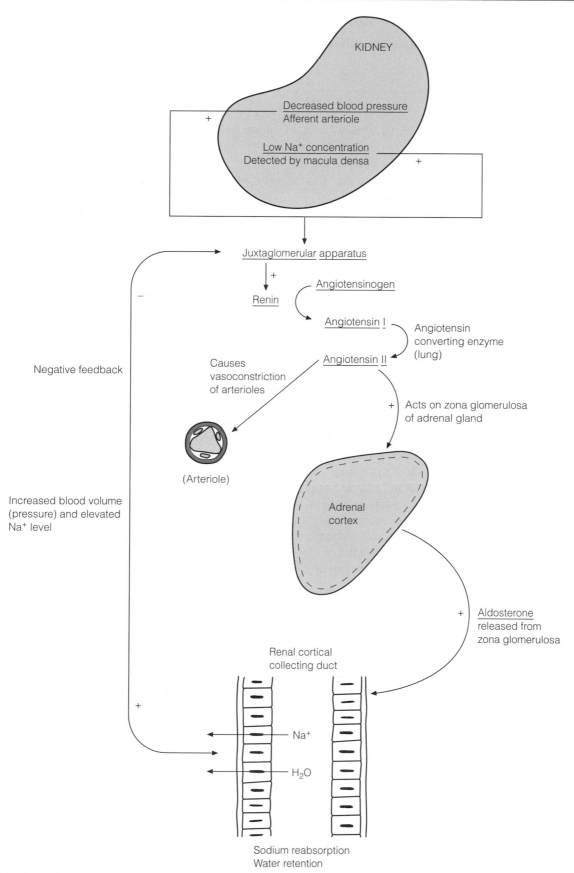

Figure 23-1 Renin-angiotensin system (RAS). Diagram summarizes the regulation of aldosterone secretion by the RAS. Aldosterone acts to increase sodium and water uptake from the renal collecting tubules.

Table 23-1 Primary versus secondary hyperaldosteronism

	Plasma aldosterone	Plasma renin	Plasma Na+	Plasma K+
Primary hyperaldosteronism	↑	↓	↑	↓
Secondary hyperaldosteronism	↑	↑	↑	↓

Secondary Hyperaldosteronism   In contrast to primary hyperaldosteronism, which is due to an abnormality in the adrenal gland itself, **secondary hyperaldosteronism** occurs as a result of a peripheral abnormality that causes the kidney to misperceive a fall in BP. These peripheral abnormalities can include renal artery stenosis, chronic renal failure, cirrhosis, or nephrotic syndrome. In these instances, the kidney's BP regulation system is fooled into thinking that the BP is abnormally low. In response, the RAS is inappropriately activated and excess aldosterone is produced. Patients with secondary hyperaldosteronism can present in an identical manner as patients with Conn's syndrome. However, patients with secondary forms of hyperaldosteronism will have **high plasma renin** in addition to high aldosterone levels (Table 23-1).

Clinical Presentation   Clinically, patients with Conn's syndrome most commonly present with a history of HTN, often not responsive to medications. The excess aldosterone stimulates sodium and water retention, as well as potassium wasting. Low potassium levels are responsible for the associated symptoms of muscle weakness, neurologic changes, thirst, polydipsia, polyuria, and/or nocturia. Tachycardia can also occur without the patient feeling palpitations. Patients will have metabolic alkalosis with increased serum HCO_3^- because aldosterone also stimulates the loss of hydrogen ion from the distal tubule through the Na^+-H^+ pump. Although sodium and water retention are key features of primary hyperaldosteronism, patients remain euvolemic due to the renal escape phenomenon.

Diagnosis   Diagnosis of primary hyperaldosteronism must be made with the patient not taking any usual antihypertensive medications, which can invalidate the results. Important laboratory findings include decreased plasma renin, increased plasma aldosterone, low serum potassium, and high 24-hour urine potassium. Additional confirmatory indicators are a mild metabolic alkalosis (HCO_3^- >30 mmol/L) and a mildly elevated serum glucose level due to the hypokalemia interfering with insulin secretion and glucose regulation. CT or MRI scan of the adrenal glands can then be used to demonstrate presence of adrenal tumors or hyperplasia.

Treatment   Treatment of primary hyperaldosteronism due to an adrenal adenoma consists of removal of the affected gland (adrenalectomy). When possible, selective excision of the adenoma is attempted to preserve any functioning adrenal tissue. Medical therapy can be used as an adjunct to surgery to control BP and replenish potassium stores prior to surgery. Possible medications include spironolactone, an aldosterone antagonist, and amiloride, a potassium-sparing diuretic. These medications are also used when the source of the aldosterone excess is due to idiopathic bilateral zona glomerular hyperplasia or if the tumor is inoperable.

Case Conclusion   With the clinical findings of uncontrolled HTN, hypokalemia, elevated plasma aldosterone, and decreased plasma renin levels, LW's physician suspects primary hyperaldosteronism. The doctor orders an abdominal CT, which confirms the presence of a 6-cm round mass in the outer cortex of her left adrenal gland. LW is started on spironolactone therapy for 4 weeks before surgical excision of her tumor.

Thumbnail: Conn's Syndrome

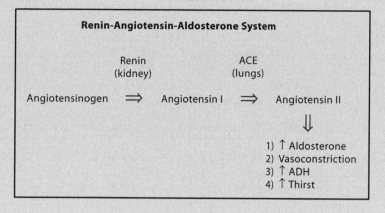

Renin-Angiotensin-Aldosterone System

Angiotensinogen $\Longrightarrow$ Angiotensin I $\Longrightarrow$ Angiotensin II

Renin (kidney)　　ACE (lungs)

$\Downarrow$

1) ↑ Aldosterone
2) Vasoconstriction
3) ↑ ADH
4) ↑ Thirst

Key Points

Functions of Aldosterone
▶ ↑ renal Na$^+$ reabsorption
▶ ↑ renal K$^+$ secretion
▶ ↑ renal H$^+$ secretion

Primary Hyperaldosteronism
▶ Due to adrenal adenoma, hyperplasia, or carcinoma producing excess aldosterone
▶ ↑ plasma aldosterone
▶ ↓ plasma renin
▶ ↑ plasma Na$^+$, ↓ plasma K$^+$

Secondary Hyperaldosteronism
▶ Due to renal artery stenosis, cirrhosis, nephrotic syndrome, or CHF causing overactivity of the RAS
▶ ↑ plasma aldosterone
▶ ↑ plasma renin
▶ ↑ plasma Na$^+$, ↓ plasma K$^+$

Questions

1. A 33-year-old man complains of increased thirst, fatigue, and occasional heart palpitations unrelated to activity for the past 2 months. In the past, he has been healthy and has had no known medical conditions. BP on this visit is elevated at 158/96 mm Hg. Initial ECG evaluation is within normal limits. Key features in the diagnosis of primary hyperaldosteronism do not include:

   A. Metabolic acidosis
   B. Unprovoked hypokalemia
   C. Low plasma renin activity
   D. High aldosterone
   E. HTN

2. A 50-year-old woman with a history of HTN is incidentally found to have bilateral adrenocortical hyperplasia on abdominal CT workup for kidney stones. She is currently taking atenolol for treatment of her HTN. Appropriate treatment choices for a patient with bilateral adrenocortical hyperplasia causing primary hyperaldosteronism include:

   A. Bilateral adrenalectomy
   B. Loop diuretics
   C. Spironolactone
   D. ACE inhibitors
   E. C and D

HPI: JF is a 42-year-old white man who presents to his primary care physician for repeat BP measurement after elevated BPs were found on two previous office visits. On this day, JF's BP remains elevated at 192/118 mm Hg. JF states that work has been especially stressful recently, and the stress may be contributing to his elevated pressures. Although he would describe himself as a generally relaxed type of guy, JF complains of recurrent "anxiety attacks" which he has noticed increasing in frequency over the past 6 months. The anxiety attacks occur sporadically, consisting of episodes of severe headache, flushing, sweating, palpitations, and a sense of impending doom. According to JF, the episodes usually last for less than 15 minutes and were not relieved with a trial of antianxiety medications from another doctor.

PE: Physical exam is within normal limits, except for the elevated BP measurements. Cardiac evaluation of the palpitations with resting ECG is also normal.

With the diagnosis of new-onset HTN and a history of paroxysmal attacks of anxiety-like symptoms, JF's physician suspects pheochromocytoma as a possible explanation for JF's symptoms.

Thought Questions

- What is the function of the adrenal medulla?

- How does the blood supply to the adrenal medulla regulate synthesis of its secretory products?

- What is pheochromocytoma? What are the typical signs and symptoms?

- How is pheochromocytoma diagnosed? What are the treatment options?

Basic Science Review and Discussion

The **adrenal medulla** comprises the inner 10% to 20% of the adrenal gland and is responsible for catecholamine synthesis. In response to stress, the adrenal medulla synthesizes and secretes **norepinephrine** and **epinephrine** into the circulation, binding adrenergic receptors on target cells. The end-organ effect of this binding is comparable with direct stimulation by sympathetic nerves and is important as part of the body's "fight or flight" response mechanism to stress.

Adrenal Medulla Histology   The primary cell type in the adrenal medulla is the chromaffin cell, also known as a pheochromocyte. Chromaffin cells are derived from the neural crest and can be found in sites other than the adrenal gland, such as the sympathetic ganglia, the carotid body, the pericardial sac, and the aortic bifurcation. These cells are named for their characteristic brown color under a microscope ("phios" = dusky and "chroma" = color) due to their *affinity* for *chromic* acid, which oxidizes the catecholamines stored within the cell granules into melanin.

Catecholamine Synthesis   The adrenal medulla has a dual arterial supply, but a single venous drainage. Most of the medullary blood supply goes through the cortex first, but about 20% of the blood supply passes directly into the medulla, without exposure to cortical secretory products. The blood that goes through the cortex is bathed in glucocorticoids produced in the zona fasciculata and is thus rich in the enzyme phenylethanolamine-N-methyltransferase (PNMT). PNMT converts norepinephrine to epinephrine in the cytosol of chromaffin cells. The less than 20% of cells supplied with blood that has not passed through the cortical circulation produce mainly norepinephrine, since they have low levels of PNMT. The ratio of secretory products from the adrenal medulla is thus a direct consequence of the dual medullary blood supply. Typically, the output of the medulla is greater than 80% epinephrine and less than 20% norepinephrine.

Secretion of catecholamines is regulated by the limbic system and the hypothalamus. Activation of the sympathetic nervous system by "emergency" conditions stimulates catecholamine secretion within seconds to minutes of stress exposure. These stressors include exercise, hypoglycemia, hypovolemia, hypotension, and pain. The release of catecholamines occurs much more rapidly than the slower increase in blood cortisol, which can take up to 1 hour.

Pheochromocytoma   The most common tumor of the adrenal medulla in adults is **pheochromocytoma.** Pheochromocytomas are catecholamine-secreting tumors derived from chromaffin cells. These rare tumors cause HTN by releasing large amounts of catecholamines into the circulation. About 98% of the tumors occur in the abdomen, especially in the adrenal medulla (90%), but they may develop in any chromaffin tissue. The tumors produce norepinephrine, epinephrine, or, more commonly, both. Predominant production of epinephrine, when present, suggests an adrenal location.

Pheochromocytoma occurs in about 1/1000 hypertensive individuals. The incidence is higher in patients with moderate to severe HTN. Though often sporadic, pheochromocytomas may also be associated with other familial neuroendocrine disorders such as neurofibromatosis, von Hippel-Lindau disease, and MEN II and III. Pheochromocytomas are characterized by a rough rule of tens; that is, about 10% of cases are malignant, 10% occur bilaterally in the adrenals, 10% are extra-adrenal, 10% calcify, 10% occur in children, and 10% are familial.

Clinical Presentation   The most prominent clinical feature of pheochromocytoma is HTN, which is usually constant (50%-60%) and may be severe. Classically, patients describe **paroxysms of severe HTN** with pallor and headache (norepinephrine effects); this constellation of symptoms occurs in about 30% to 60% of patients. Paroxysms can last from a few seconds to a few days, but usually last less than 15 minutes. They are also associated with flushing, sweating, palpitations, and hyperglycemia (epinephrine effects). In addition, patients may complain of tachycardia, tachypnea, cold and clammy skin, angina, nausea, vomiting, or epigastric pain. Attacks are similar to anxiety attacks in that patients may also experience a sense of impending doom. Paroxysmal attacks may be provoked by palpation of the tumor, postural changes, abdominal compression or massage, induction of anesthesia, emotional trauma, or beta-blockers. Physical examination of a patient with pheochromocytoma is usually normal with the exception of HTN, unless the exam is performed during a paroxysmal attack.

Diagnosis   The diagnosis of pheochromocytoma is based on detection of elevated levels of serum catecholamines or their metabolic breakdown products in the urine. The principal urinary metabolic products of epinephrine and norepinephrine are the metanephrines **vanillylmandelic acid (VMA)** and **homovanillic acid (HVA)**. Normal persons excrete only very small amounts of these substances in the urine. Patients with pheochromocytoma, however, have intermittent increases in excretion of epinephrine, norepinephrine, and their metabolic products. If the patient is examined during a hypertensive paroxysm, 2- or 3-hour timed urine or blood collection for catecholamines is the best test. With constant HTN, complete 24-hour urine collection for catecholamines and metanephrines is diagnostic if urinary excretion of these substances is elevated in the absence of coma, dehydration, or extreme stress states.

Treatment   The only definitive treatment for pheochromocytoma is surgical resection of the tumor. Stringent perioperative BP and cardiac monitoring is imperative because surgical manipulation of the tumor can potentially cause release of stored catecholamines into the circulation, precipitating a life-threatening hypertensive crisis during surgery. These crises can be prevented by preoperative administration of α-adrenergic blockers and beta-blockers, which will maintain BP and cardiac function at normal physiologic levels.

Case Conclusion   JF undergoes a 24-hour timed urine collection for evaluation of possible pheochromocytoma. Urinary levels of free epinephrine, norepinephrine, VMA, and HMA are all elevated. Follow-up T2-weighted abdominal MRI localizes a hyperintense 4-cm mass in the region of the left adrenal gland.

Thumbnail: Pheochromocytoma

Synthesis of catecholamines in the adrenal medulla	Actions of catecholamines
Tyrosine	Increased rate and force of contraction of heart muscle
↓ *Tyrosine hydroxylase*	Constriction of blood vessels
Dihydroxyphenylalanine (DOPA)	Dilation of bronchioles
↓ *DOPA decarboxylase*	Stimulation of lipolysis in adipocytes
Dopamine	Increased metabolic rate
↓ *Dopamine-β-hydroxylase*	Dilation of pupils
Norepinephrine	Inhibition of parasympathetic "rest and rumination" processes
↓ *Phenylethanolamine-N-methyltransferase (PNMT)*	
Epinephrine	

Key Points

- Tumor of chromaffin cells, most commonly in the adrenal medulla.
- Excess synthesis of norepinephrine and epinephrine results in overactivation of the sympathetic nervous system.
- Characterized by paroxysms of HTN, headache, sweating, pallor, tachycardia, anxiety, and tremor.
- Diagnosis confirmed by elevated urinary catecholamines, VMA, and HMA.

- Definitive treatment is surgical resection of the adrenal tumor.
- Associated neuroendocrine disorders: neurofibromatosis, von Hippel-Lindau disease, MEN syndromes.
- Ten percent rule: 10% malignant, 10% bilateral, 10% extra-adrenal, 10% calcified, 10% in children, and 10% familial.

Questions

1. A 32-year-old woman with a history of chronic HTN is evaluated for pheochromocytoma after complaining of multiple episodes of headache and palpitations. A 24-hour urine specimen is significant for greater than 135 mg total catecholamines per gram of creatinine. Which of the following is not an appropriate option for the management of pheochromocytoma?

   A. Surgery
   B. Dopamine
   C. Phenoxybenzamine
   D. Propranolol
   E. Phentolamine

2. A 22-year-old woman experiences sudden onset of nausea, headache, tachycardia, sweating, and chest pain. Her family calls 911 and she is immediately rushed to the nearest emergency room. Upon arrival, BP is significantly elevated at 208/136 mm Hg. She states that she has had similar episodes in the past, but they have usually resolved within a few minutes. What is the best test for diagnosis of her condition?

   A. 24-hour timed urine collection for catecholamines.
   B. Repeat BP measurements three times.
   C. 2-hour timed urine collection for metanephrines.
   D. Abdominal CT.
   E. Serum TSH, free T_4.

> **HPI:** KP is a 25-year-old white woman who has just delivered a full-term infant via normal spontaneous vaginal delivery. Immediately after delivery, the obstetrician notices ambiguous genitalia on the baby and consults the pediatricians for an evaluation.
>
> **PE:** On physical exam, the infant appears to be female, however, there is moderate clitoromegaly and fusion of the labioscrotal folds. The baby is further evaluated for possible congenital adrenal hyperplasia.

Thought Questions

- What is congenital adrenal hyperplasia?

- What mechanisms regulate cortisol and aldosterone production?

- What is the common precursor to all steroid hormones? Which enzymes are important in the steroidogenic pathway?

Basic Science Review and Discussion

Congenital adrenal hyperplasia (CAH) refers to a group of autosomal-recessive disorders caused by deficiencies in the adrenal enzymes that are required for cortisol or aldosterone synthesis. As a result, precursors proximal to the enzyme block accumulate and are shunted toward the formation of adrenal androgens. Affected individuals can present with a wide spectrum of clinical disease phenotypes resulting from the androgen excess. Mild enzyme deficits may be clinically unapparent, whereas complete enzyme absence can result in severe adrenal insufficiency with virilism and salt-wasting in infancy. Since the affected enzyme can be totally or partially impaired, the degree of enzyme deficiency determines the severity of the condition.

Adrenal Cortex Review The adrenal cortex is divided into three functionally distinct areas for hormone synthesis. The zona glomerulosa, fasciculata, and reticularis are each responsible for the production of specific endocrine products. These are mineralocorticoids (aldosterone), glucocorticoids (cortisol), and androgens, respectively. Hormone synthesis in the zona fasciculata and zona reticularis is regulated by the hypothalamic-pituitary axis. More specifically, the hypothalamus secretes CRH, which subsequently stimulates the production of ACTH from the anterior pituitary. ACTH then acts on the adrenal cortex to promote synthesis of cortisol and androgens. In contrast, synthesis in the zona glomerulosa is primarily regulated via the renin-angiotensin system. ACTH and CRH have minimal regulatory effects on the zona glomerulosa.

Steroid Hormone Synthesis Cortisol and aldosterone are steroid hormones synthesized from a common precursor molecule, cholesterol. The steroid hormone synthesis pathway is depicted in Figure 25-1. Many of the enzymes involved in cortisol and aldosterone synthesis are cytochrome P450 enzymes. Congenital adrenal hyperplasia is most commonly due to **21-hydroxylase deficiency,** accounting for more than 90% of cases of adrenal hyperplasia. Less commonly involved enzymes are **11β-hydroxylase** and **3β-hydroxysteroid dehydrogenase** (Table 25-1).

Clinical Presentation The hallmark of CAH is **inadequate production of glucocorticoids.** The "classical" form of CAH occurs when cortisol synthesis is extremely low or absent, with the deficiency manifesting as ambiguous genitalia at birth. In affected female infants, examination of the external genitalia will reveal a phallus-like structure (smaller than a penis, but larger than a clitoris), a single opening at the base corresponding to the urogenital sinus, and varying degrees of incomplete fusion of the labioscrotal folds. Males with 21-hydroxylase deficiency are generally not diagnosed immediately after birth because their genitalia will appear normal. Rather, these male infants will present at 1 to 4 weeks of age with symptoms resulting from severe salt wasting and deficient cortisol. These may include failure to thrive, recurrent vomiting, dehydration, and shock.

Milder, "non-classical" forms of the condition (late-onset 21- or 11β-hydroxylase deficiency) may not present until childhood or adolescence. In these instances, children will have precocious puberty in association with the laboratory abnormalities of hyponatremia and hyperkalemia. Premature closure of the epiphyseal growth plates results in short stature, even though these children grow at an accelerated rate when young. Often these children lack sufficient amounts of cortisol to mount an adequate stress response and are thus prone to frequent illnesses. Adult women with CAH may have associated signs and symptoms of androgen excess such as hirsutism, amenorrhea, acne, and infertility.

Genetics The defects causing congenital adrenal hyperplasia are autosomal-recessive disorders caused by abnormal-

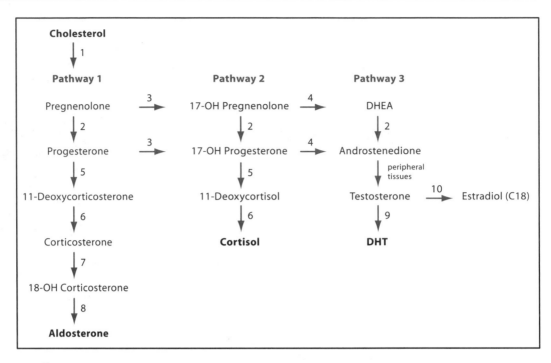

Key enzymes
  1 = Desmolase
  2 = 3β-hydroxysteroid dehydrogenase (3βHSD)
  3 = 17α-hydroxylase
  4 = C-17 Lyase
  5 = 21-hydroxylase
  6 = 11β-hydroxylase
  7 = 18-hydroxylase
  8 = 18-oxidase
  9 = 5α-reductase
  10 = Aromatase

Pathway 1 = Aldosterone synthesis (C21 Mineralocorticoids)
Pathway 2 = Cortisol synthesis (C21 Glucocorticoids)
Pathway 3 = Testosterone synthesis (C19 Androgens)

Figure 25-1 Pathways of steroid hormone production in the adrenal gland.

ities of the gene that codes for the enzyme involved. These abnormalities include insertions, deletions, missense/nonsense codons, and point mutations. Some of these defects result in severe dysfunction of the enzyme, while others result in only partial impairment. Because the condition is inherited in a recessive fashion, both genes must carry the

same mutation or deletion in order for the condition to be expressed. Carriers or heterozygotes that carry only one abnormal gene are asymptomatic.

Diagnosis   The diagnosis of CAH is suggested by clinical presentation and confirmed with laboratory evaluation to

Table 25-1 Congenital adrenal hyperplasia syndromes

Enzyme deficiency	Accumulated precursors	Missing hormones
21-hydroxylase	Progesterone, 17OH-progesterone	Cortisol, aldosterone
11β-hydroxylase	11-deoxycortisol, 11-deoxycortisosterone	Cortisol, aldosterone
3βHSD	DHEA	Cortisol
Desmolase	Cholesterol	Cortisol, aldosterone, testosterone
17α-hydroxylase	Pregnenolone, progesterone	Cortisol, testosterone

identify the deficient enzyme. For example, because 21-hydroxylase functions in both glucocorticoid and mineralocorticoid synthesis, patients may show signs of virilization and "salt wasting" such as hyponatremia, hypovolemia, hyperkalemia, and hypotension. Without 21-hydroxylase, there is increased production of progesterone, 17-OH-progesterone (17-OHP), and dehydroepiandrosterone (DHEA). Serum cortisol and aldosterone will be low or absent, while urinary metabolites of cortisol and aldosterone precursors (17-ketosteroids and pregnanetriol) will be increased. In addition, both plasma ACTH and renin levels will be increased due to the loss of negative feedback by cortisol and aldosterone. If the cause of CAH is 11β-hydrogenase deficiency, deoxycortisol accumulates. Deoxycortisol and its metabolites have mineralocorticoid properties and may cause pronounced HTN. An ACTH stimulation test can help identify the defective enzyme. Levels of adrenal hormone precursors are measured before and 30 minutes after 250 μg of synthetic ACTH is injected IV. The rise and ratio of the various precursors in response to ACTH aids in the identification of the defective enzyme.

Treatment Treatment of CAH involves glucocorticoid replacement and possible mineralocorticoid replacement to restore associated electrolyte abnormalities. Early recognition and treatment of CAH is important for severe enzyme deficiencies to prevent metabolic complications and irreversible growth patterns. In milder cases with few or no symptoms, the risks and benefits of long-term glucocorticoid therapy (i.e., iatrogenic Cushing's syndrome) should be balanced. Affected female infants may require surgical reconstruction to reverse the effects of virilization (Table 25-2).

Table 25-2 Steroid treatment: balance of risks and benefits for treatment of CAH

Insufficient cortisol	Excess cortisol
Hairiness	Increased appetite
Acne	Weight gain
Greasy skin	Muscle weakness
Irregular periods	Thin skin, easy bruising
Reduced fertility	High BP
Tiredness	Osteoporosis
Fatigue	Diabetes

Case Conclusion A karyotype analysis identifies the infant as a 46XX female. Laboratory studies confirm the diagnosis of CAH and are significant for elevated serum 17-OHP and DHEA, with excess urinary pregnanetriol excretion. Metabolic abnormalities include hyponatremia and hyperkalemia, with undetectable levels of plasma cortisol and aldosterone. The family is counseled regarding treatment options and surgical correction for their daughter's ambiguous genitalia.

Thumbnail: Congenital Adrenal Hyperplasia

21-hydroxylase deficiency
Accounts for 90% of cases of CAH
Accumulation of progesterone and 17-OHP

11β-hydroxylase deficiency
Accounts for fewer than 10% of cases of CAH
Accumulation of 11-deoxycorticosterone and 11-deoxycortisol

Signs and symptoms of CAH
Decreased or absent plasma cortisol and aldosterone
Androgen excess can result in virilism, hirsutism, and salt-wasting

Key Points

▶ Autosomal-recessive disorders resulting from the absence of enzymes necessary for cortisol and/or aldosterone synthesis.

▶ Symptoms and signs of androgen excess result from accumulation of testosterone precursors.

▶ Treatment includes glucocorticoid and/or mineralocorticoid replacement to correct electrolyte abnormalities.

Questions

1. A 14-year-old girl is brought in to see her pediatrician because her parents are concerned that her growth is stunted. Her parents state that she grew quite rapidly as a child, but has remained at the same height of 4 feet 8 inches for the past 3 years. Her mother and father are 5 feet 9 inches and 6 feet 4 inches, respectively. In addition, the girl has not reached menarche yet. On physical exam, the girl is mildly obese with a husky voice and some evidence of increased facial hair. Which of the following is mostly likely to be elevated in this patient?

   A. 21-hydroxylase
   B. 11β-hydroxylase
   C. DHEA
   D. Cortisol
   E. Aldosterone

2. A 1-month-old baby boy is brought in to see his pediatrician for his regularly scheduled well-child check. Despite an uncomplicated delivery and uneventful first 2 weeks at home, his mother states that the child has become increasingly fussy and is not feeding well. He often immediately vomits up most of what he has just taken in. On physical exam, the child appears dehydrated with poor skin turgor and muscle tone. The pediatrician admits the child to the hospital on the basis of dehydration and failure to thrive. Deficiencies in which of the following could account for this child's symptoms?

   A. Testosterone
   B. Aldosterone
   C. Growth hormone
   D. Epinephrine
   E. DHEA

HPI: AC is a 38-year-old gravida 5 para 4 woman who presents to the emergency department (ED) with a 2-day history of nausea, vomiting, diarrhea, dizziness, and fatigue. Ten days earlier, AC delivered a viable male infant at term via normal spontaneous vaginal delivery. Immediately after the delivery, however, AC's uterus remained soft and boggy. Postpartum bleeding was treated with aggressive fundal massage and oxytocin. AC continued to hemorrhage despite these interventions and was taken to the operating room for uterine artery embolization. During the procedure, she received 2 units of packed RBCs and 3 units of fresh frozen plasma. The embolization finally stopped the bleeding. AC remained in the hospital for a total of 7 days until her electrolyte abnormalities and coagulopathy stabilized. She had been home for 3 days when she came to the ED.

PE: In the ED, AC appears dehydrated with significant orthostatic hypotension. AC states that she has been unable to breast-feed her baby because she has felt too weak and has not produced any milk. With a history of failure of lactation and significant postpartum hemorrhage, ED physicians express concern over the possibility of Sheehan's syndrome. She is admitted to the hospital for IV rehydration and further evaluation of her symptoms.

Thought Questions

- Describe the anatomy of the pituitary gland.
- What hormones are synthesized in the anterior pituitary? In the posterior pituitary?
- What is Sheehan's syndrome? How does it usually present?

Basic Science Review and Discussion

The pituitary gland is a structural and functional extension of the hypothalamus that secretes a variety of hormones. These hormones act on nonendocrine tissues and modulate the activity of other endocrine glands. Because the secretion of these hormones is directly controlled by the hypothalamus, the pituitary gland plays a central role in integrating the nervous and endocrine systems.

Pituitary Anatomy The pituitary gland (Figure 26-1) is located within a bony enclosure called the sella turcica. It lies immediately beneath the brain, hypothalamus, and optic chiasm, and is partially overlain by a reflection of the dura mater known as the diaphragma sella. The gland itself is divided into anterior and posterior divisions, based on their embryologic derivations. The anterior pituitary, which is composed of the **pars distalis, pars intermedia,** and **pars tuberalis,** is derived from Rathke's pouch (oral ectoderm). In contrast, the posterior pituitary (pars nervosa) and infundibular stem are derived from neural tissue.

The pars distalis portion of the anterior pituitary is responsible for the majority of pituitary hormone secretion. It has a unique blood supply in that the pars distalis lacks nutrient arteries. Instead, the pars distalis receives its nutritive blood supply through a **portal system** of capillaries that connects the hypothalamus to cells within the anterior pituitary. The portal system is also the link by which neurohormones synthesized by the tuberal nuclei of the hypothalamus [gonadotropin-releasing hormone (GnRH), CRH, TRH, and GHRH] reach the pars distalis. Without this vascular link, most of the cells within the pars distalis are unstimulated and will atrophy. Levels of neurohormones vital to the normal maintenance of pars distalis function must be high and are only present at these high levels within the portal system, not within the systemic circulation.

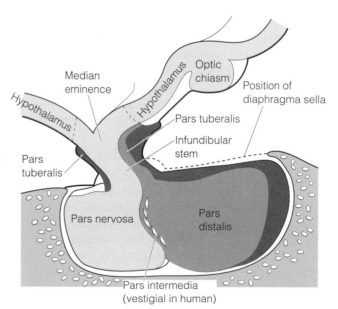

Figure 26-1 Diagram of the adult pituitary gland, mid-saggital view. The anterior pituitary is derived from oral ectoderm, while the posterior pituitary is neural tissue. (Image courtesy of Joel Schechter, PhD, Keck School of Medicine at the University of Southern California.)

Anterior Pituitary Cells and Their Products There are a variety of cell types within the pars distalis. The names of cells are related to the primary function of their hormonal secretions. **Acidophils** are cells whose hormonal secretory granules stain red with acidic stains. Acidophils are therefore somatotrophs that secrete GH, lactotrophs that secrete prolactin (PRL), and mammosomatotrophs that secrete both GH and PRL. **Basophils** are cells whose hormone secretory granules stain blue with basic stains. Basophils are therefore thyrotrophs that secrete TSH, gonadotrophs that secrete FSH and LH, and corticotrophs that secrete ACTH. With the exception of lactotrophs that are tonically inhibited by dopamine, the secretory cells of the pars distalis are stimulated to produce their hormone products via neurohormones from the hypothalamus. These neurohormones include TRH, GnRH, GHRH, and CRH.

The hormones of the anterior pituitary act on a wide variety of target organs. GH stimulates growth processes throughout the body and acts on long bones to stimulate bone growth. PRL released after pregnancy acts on the mammary glands to stimulate lactation. TSH causes the thyroid gland to synthesize thyroid hormone, while ACTH controls the activity of the adrenal cortex to release glucocorticoids. Finally, FSH and LH signal the testes and ovaries to synthesize both testosterone and estrogen.

Sheehan's Syndrome In normal pregnancy, the pituitary gland enlarges to roughly twice its normal size. As a result of the increased size and delicate vascular structure, the pituitary is especially vulnerable to infarction during this time. When ischemic necrosis of the pituitary gland occurs, it is known as **Sheehan's syndrome.** Sheehan's syndrome was first described in association with postpartum hemorrhage in 1939. Classically, the syndrome involves total destruction of the anterior pituitary with resultant clinical panhypopituitarism. Risk factors for pituitary infarction include diabetes, temporal arteritis, sickle-cell disease, atherosclerosis, eclampsia of pregnancy, and coagulopathy. The posterior pituitary is rarely affected because it is more resistant to ischemic damage.

The incidence of Sheehan's syndrome is about 1 per 10,000 deliveries. Clinical manifestations of hypopituitarism are usually not seen until 70% to 75% of the pituitary tissue is lost. In reality, the extent of tissue loss is variable, and partial or complete spontaneous recoveries can occur. Thus, Sheehan's syndrome can involve only selective defects of pituitary function. Panhypopituitarism is most often associated with postpartum hemorrhage, but other causes

include disseminated intravascular coagulation (DIC), sickle-cell anemia, cavernous sinus thrombosis, giant cell arteritis, and trauma to the pituitary. The loss of hormone secretion from the pituitary follows a specific sequence. Namely, FSH and LH are usually lost first, followed by GH, TSH, ACTH, and PRL.

Clinical Presentation Patients with Sheehan's syndrome present with a variety of signs and symptoms related to the loss of normal endocrine function. The most common presentation is failure to lactate, usually within the first 7 days postpartum. Hypothyroidism from lack of TSH causes fatigue, slow speech, cold intolerance, dry skin, and constipation. Low ACTH results in adrenal insufficiency and is responsible for hypotension, poor stress and infection tolerance, hypoglycemia, nausea, and vomiting from the absence of both cortisol and aldosterone. Loss of sexual function occurs as a result of the lack of gonadotropins. Hypogonadism can also present as amenorrhea in women and loss of muscle mass in men. GH deficiency causes fatigue, loss of bone and muscle, and dyslipidemia. Rarely, diabetes insipidus can occur secondary to the loss of antidiuretic hormone (ADH) if the posterior pituitary is infarcted as well.

Diagnosis Diagnosis of panhypopituitarism is usually quite obvious, but partial deficiencies are often difficult to elicit. A woman with panhypopituitarism will have low levels of pituitary hormones (LH, FSH, PRL, ACTH, TRH, GH) as well as target hormones (aldosterone, cortisol, testosterone, estrogen, thyroid hormone). Thus, patients with hypothyroidism caused by Sheehan's syndrome will have low T_3 and T_4 levels with normal or inappropriately low TSH levels. Stimulation tests (insulin tolerance test) or pituitary testing for measurement of pituitary hormone secretion following administration of hypothalamic releasing hormones are often required for confirmation of the diagnosis.

Treatment Treatment for panhypopituitarism is with appropriate replacement of target hormones as needed. This may include estrogen/testosterone, thyroid hormone, and glucocorticoids. In patients with both hypothyroidism and adrenal insufficiency, glucocorticoids are replaced first because T_4 therapy can exacerbate glucocorticoid deficiency and theoretically induce an adrenal crisis. Replacement of growth hormone is necessary in children with hypopituitarism to ensure normal growth and development, but is controversial in adults because its replacement has not proved to be beneficial. Prognosis is good if the pituitary deficiencies are detected and treated early.

Case Conclusion Serum measurements of AC's hormone levels reveal low T_3 and T_4 with an undetectable TSH level. In addition, AC also undergoes an insulin tolerance test to measure pituitary function. The insulin tolerance test induces transient hypoglycemia, which in patients with a normal pituitary gland stimulates ACTH and subsequent cortisol release. Normal stimulated levels of cortisol range in the hundreds, but AC's cortisol level remains less than 10 µg/mL. She is diagnosed with pituitary failure caused by Sheehan's syndrome and is immediately started on hydrocortisone, mineralocorticoid, levothyroxine, and estrogen/progesterone replacement.

Thumbnail: Panhypopituitarism (Sheehan's Syndrome)

Pars distalis

Acidophils:

Somatotrophs: GH stimulates growth processes throughout the body.

Lactotrophs: PRL stimulates "prepared" mammary gland to secrete milk and causes smooth muscle contraction of the uterus.

Mammosomatotrophs: GH and PRL.

Basophils:

Thyrotrophs: TSH stimulates the thyroid gland to produce thyroid hormone.

Gonadotrophs: FSH and LH are required for normal maturation of germ cells and production of sex hormones in the ovary and testes.

Corticotrophs: ACTH controls the activity of the adrenal cortex, especially glucocorticoids.

Key Points

▶ Ischemic necrosis of the anterior pituitary gland, classically following postpartum hemorrhage.

▶ Clinical presentation: failure of lactation, hypothyroidism, loss of sexual function, nausea/vomiting, hypotension, fatigue.

▶ Order of pituitary loss of function: FSH and LH, GH, TSH, ACTH, and PRL.

▶ Treatment: replacement of necessary hormones.

Questions

1. A 24-year-old G2P2 woman gives birth to a viable female infant weighing 3832 g. Her delivery was complicated by 600 mL of postpartum hemorrhage secondary to uterine atony. She presents to the ED complaining of nonspecific signs of fatigue, nausea, and vomiting. She appears pale and mucous membranes are dry. She has a history of gestational DM and is not currently on insulin therapy. Which of the following signs and symptoms would she not be expected to have?

   A. Cold intolerance
   B. Failure of lactation
   C. Stress intolerance
   D. Increased skin pigmentation
   E. Sparse axillary and pubic hair

2. An 8-year-old boy complains of frequent headaches, constipation, and fluctuating loss of vision while at school. His parents state that the boy has been unusually fatigued and lethargic. Physical exam reveals a pale-skinned, short-statured boy at the 20th percentile for height and 75th percentile for weight. Visual field testing reveals a bitemporal hemianopsia. CT scan of the head reveals an enlarged sella turcica. What is this boy's most likely diagnosis?

   A. Craniopharyngioma
   B. Dwarfism
   C. Prolactinoma
   D. Cushing's disease
   E. Addison's disease

HPI: RB is a 23-year-old Latino man who is brought to the ER by paramedics after being involved in an automobile versus motorcycle accident. RB was thrown off his motorcycle, landing about 10 feet away with his helmet cracked, but still in place.

PE: On arrival to the ER, he appears stuporous, but arousable. RB is intubated secondary to signs of agonal breathing. Following intubation, vital signs are stable. Primary survey reveals a dislocated right shoulder joint and numerous lacerations on his face and right upper extremity. There is no evidence of acute blood loss; mucous membranes are pink and moist. Radiologic evaluations, including those of the cervical spine, chest, and pelvis, are noncontributory. Head CT is significant for cerebral edema with slight narrowing of the ventricles.

Labs: Laboratory tests are significant for hyponatremia with sodium at 124 mEq/L.

Thought Questions

- What is the function of ADH? Where is it produced and what regulates its secretion?

- What are the clinical consequences of ADH excess? ADH deficiency?

- What are common causes of the syndrome of inappropriate ADH (SIADH)? How is it treated?

- What is the difference between central diabetes insipidus (CDI) and nephrogenic diabetes insipidus (NDI)?

Basic Science Review and Discussion

Pituitary Anatomy   The pituitary gland sits within a bony enclosure called the sella turcica, immediately beneath the brain, hypothalamus, and the optic chiasm. It is functionally and embryologically divided into two distinct regions: the anterior pituitary and the posterior pituitary. While the anterior pituitary is derived from oral ectoderm and synthesizes multiple tropic hormones, the posterior pituitary gland is derived from neural tissue and is responsible for the production of ADH (or vasopressin) and oxytocin.

This posterior pituitary is also known as the **pars nervosa** and is part of the hypothalamo-neurohypophyseal system (Figure 27-1). That is, hormones are synthesized by neurons in the tuberal nuclei of the hypothalamus and transported down axons for storage in the posterior pituitary. Prior to their release, ADH and oxytocin are stored within neurohormonal secretory granules with their respective neurophysins and are released by exocytosis at the neuroendocrine synapse. The hormones then diffuse through the tissue fluid in the perivascular space to adjacent capillaries where they enter the circulation; from there, they are distributed to target organs. The tuberal nuclei in the hypothalamus are known as the **supraoptic nucleus (SON)** and the **paraventricular nucleus (PVN)**. The SON primarily produces ADH,

while the PVN primarily produces oxytocin. ADH acts on the kidney to preserve water content, while oxytocin causes contraction of the smooth muscle of the uterus and the myoepithelial cells of the mammary gland.

Syndrome of Inappropriate Antidiuretic Hormone Secretion
Water balance in the body is maintained by two primary mechanisms: thirst and ADH secretion. These two mechanisms act to maintain normal plasma osmolality in the range of 280 to 290 mOsm/kg. ADH acts on the collecting tubules in the kidneys to increase water reabsorption. It is released in response to decreased blood volume (hemorrhage) or an increase in serum osmolality. In addition, stress can also promote ADH secretion. While serum osmolality is a more sensitive stimulator of ADH release, acute blood loss is a more powerful stimulator of ADH secretion. Because baroreceptors are less sensitive than osmoreceptors, a 5% to 10% decrease in blood volume must occur before ADH is released. Thirst is stimulated at 290 mOsm/kg, while ADH is released with increases in plasma osmolality of less than 1%. Severe hypovolemia, however, can cause exponential increases in ADH, magnitudes greater than that stimulated by elevated plasma osmolality.

ADH acts on the kidney to preserve water content. It does this through a G protein adenylate cyclase coupling system that increases cyclic AMP and activates protein kinase A. This system leads to the insertion of the aquaporin protein into the tubule cell plasma membrane. Aquaporin serves as a channel that allows water to enter the cell from the lumen. Without aquaporin, free water is lost in the urine.

SIADH is characterized by abnormal secretion of excess ADH despite euvolemia and serum hypo-osmolality. SIADH causes a clinical state of *euvolemic hyponatremia* (serum sodium <135 mEq/L) because the retention of free water dilutes serum sodium. Urine is highly concentrated in cases of SIADH because of the inability to transport free water into the collecting tubules. There is no evidence of edema, ascites, or CHF due to volume overload because most of the

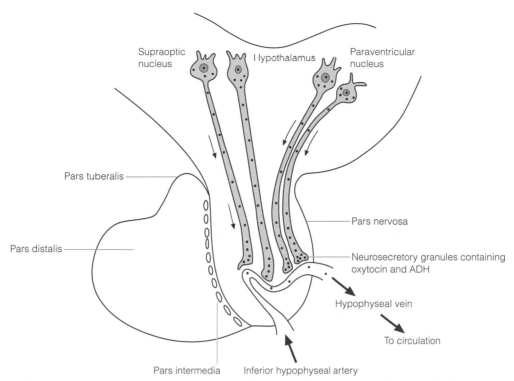

Figure 27-1 Diagram of the neurosecretory neurons in the supraoptic and paraventricular nuclei of the hypothalamus. Axons from these neurons extend into the pars nervosa of the pituitary. ADH and oxytocin are released from the neurosecretory granules into the blood vessels of the pars nervosa for release into the circulatory system.

excess body water accumulates intracellularly, not within the intravascular space. The intracellular edema is clinically significant because of the potential to alter cell functions, the CNS being most sensitive to these changes.

The signs and symptoms of SIADH are usually not clinically apparent unless serum sodium is less than 120 mEq/L. The earliest symptoms include anorexia, nausea, and vomiting. CNS changes may be evident, including headache, irritability, and disorientation. As the serum sodium concentration falls below 110 mEq/L, more serious CNS alterations resulting from brain edema will be present. These include delirium, psychosis, ataxia, seizures, and/or coma. On physical exam, papilledema, hypoactive reflexes, and focal neurologic signs may be present as well.

There are numerous causes of SIADH, including CNS disorders, malignancy, pulmonary disease, endocrine disorders, and drugs. Stress-inducing states such as extreme nausea, pain, or surgery can also trigger excess ADH production from the hypothalamus. CNS disorders range from head trauma, as in this patient, to stroke and brain tumor. Malignancies can cause SIADH through ectopic ADH production from the tumor itself; the most common association is with small cell carcinoma of the lung. Other lung diseases such as

pneumonia, tuberculosis, and COPD are also possible causes of SIADH. A multitude of drugs have been associated with the syndrome, the most common of which are the nonsteroidal anti-inflammatory drugs (NSAIDs). Narcotics, antidepressants, diuretics, oral hypoglycemics, and several antibiotics have also been implicated in the condition. It is important to examine all of these possible causes of SIADH in order to identify and correct the underlying pathology.

SIADH usually goes unrecognized until patients become symptomatic and laboratory studies reveal significant hyponatremia. Serum osmolality will be low (<280 mOsm/kg) while urine osmolality will be inappropriately high (>100 mOsm/L). The primary treatment for mildly symptomatic hyponatremia is water restriction until the cause of the condition can be identified and corrected. Demeclocycline may be given to patients who are not responsive to water restriction. Severe hyponatremia (serum sodium < 110 mEq/L) can be treated with isotonic or hypertonic saline to prevent seizures or coma. Hyponatremia must be corrected slowly to avoid the complication of central pontine myelinosis (CPM) from overly rapid correction. In all instances, serum and urine electrolytes should be followed appropriately and patients should be monitored frequently for acute neurologic changes.

Diabetes Insipidus While an excess of ADH can be hazardous because of complications from hyponatremia, an absence or unresponsiveness to ADH is life threatening due to dehydration and hypernatremia. **CDI** differs from **NDI** in that CDI is characterized by the absence of ADH production, while NDI is characterized by unresponsiveness to ADH in the collecting tubules of the kidney. Whether there is no ADH or there is no response to ADH, the net effect of these defects is excessive amounts of dilute urine, resulting in hypernatremia and dehydration.

Both central and nephrogenic forms of diabetes insipidus (DI) can occur as sporadic or inherited conditions. CDI most commonly occurs secondary to tumors, infiltrative lesions, or neurosurgical destruction of the posterior pituitary or hypothalamus. Less commonly, CDI may be idiopathic or inherited as either an autosomal dominant or an autosomal recessive trait. NDI occurs as an X-linked recessive hereditary disease or as a secondary result of a defect within the kidney itself that makes the nephrons insensitive to ADH. The defect may be related to either defective or absent ADH receptors on the cortical collecting ducts or abnormal aquaporin protein. Renal diseases such as polycystic kidney disease, sickle-cell nephropathy, and pyelonephritis can cause ADH insensitivity, as well as nephrotoxic drugs like the aminoglycosides, lithium, and demeclocycline.

The onset of symptoms in DI can be either abrupt or insidious in patients of any age. Patients will complain of increased thirst, drinking large amounts of fluids, and urinating frequently. Enormous quantities of fluid may be ingested and large volumes of very dilute urine are excreted. If fluid intake is not sufficient enough to maintain plasma volume, hyperosmolar dehydration, hypernatremia,

hyperchloremia, and prerenal azotemia may ensue. Possible complications of this extremely dehydrated state include seizures and death from hypovolemic shock. Young children are especially at risk for failure to thrive, dehydration, and mental retardation from CNS damage because they are not able to communicate increased thirst or voluntarily increase their water intake.

The diagnosis of DI can be confirmed by measuring the urine specific gravity in the first morning urine. Dilute urine associated with high serum sodium and high plasma osmolality establishes the diagnosis. The serum sodium may be as high as 170 mEq/L (normal 140 mEq/L) while the serum osmolality is greater than 300 mOsm/kg (normal 280–290 mOsm/kg). Central and nephrogenic forms of diabetes insipidus are further distinguished based on the water deprivation test. In this test, the response to exogenously administered desmopressin (DDAVP, a synthetic analogue of vasopressin) in a patient with DI following water deprivation is observed. Patients with CDI will be able to appropriately concentrate their urine with the addition of DDAVP, while patients with NDI will continue to produce large amounts of dilute urine because their nephrons are still unable to respond.

For CDI, the treatment of choice is DDAVP to replace the missing endogenous ADH. This approach is not helpful for NDI because the kidney cannot respond to endogenous or exogenous ADH. These patients should be treated with thiazide diuretics or amiloride. These medications impair salt absorption along the distal tubule, reducing free water loss to the collecting system and thereby decreasing urine volume and increasing urine concentration. Adequate fluid intake and close observation for signs of dehydration are essential for long-term management of all DI.

Case Conclusion RB is admitted to the intensive care unit (ICU) for frequent monitoring and stabilization of his injuries. His water intake is limited as physicians evaluate his cerebral edema and neurologic deficits. RB is weaned off the ventilator by day 3 and his condition slowly improves over the next few days. By hospital day 6 he is alert and awake, though amnesic to the events of his accident. His hyponatremia normalizes to 142 mEq/L and he is transferred to the floor for further recovery.

Thumbnail: SIADH/Diabetes Insipidus

SIADH

Defect: Excess ADH production

Causes: CNS disorders (head trauma, stroke, brain tumor, meningitis, subarachnoid hemorrhage), malignancy (lung, brain, pancreas, prostate, ovary), pulmonary disease (TB, pneumonia, empyema), endocrine disorders (hypothyroidism, glucocorticoid deficiency), drugs (NSAIDs, antidepressants, diuretics)

Laboratory abnormalities: euvolemic hyponatremia (serum sodium < 135 mEq/L), hypotonicity (plasma osmolality <280 mOsm/kg water), inappropriately concentrated urine (>100 mOsm/kg water), elevated urine sodium concentration (>20 mEq/L)

Treatment: water restriction, followed by treatment of the underlying condition

CDI

Defect: deficiency of ADH production

Cause: most commonly due to destruction of PVN, SON, or posterior pituitary by tumor, pressure, or surgical ablation

Treatment: DDAVP

NDI

Defect: renal tubule unresponsiveness to ADH

Cause: due to defective/absent ADH receptors on the cortical collecting duct or defective/absent aquaporin protein

Treatment: thiazide diuretics, amiloride

Key Points

▸ ADH increases water reabsorption, released in response to severe hemorrhage, increased serum osmolality, or stress.

▸ SIADH results in euvolemic hyponatremia; treat with water restriction.

▸ Symptoms and signs of CDI and NDI include copious amounts of dilute urine, hypernatremia, and dehydration.

▸ Treat CDI with DDAVP to replace endogenous ADH.

▸ NDI will not respond to DDAVP.

Questions

1. A previously healthy 3-day-old boy is brought in to see his pediatrician for a history of irritability and failure to thrive. His mother states that his diapers are constantly soaking wet, forcing her to change them some 20 times a day. The baby is also breast-feeding poorly and when he cries, no tears are visible. On physical exam, the baby is limp with tachycardia. His mucous membranes are pale and dry. Of note, his diaper is wet and bulging. Which of the following is a potential complication of this condition?

   A. CHF
   B. Central pontine myelinosis
   C. Diarrhea
   D. Mental retardation
   E. Psychosis

2. A 62-year-old man with a 40-pack per year history of smoking has just been diagnosed with carcinoma of the lung. Lung cancers are often associated with paraneoplastic conditions. Which of the following types of cancer is not correctly associated with the ectopic hormone it produces?

   A. Squamous cell carcinoma and PTH-related peptide
   B. Squamous cell carcinoma and ADH
   C. Renal cell carcinoma and erythropoietin
   D. Small cell lung carcinoma and ACTH
   E. Breast carcinoma and PTH-related peptide

HPI: DK is a 33-year-old white man who presents for the first time with a long history of "heartburn" not relieved by over-the-counter medications. DK states that the heartburn occurs intermittently, is not related to meals, and is often associated with abdominal pain and diarrhea. He is concerned that he might be developing an ulcer because "ulcers tend to run in his family."

PE: On physical exam, DK is an anxious-appearing man who appears older than his stated age. His facial features appear unusually coarse, including a prominent brow and jawbone. Physical exam is significant for a palpable liver edge, 4 cm below the costal margin. DK denies smoking or excessive alcohol use.

Labs: Serum laboratory evaluation reveals elevated serum Ca^{2+} levels, but DK denies any history of kidney stones or bone pain. Other routine labs are noncontributory, and the remainder of the physical exam is within normal limits.

Thought Questions

- What endocrine abnormalities could account for DK's signs and symptoms? What is his most likely diagnosis?

- How are the MEN syndromes inherited? What organs are affected in each syndrome?

- What are the common clinical manifestations of a patient with MEN I? MEN IIa? MEN IIb?

Basic Science Review and Discussion

The **multiple endocrine neoplasias** are inherited autosomal-dominant cancer syndromes. They are categorized into MEN I and MEN II. MEN II is further subdivided into MEN IIa and MEN IIb. (Note: Some texts refer to MEN I, IIa, and IIb as MEN I, II, and III, respectively.)

MEN I involves neoplasia of the **p**arathyroid glands, **p**ancreatic islets, and **p**ituitary gland. A good mnemonic is the "**3 P's.**" MEN II syndromes both consist of medullary thyroid cancer and pheochromocytoma. Subtypes IIa and IIb differ in that IIa also has parathyroid involvement while IIb is associated with mucosal neuromas.

Genetics The MEN syndromes arise from germline mutations in either tumor suppressor genes or oncogenes. Recently, it was discovered that the mutation for MEN I occurs in a gene on chromosome 11 that codes for the protein menin. This gene is ubiquitously expressed in all cells and functions as a tumor suppressor. As a result, mutations within this gene cause loss of tumor suppressor function and uncontrolled cell cycle regulation. The gene responsible for MEN II syndromes is a proto-oncogene called *RET* on chromosome 10. In contrast to the *menin* gene of MEN I, *RET* is specifically expressed in cells derived from the neural crest. These include the C cells in the thyroid gland and the chromaffin cells of the adrenal medulla. As an oncogene, activation of *RET* leads to increased cell division and subsequent tumor formation.

MEN I The patient described in this case presents with multiple endocrine-related findings, including a history of peptic ulcer disease, asymptomatic hypercalcemia, and evidence of GH excess (coarse facial features, enlarged liver). In a young patient with multiple endocrine abnormalities, the diagnosis of a MEN syndrome should be considered. In this case, MEN I is most likely because of the associated pituitary symptoms, parathyroid-related hypercalcemia, and excessive acid secretion from a pancreatic islet gastrinoma. The history is also suggestive because the patient mentions a positive family history of chronic ulcer disease.

Primary hyperparathyroidism is present in up to 90% of patients with MEN I. In contrast to the single adenomas found in idiopathic primary hyperparathyroidism, the genetic condition usually involves diffuse hyperplasia or multiple adenomas in all four parathyroid glands. Asymptomatic hypercalcemia, as in this patient, is the most common manifestation; about 25% of patients have evidence of kidney stones. Pancreatic islet cell tumors occur in about 30% to 75% of affected patients. Islet cell tumors can arise from a variety of cell types within the islet; these tumors may secret insulin, gastrin, somatostatin, ACTH, vasoactive intestinal polypeptide (VIP), serotonin, or prostaglandin. Also known as **Zollinger-Ellison syndrome,** gastrinomas are the most common islet tumor and are associated with intractable and complicated peptic ulceration. Over half of all MEN I patients have peptic ulcer disease, and the ulcers are often multiple and atypical in location. Although Zollinger-Ellison syndrome can also occur sporadically, some 20% to 60% of patients who first present with this condition will prove to have MEN I.

Pituitary tumors associated with MEN I arise from a variety of cells within the anterior pituitary. Pituitary adenomas are found in 50% to 65% of MEN I cases. The most common form is a hypersecreting prolactinoma, but other common products include growth hormone that results in the signs and symptoms of acromegaly noted in DK. These include coarsening of facial features, deepening of the voice, and enlargement of internal organs (heart, spleen, liver, etc.). Like sporadic pituitary tumors, these neoplasms can cause visual disturbance, headache, and hypopituitarism if the surrounding normal tissue becomes compressed and is rendered nonfunctional.

MEN IIa MEN IIa consists of medullary cancer of the thyroid, pheochromocytoma, and parathyroid hyperplasia. Medullary cancer of the thyroid is the most consistent and most life-threatening feature of the syndrome, followed by pheochromocytoma. In contrast to sporadic cases of pheochromocytoma, the inherited form associated with the MEN syndromes is usually bilateral and presents with paroxysmal rather than sustained HTN.

MEN IIb Like MEN IIa, MEN IIb includes medullary cancer of the thyroid and pheochromocytoma. However, MEN IIb patients are distinguished by the presence of mucosal neuromas, which give these patients a characteristic appearance. All MEN IIb patients exhibit a marfanoid phenotype (slender body, long and thin extremities, abnormally lax ligaments), thick eyelids, and diffusely hypertrophied lips. The neuromas appear as small, shiny bumps on the lips, tongue, and buccal mucosa.

Diagnosis Diagnosis of the MEN syndromes depends on the presentation of symptoms and the organs involved. Almost any combination of tumors and symptom complexes described is possible, and involvement of all three conditions associated with each syndrome is not necessarily required for diagnosis. For example, only 40% of patients diagnosed with MEN I actually have the complete combination of parathyroid hyperplasia, pituitary adenoma, and a pancreatic islet tumor. Diagnosis can be confirmed with genetic screening consisting of restriction fragment length polymorphism DNA analysis. Tests for the diagnosis of specific endocrine abnormalities include a 24-hour urine collection for catecholamines identifying pheochromocytoma, serum calcium and PTH levels to detect hypercalcemia, and measurement of IGF-1 to confirm acromegaly. Zollinger-Ellison syndrome is the major cause of morbidity and mortality in MEN I, while mortality in MEN II is due to the aggressive nature of medullary thyroid carcinoma. Relatives of MEN patients should be screened annually with an accurate medical history and physical examination with pertinent laboratory tests to detect early manifestations of the condition.

Treatment Treatment of parathyroid and pituitary lesions is primarily surgical. Pancreatic islet cell tumor excision is more complex because the tumors are often small and multiple. While attempts to localize and remove the specific tumor should be made in all patients, symptomatic treatment for gastrinomas can be achieved with proton pump inhibitors and histamine-2 (H_2) blockers. Prophylactic thyroidectomy should be considered in identified gene carriers of MEN II to avoid morbidity and mortality. MEN II patients undergoing surgery for medullary thyroid cancer or hyperparathyroidism should have any associated pheochromocytoma removed first because of the risk of a hypertensive crisis during surgical resection. Prognosis for patients with MEN syndromes is good if the tumors are identified and removed early in the course of the disease process.

Case Conclusion DK is diagnosed with MEN I after further investigation confirms elevated serum IGF-1 and basal gastrin levels in association with his asymptomatic hypercalcemia. Head CT scan is significant for an enlarged sella turcica, indicative of a pituitary neoplasm. He is started on a trial of omeprazole for relief of his peptic ulcer disease symptoms while awaiting surgical excision of his pituitary and parathyroid neoplasms.

Thumbnail: MEN Syndromes

MEN I—"the 3 P's":
Parathyroid hyperplasia
Pituitary adenoma
Pancreatic islet cell tumors

MEN IIa
Medullary thyroid carcinoma
Pheochromocytoma
Parathyroid hyperplasia

MEN IIb
Medullary thyroid carcinoma
Pheochromocytoma
Mucosal neuromas

Key Points

▶ All syndromes are autosomal dominant.

▶ MEN I is characterized by a germline mutation in the menin gene and a tumor suppressor gene on chromosome 11. *Menin* is normally expressed in all cells. Mutations in tumor suppressor genes cause cancer through loss of function and cell cycle regulation.

▶ MEN II is characterized by a germline mutation in the *RET* proto-oncogene, which is expressed in neural crest-derived cells. Mutations in oncogenes cause cancer through activation of the oncogene, stimulating uncontrolled cell division.

Questions

1. A 23-year-old African-American woman is advised to undergo genetic screening because her mother was recently diagnosed with a MEN syndrome. Her mother's medical history includes chronic headaches, DM, asthma, multiple kidney stones, and HTN. Screening tests to identify her mother's specific type of MEN syndrome should include:

   A. *RET* germline mutation evaluation
   B. *Menin* germline mutation evaluation
   C. Serum Ca and intact PTH measurement
   D. 24-hour urinary free catecholamines
   E. Basal and stimulated plasma calcitonin

2. An 18-year-old male college student complains of numerous episodes of headache, sweating, palpitations, and tachycardia lasting about 60 minutes each while in class. A visit to the student health center during one of these episodes reveals a BP of 200/120 mm Hg; 24-hour urinary catecholamine secretion is greater than 200 μg. The patient is tall and slender with exceptionally long fingers and toes. For which of the following conditions does this patient have the highest risk?

   A. Peptic ulcer disease
   B. Hyperthyroidism
   C. Osteoporosis
   D. Galactorrhea
   E. Thyroid carcinoma

HPI: TM is a 61-year-old white man who complains of increasing fatigue and decreased libido for the past 2 years. He states that his marriage has been strained because he has had problems with impotence in the past and has since lost interest in being intimate with his wife. Recently, he has noticed that he tends to urinate more frequently, but reasons that he is often thirsty and drinks a lot of water. TM explains that as he gets older, his body "just isn't like it used to be anymore." He used to enjoy jogging on a daily basis, but is now limited by fatigue and joint pain in his knees. TM admits to drinking about a 6-pack of beer every week and smoking half a pack of cigarettes per day for the past 20 years.

PE: Physical exam reveals a tanned-skin male who appears older than his stated age. Abdominal exam reveals mild nontender hepatomegaly. Musculoskeletal exam shows decreased range of motion of the bilateral wrists and knees. The remainder of the physical exam is noncontributory.

Labs: Relevant laboratory tests are sent for the workup of fatigue and possible DM.

Thought Questions

- What hereditary metabolic condition could explain TM's symptoms and physical exam findings?

- What organs are affected in hemochromatosis? In Wilson's disease?

- What are the chronic complications of hemochromatosis? Of Wilson's disease?

Basic Science Review and Discussion

Iron Metabolism The iron content of a healthy adult male is roughly 4 g, with 2.5 g in the red cell mass (1 g of Hb contains 3.4 mg of iron). In women, iron content is slightly lower because of smaller body size, lower red cell mass, and depletion of iron reserves through the menstrual cycle. Iron is stored in the body as both water-soluble **ferritin** and water-insoluble **hemosiderin.** Iron derived from the destruction of erythrocytes is recycled through the cells of the reticuloendothelial (RE) system. From the RE system, iron re-enters the circulation pool bound to the carrier molecule **transferrin.** Each transferrin molecule can bind two iron ions and transports the iron through the circulation for re-incorporation into heme or other proteins. The serum ferritin concentration indirectly reflects the size of the iron stores, and increases rapidly as transferrin becomes saturated.

Iron homeostasis in the body is regulated by a combination of absorption and excretion mechanisms. About 1 to 2 mg per day of iron is absorbed from the diet to maintain a constant iron balance within the body. Dietary iron is normally absorbed in the GI tract as ferrous ion (Fe^{2+}), but must be converted to the ferric form (Fe^{3+}) for binding to transferrin. Iron is most efficiently absorbed in the duodenum. At the same time, iron is lost through secretions from the gut, desquamation from the skin, blood loss (menstruation), and in the feces and urine. Average iron loss in a 70 kg male is about 1 mg per day. Women tend to lose more iron on average because of their regular menstrual cycles. Iron requirements and subsequent excretion are also increased during pregnancy.

Hemochromatosis **Hereditary hemochromatosis** is an autosomal recessive disease that results in the abnormal accumulation of iron within multiple organs of the body. It is the most common autosomal recessive genetic order and affects about 1 in 300 whites of Northern European descent. African Americans, Asian Americans, and other minorities are rarely affected. Secondary hemochromatosis can arise from chronic transfusion therapy, as in patients with thalassemia.

The primary defect in hereditary hemochromatosis consists of a mutation in the *HFE* gene on chromosome 6. Specifically, the mutation substitutes tyrosine for cysteine at position 282 (C282Y mutation) and results in impaired transferrin-mediated uptake of iron from the circulation and increased iron absorption from the intestine. Iron absorption continues despite elevation of body stores, eventually resulting in iron toxicity. Excess iron is hazardous because it produces free radical formation and can result in damage to cell membranes and DNA cleavage. The excess iron deposits in the liver, pancreas, heart, adrenal glands, testes, pituitary, joints, kidneys, and skin. Iron overload can then lead to hepatic, pancreatic, and cardiac insufficiency as well as hypogonadism from the loss of LH and FSH secretion from the pituitary.

Hemochromatosis is a chronic disease that usually does not manifest until after the fifth decade, at which point the symptoms of iron overload and organ malfunction secondary to iron deposition become clinically apparent. Early symptoms of hemochromatosis include severe fatigue, impotence in men, and arthralgia. Later, skin hyperpigmentation (bronzing) and DM can occur as a result of iron deposits combining with melanin in the skin and progressive accumulation of iron in the pancreas. The iron accumulation destroys beta cells within the pancreas and leads to insufficient insulin production. This combination of skin hyperpigmentation and insulin deficiency is classically known as "bronze diabetes."

A late finding in hereditary hemochromatosis is the presence of micronodular liver cirrhosis secondary to progressive iron deposition in the liver parenchyma. This tissue damage may lead to hepatocellular carcinoma years later and is the most common cause of death in patients with hereditary hemochromatosis.

Most patients with hemochromatosis are asymptomatic and are diagnosed when elevated serum iron levels are noted on a routine chemistry screening panel. Often patients will also have elevated liver enzymes. While elevated serum iron level and liver enzymes are not diagnostic, an elevated fasting transferrin saturation of greater than 60% in men and 50% in women is definitively diagnostic. Serum ferritin levels higher than 200 μg/L in premenopausal women and 300 μg/L in men are also indicative of hemochromatosis. However, ferritin levels are less sensitive than transferrin saturation as a screening test for hemochromatosis. Genetic screening in all first-degree relatives of patients with hemochromatosis is indicated to identify patients at risk for future irreversible organ damage.

Treatment for hemochromatosis consists of weekly phlebotomy to remove excess iron from the body and maintain normal iron stores. A normal life span can be expected if iron reduction is initiated before the development of cirrhosis and liver carcinoma, the most serious complications of the disease. Dietary intake of iron-rich foods (red meat, alcohol, raw shellfish, etc.) should be limited. Medical therapy with the iron-chelating agent **deferoxamine** is possible in patients who cannot tolerate phlebotomies. However, chelation therapy is time consuming, painful, and not nearly as effective as phlebotomy.

Copper Metabolism Copper is an essential trace element, serving as a cofactor for numerous systemic enzymes. In this capacity, it is necessary for bone formation, absorption and utilization of iron, hormone production, and erythropoiesis. The highest concentration of copper is found in the kidney and liver, followed by the brain, heart, and bone in decreasing order. All the fluids of the body contain copper complexes; total serum levels normally range from 1.1 to 1.5 μg/mL, depending on age and health condition. About 95% of the copper in the plasma is bound to the binding protein **ceruloplasmin**. The other 5% is found in association with plasma albumin and amino acids.

Dietary intake of copper is usually about 1.5 to 2.5 mg copper per day. Copper is primarily absorbed in the acidic environment of the stomach and upper intestine. The main excretory route for copper is through bile.

Wilson's Disease Like hemochromatosis, Wilson's disease is an autosomal-recessive inherited disorder of mineral toxicity. In contrast to the iron overload of hemochromatosis,

Wilson's disease is characterized by copper overload, with deposits in the liver, brain, cornea, and kidney.

The genetic defect in Wilson's disease is caused by a variety of different mutations on chromosome 13 that result in loss of ability to export copper from liver into the bile and to incorporate copper into ceruloplasmin, the copper-carrying protein. Without a mechanism for copper removal from the liver, copper leaks into the plasma and collects in extrahepatic tissues. Wilson's disease is also known as **hepatolenticular degeneration** because of the propensity for copper to accumulate in the liver and basal ganglia.

In contrast to patients with hemochromatosis who do not present clinically until after age 50, patients with Wilson's disease are usually symptomatic before age 30. Liver disease (hepatitis) is the most common initial presentation in children, while adults tend to present with neuropsychiatric symptoms. The pathognomonic finding in Wilson's disease is the presence of a brownish or gray-green **Kayser-Fleischer ring** in the cornea visible on slit-lamp examination. Kayser-Fleischer rings result from the deposition of copper within Descemet's membrane of the cornea. They are almost always present by the time neuropsychiatric symptoms become evident.

Numerous physical findings involving multiple organ systems can be present with Wilson's disease. Neurologic signs include parkinsonian symptoms (bradykinesia, resting tremor, rigidity), dementia, dysarthria, dystonia, asterixis, and abnormal eye movements. Psychiatric symptoms include personality changes, psychosis, mania, depression, or even schizophrenia. Skeletal abnormalities can also occur and range from osteoporosis to osteoarthritis. Cirrhosis in Wilson's disease may be micronodular or macronodular. Like hemochromatosis, a serious complication of Wilson's disease is the increased risk for hepatocellular carcinoma following hepatitis and cirrhosis.

Diagnosis of Wilson's disease involves a high index of suspicion followed by confirmation with laboratory abnormalities. The diagnosis should be considered in any young patient who presents with hepatitis, hepatosplenomegaly, portal HTN, and neurologic or psychiatric abnormalities. Laboratory findings consistent with Wilson's disease include low serum ceruloplasmin levels (<20 μg/dL), increased urinary copper excretion (>100 μg/24 hours), and elevated hepatic copper concentration (>250 μg/g of dry liver) found on liver biopsy. CT or MRI imaging studies of the brain may demonstrate signal abnormalities in the basal ganglia, but are not required for diagnosis.

Early diagnosis and treatment of Wilson's disease is critical, because it is fatal if left untreated. Treatment of choice is the chelating agent **penicillamine** to facilitate urinary excretion of chelated copper. Treatment should be continued indefinitely and family members should be screened with serum ceruloplasmin, liver function tests, and slit-lamp examination.

Case Conclusion   TM's laboratory evaluation reveals mildly elevated liver enzymes [aspartate transaminase (AST), alkaline phosphatase] in association with an elevated plasma iron level. Serum glucose is also elevated at 300 mg/dL. Subsequent transferrin and ferritin studies show a transferrin saturation of 65% and serum ferritin levels of 350 μg/L. TM is diagnosed with hemochromatosis and subsequently placed on a biweekly phlebotomy schedule. He is started on insulin therapy for DM secondary to pancreatic insufficiency. In addition, TM's brother and sister are recommended to undergo *HFE* mutation testing.

Thumbnail: Hemochromatosis/Wilson's Disease

Hemochromatosis

Genetics: autosomal recessive

Defect: iron overabsorption

Presentation: onset after age 50 with fatigue, impotence, joint pain

Organs affected: liver, pancreas, heart, adrenals, testes, pituitary, joints, skin, kidneys

Also known as: "bronze diabetes"

Laboratory abnormalities: high transferrin saturation, high serum ferritin

Treatment: weekly phlebotomy, deferoxamine

Wilson's disease

Genetics: autosomal recessive

Defect: abnormal copper transport and excretion

Presentation: onset before age 30 with hepatitis, neuropsychiatric symptoms, Kayser-Fleischer rings

Organs affected: liver, basal ganglia, cornea, kidney

Also known as: "hepatolenticular degeneration"

Laboratory abnormalities: low serum ceruloplasmin, high urinary copper excretion

Pathognomonic finding: Kayser-Fleischer ring

Treatment: penicillamine

Key Points

▶ Autosomal recessive inherited disorders of mineral toxicity.

▶ Iron carrying protein is transferrin, copper-carrying protein is ceruloplasmin.

▶ Hemochromatosis results in micronodular liver cirrhosis leading to hepatocellular carcinoma.

▶ Wilson's disease results in liver cirrhosis and neurologic disorders.

Questions

1. A 23-year-old man complains of new-onset right hand tremor for the past 3 weeks. The tremor occurs at rest and is also associated with unsteady gait and poor coordination. The patient has a history of asymptomatic elevated liver enzymes in the past (ALT > AST). Which of the following is not consistent with this patient's most likely diagnosis?

   A. Autosomal recessive
   B. Treatment with penicillamine
   C. Treatment with deferoxamine
   D. Kayser-Fleischer rings
   E. Increased risk of hepatocellular carcinoma

2. A 55-year-old woman visits her primary care physician because she is concerned about the possibility of hemochromatosis. Her older brother has recently been diagnosed with the disease. The initial test of choice for diagnosis of hemochromatosis is:

   A. Serum transferrin saturation
   B. Serum iron level
   C. Serum ferritin level
   D. 24-hour urine iron level
   E. Liver biopsy

Case 15

1. D
2. B

Case 16

1. C
2. B
3. D

Case 17

1. C
2. E

Case 18

1. B
2. D

Case 19

1. B
2. E

Case 20

1. B
2. A

Case 21

1. A
2. E

Case 22

1. E
2. D

Case 23

1. A
2. E

Case 24

1. B
2. C

Case 25

1. C
2. B

Case 26

1. D
2. A

Case 27

1. D
2. B

Case 28

1. B
2. E

Case 29

1. C
2. A

Part III

Reproduction

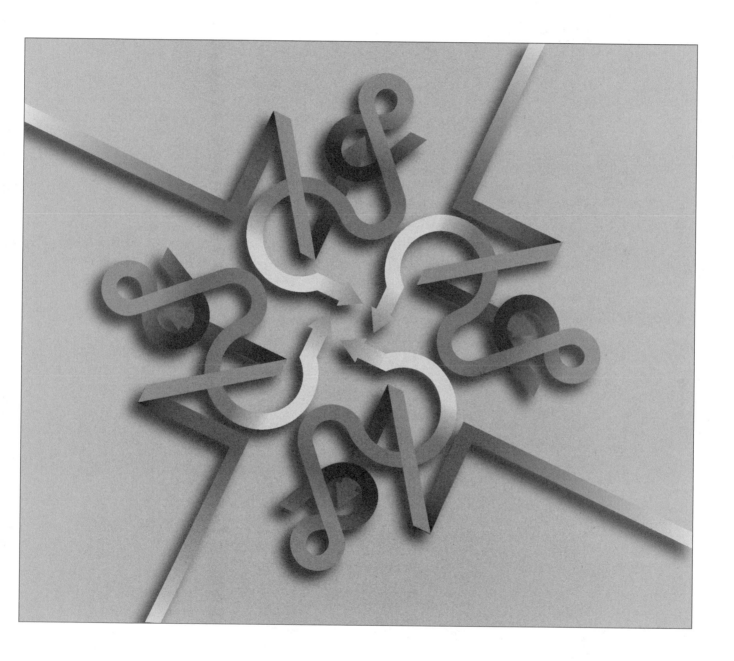

HPI: GA is a 14-year-old female who presents for a physical exam because her mother is concerned that she has not begun to develop breasts or menstruate yet. Her mother reports that she has had a relatively normal childhood, complicated only by hearing impairment requiring a hearing aid. She was the product of a normal birth without any complications during the prenatal course, although at birth she was swollen.

PE: On physical exam she is 58 inches tall and weighs 108 pounds with normal vital signs. Her HEENT exam reveals slightly low-set ears and webbing of the neck. Her cardiac exam is RRR with a II/VI SEM, and her chest exam reveals wide-set nipples and Tanner stage I breasts. A pelvic exam reveals no pubic hair and prepubertal external genitalia. A speculum exam reveals a cervix.

Thought Questions

- What are the steps of gonadal development in males and females?

- What abnormalities of gonadal development can affect males? Females?

- What is this patient's most likely diagnosis?

Basic Science Review and Discussion

The genetic sex of an embryo is determined at the time of fertilization by the composition of the sex chromosomes. However, gonadal development into **testes** or **ovaries** does not begin until the fourth embryonic (sixth menstrual) week. At this time, undifferentiated **primordial germ cells** derived from endoderm migrate from the yolk sac to the **genital ridges** to form **primitive sex cords,** which collectively form the **indifferent gonads.**

If a Y chromosome is present, a gene located in the **sex-determining region of the Y chromosome (SRY)** activates genes on several other chromosomes to assist with testicular development. As a result, the undifferentiated sex cords enlarge, split, and develop into **testis or medullary cords,** and the primordial germ cells differentiate into immature **spermatogonia.** The medullary cords eventually give rise to the tubules of the **rete testis.** The supporting cord cells, **Sertoli and Leydig cells,** arise from the testicular surface epithelium and the original mesenchyme of the gonadal ridge, respectively. By puberty, the medullary cords develop a lumen and form the **seminiferous tubules,** which ultimately join the rete testis tubules and **efferent ductules.**

If the embryo is female and therefore does not contain a Y chromosome, the sex cords continue to develop into medullary cords since ovarian differentiation occurs about 2 weeks later than testicular development. However, in the absence of SRY and its gene products, the medullary cords degenerate and **cortical cords** develop. The germ cells differentiate into **primordial oocytes (oogonia)** within follicles, and the surrounding epithelium differentiates into **granulosa cells,** which are analogous to the Sertoli cells in the male. The follicles are then separated by growth of subepithelial mesenchymal tissue that later forms the **ovarian stroma or thecal cells.** By the eighth embryonic week, the male and female gonads are histologically distinct.

Chromosomal Abnormalities Leading to Gonadal Dysgenesis
Abnormalities in gonadal development occur when chromosomal abnormalities exist. Males who have a 47,XXY karyotype have **Klinefelter's syndrome.** While testicular development is initially normal in these individuals, the presence of at least two X chromosomes causes the germ cells to die off when they enter meiosis, eventually resulting in small, firm testes and hyalinization of the seminiferous tubules. Other classic findings in Klinefelter's syndrome include infertility, gynecomastia, mental retardation, and elevated gonadotropin levels due to the decreased levels of circulating androgens.

Females who have a 45,X (also designated 45, XO) karyotype have gonadal dysgenesis, or **Turner's syndrome.** Because normal oocyte growth requires the activity of both X chromosomes, oocyte death ensues and follicles do not develop, resulting in **streak ovaries** that do not produce sex hormones necessary for puberty. As described in this case, the classic findings include short stature, primary amenorrhea, sexual infantilism, webbed neck, low-set ears, low posterior hairline, epicanthal folds, wide carrying angle of the arms, shield-like chest, wide-set nipples, short fourth metacarpal, renal anomalies, lymphedema of the extremities at birth, and cardiovascular anomalies, especially coarctation of the aorta.

Case Conclusion   Given the patient's physical findings, your suspicion for Turner's syndrome is high and you send the patient for chromosomal analysis, which confirms a karyotype of 45,X. The patient is diagnosed with Turner's syndrome and prescribed hormone replacement to induce secondary sexual development. Of note, a cardiac echocardiogram reveals a patent ductus arteriosus, RVH, and pulmonary HTN. She is referred to a cardiac surgeon for repair.

Thumbnail: Gonadal Development

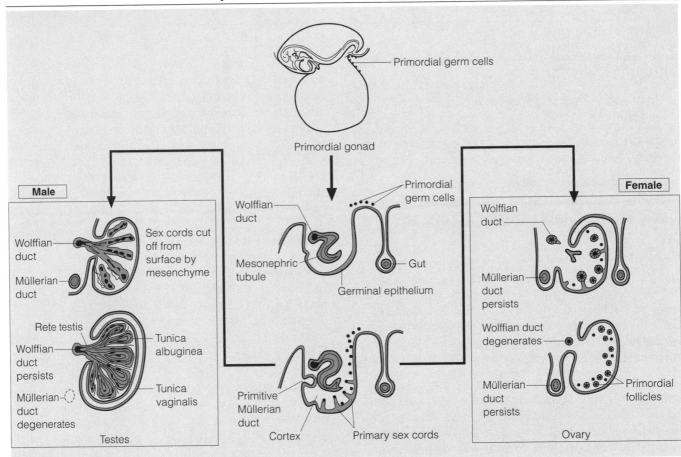

Key Points

▶ The sex of an embryo is determined at the time of fertilization by the chromosome composition.

▶ Testicular development occurs under the influence of the sex-determining region of the Y chromosome and its various gene products. In the absence of these factors, ovarian development occurs.

▶ Klinefelter's syndrome (47,XXY) is a disorder of gonadal development that occurs in 1 in 500 new-

borns and results in abnormal testes, infertility, gynecomastia, and mental retardation.

▶ Turner's syndrome (45,X) is a disorder of gonadal development characterized by streak ovaries, short stature, primary amenorrhea, sexual infantilism, webbed neck, wide carrying angle of the arms, shield-like chest, wide-set nipples, and cardiovascular anomalies.

Questions

1. Normal male gonadal development is dependent on the presence of which of the following?
   A. Sex-determining region of the Y chromosome
   B. Sex-determining region of the Y chromosome, mullerian inhibiting substance
   C. One or more X chromosomes, adrenal androgens
   D. Adrenal androgens, mullerian inhibiting substance
   E. Mullerian inhibiting substance

2. A baby is born with a 46,XY karyotype, but does not develop testes. What other phenotypic feature will be seen?
   A. Normal breast development
   B. Scrotal sac
   C. Penis
   D. Uterus
   E. Facial hair

HPI: HS is a newborn boy who was born at 39 2/7 weeks gestational age. On routine newborn examination, he is found to have a small defect on the ventral surface of the distal penis. His prenatal and labor histories are both unremarkable. The patient's parents are quite disturbed by the penile defect and are concerned about his ability to have sex and conceive when he grows up.

PE: On physical exam, he is a 3725-g male infant. On inspection of his genitalia there is a small opening on the ventral surface of the penile shaft in the midline from which urine is expelled. He has a normal scrotum and both testes are descended and appear normal on palpation.

Thought Questions

- What are the steps of genital duct differentiation in males and females?

- What are the steps of external genitalia development in males and females?

- Discuss hypospadias.

- What abnormalities of genital duct differentiation can affect females?

Basic Science Review and Discussion

Parallel to gonadal development, the male and female internal genitalia develop from separate duct systems in the fourth embryonic week. Initially, both **wolffian (mesonephric) ducts** and **müllerian (paramesonephric) ducts** are present in the embryo (see Thumbnail). The wolffian duct is originally part of the **primordial kidney (mesonephros)** and grows toward the urogenital sinus to eventually contact the primitive sex cords. Meanwhile, the müllerian duct develops laterally to the wolffian duct from an invagination of the coelomic epithelium of the urogenital ridge. Further differentiation of the duct systems is dependent on the presence of testicular secretory products. Therefore, a female phenotype will develop in the absence of these secretory products. Depending on the genetic sex of the fetus, the other duct system disappears by the third fetal month.

In genetic males, the sex-determining region of the Y chromosome (SRY) induces the production of **müllerian-inhibiting substance (MIS)** from Sertoli cells. As its name suggests, MIS causes the mullerian ducts to regress. The Leydig cells secrete testosterone, which then induces development of the wolffian ducts to form the **epididymis, vas deferens,** and **seminal vesicles.** Under the influence of **dihydrotestosterone (DHT)** formed locally from the **5-α-reductase**–mediated conversion of testosterone, the tissue at the base of the regressing mullerian tubercle develops into the **prostate gland.**

In contrast to male embryos, the müllerian duct system persists in female embryos due to the absence of MIS and eventually gives rise to the **fallopian tubes, uterus,** and **upper one third of the vagina.** The cranial portion of the müllerian duct remains patent to the coelomic cavity and becomes the fimbria portion of the fallopian tube. The caudal portion of the müllerian duct crosses the wolffian duct ventrally and contacts the müllerian duct from the opposite side. These eventually fuse to form the uterine canal. Uterine and cervical anomalies can occur when these ducts do not develop or fuse properly. When the combined müllerian ducts reach the posterior wall of the urogenital sinus, the formation of a **paramesonephric or müllerian tubercle** is induced. The upper one third of the vagina develops from the uterine canal and the lower portion develops from the urogenital sinus. Finally, the wolffian duct system regresses in the absence of testosterone.

Development of male or female external genitalia is dependent on the presence or absence of testicular testosterone, which is locally converted to DHT by the enzyme 5-α-reductase. While the differentiation of external genitalia due to hormone exposure begins in the fifth embryonic week, it is not until the eighth embryonic week that the structures of the indifferent external genitalia become apparent. These structures include the **genital tubercle, urogenital slit, lateral genital folds,** and **labioscrotal swellings.** Under the influence of DHT, the penis develops when the genital folds fuse around the urethra and the genital tubercle develops into the glans penis. As the labioscrotal swellings enlarge, they fuse to form the **scrotum.** The **prostate gland** and **bulbourethral glands** arise from the urogenital sinus. Testicular descent into the scrotum is mediated by fetal gonadotropins and the **gubernaculum,** a fibrous cord that connects each testis to the developing scrotum. As the embryo grows, the testes are gradually pulled down toward the scrotum. Final descent of the testes through the bilateral inguinal rings occurs in the last 3 months of pregnancy. Failure of the inguinal canals to narrow after testicular descent can lead to the eventual descent of abdominal contents into the scrotum, resulting in inguinal hernias.

In the absence of testosterone and irrespective of the presence or absence of ovaries, the folds of the urogenital slit do not fuse in the female embryo. The anterior portion of the urogenital sinus becomes the urethra, above which the genital tubercle develops into the **clitoris.** Meanwhile, the posterior portion develops into the lower two thirds of the vagina. The **labia minora** and **labia majora** develop from the lateral genital folds and the labioscrotal swellings, respectively. In females, the gubernaculum attaches to the ovary and cornua of the uterus, ultimately forming the **ovarian and round ligaments.** Prior to the end of pregnancy, connective tissue obliterates the gubernacular attachments to the labioscrotal swellings.

Hypospadias results when the distal urethra does not develop appropriately and the urethral meatus is found anywhere along the ventral surface in the midline of the penile shaft, scrotum, or perineum. It is the most common congenital anomaly of the penis. Because it is associated with hernias and undescended testes, detailed examination of the genitals is important when hypospadias is identified. When hypospadias occurs proximally, curving of the penis known as **chordee** can result. Surgical repair to extend the urethral meatus to the tip of the glans penis involves usage of preputial tissue, making circumcision contraindicated in cases of hypospadias. Distal lesions have an excellent prognosis, whereas proximal lesions may require multiple revisions to create a normal-appearing penis.

As previously mentioned, vaginal, cervical, and uterine abnormalities can occur when the two müllerian ducts do not fuse properly (see Figure 31-1). This can result in a range of abnormalities, including **uterus arcuatus,** where the uterus is only slightly indented in the middle, and **uterus didelphys,** where the uterus, cervix, and sometimes vagina are duplicated entirely.

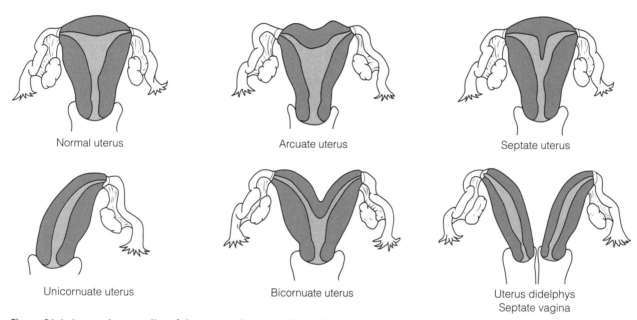

Normal uterus   Arcuate uterus   Septate uterus

Unicornuate uterus   Bicornuate uterus   Uterus didelphys Septate vagina

Figure 31-1 Anatomic anomalies of the uterus. (Reprinted from *Blueprints Obstetrics and Gynecology,* 3rd ed. Malden, MA: Blackwell Publishing, 2004.)

Case Conclusion A pediatric urologist is consulted. He examines HS and meets with his parents. He reassures them that the surgical repair should be relatively straightforward, and that HS will most likely have a normally functioning penis. The patient is discharged home on day of life 2 with his mother and given follow-up appointments for the surgical repair.

Thumbnail: Differentiation of the Male and Female Internal Genitalia

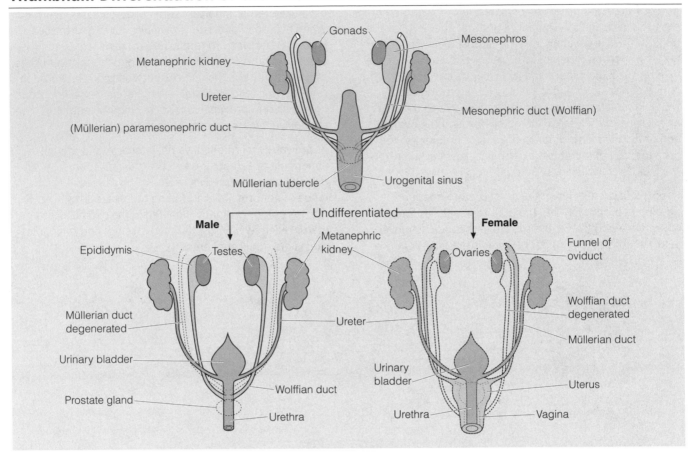

Key Points

▶ Various gene products influenced by SRY mediate wolffian duct differentiation in genetic males. Absence of these gene products leads to the development of female internal genitalia from the mullerian duct system.

▶ DHT mediates the development of male external genitalia. In its absence, female external genitalia develop.

▶ Abnormalities in fusion of the urethral folds can lead to varying degrees of hypospadias.

▶ Uterine, cervical, and vaginal anomalies can arise from absent or improper fusion of the mullerian duct system.

Questions

1. A 16-year-old girl comes to your clinic because she is concerned that she has not begun to menstruate yet. Her prenatal, birth, and childhood histories are all benign. Physical exam is significant for normal breast development, average height, a short vagina, and absence of the uterus and cervix on bimanual exam. Which of the following conditions does this patient most likely have?

   A. Hermaphroditism
   B. Turner's syndrome
   C. Klinefelter's syndrome
   D. Female pseudohermaphroditism
   E. Testicular feminization syndrome

2. Which structures arise from the wolffian duct system?

   A. Fallopian tubes, uterus, vagina
   B. Epididymis, seminal vesicle, vas deferens
   C. Fallopian tubes, uterus, vagina, clitoris
   D. Epididymis, seminal vesicle, vas deferens, gubernaculum
   E. Fallopian tubes, uterus, vagina, clitoris, Bartholin's glands

> **HPI:** MF is a 32-year-old white woman who presents to your office complaining of the inability to conceive despite regular, unprotected intercourse with her husband for 1½ years. She reports regular menses each month and had a first trimester elective termination with a previous partner. She denies a history of sexually transmitted infections (STI) or pelvic inflammatory disease (PID), prior use of an intrauterine device (IUD), pelvic surgery, or abnormal Papanicolaou (Pap) smears.
>
> **PE:** On physical exam, she has normal secondary sexual characteristics, and no hirsutism or virilization. Her pelvic exam is unremarkable, revealing a normal-sized anteverted uterus and no cervical motion or cul-de-sac tenderness.
>
> **Labs:** You send her for a series of laboratory tests including a semen analysis for her husband and schedule them for a follow-up visit.

Thought Questions

- What are the steps of meiosis?

- What are the differences between oogenesis and spermatogenesis?

- What are the causes of infertility?

- How should infertility be evaluated?

Basic Science Review and Discussion

Gametogenesis, a term used to collectively describe the production of gametes in males (spermatogenesis) and females (oogenesis), occurs via mitosis and meiosis (Figure 32-1). Both mitosis and meiosis are types of cell division. While **mitosis** duplicates the entire chromosome content of a cell, **meiosis** results in the formation of haploid cells. It is during prophase I of meiosis that genetic material is exchanged during crossover and new chromosomes are generated in the process.

Oogenesis Oogenesis is the production of female gametes wherein a diploid primary oocyte divides to ultimately produce one functional oocyte and three nonfunctional polar bodies. Females are born with all the germ cells that they will ever have contained in the ovary (700,000 to 2 million). These germ cells, or primary oocytes, are arrested in prophase I of meiosis in primordial follicles until puberty and ovulation occur. Because a large number of follicles become atretic, the number of primordial follicles at puberty falls to 400,000, of which fewer than 500 undergo ovulation. With each ovulatory cycle, several primordial follicles begin to mature but only one reaches full maturity, giving rise to one primary oocyte that resumes meiosis and ultimately results in a secondary oocyte that receives all of the cytoplasm and the first polar body that receives practically none. Because female reproductive ability lasts until menopause, primary oocytes are subject to chromosomal

abnormalities for 50 years or so, which explains the increased risk of chromosomal abnormalities with increasing maternal age. The second meiotic division, producing a mature oocyte and a total of three polar bodies (both the secondary oocyte and the first polar body divide), is only completed if the oocyte is fertilized.

Spermatogenesis Spermatogenesis is the production of male gametes wherein diploid spermatogonia that are arrested in interphase until puberty divide by mitosis to produce both a reserve of stem cells as well as primary spermatocytes. These primary spermatocytes then undergo meiosis I to form secondary spermatocytes, which then undergo the second meiotic division to ultimately produce four haploid spermatids. Spermatids must undergo **spermiogenesis** to become spermatozoa. This process includes the formation of the acrosome, condensation of the nucleus, formation of the neck, middle piece, and tail, and, finally, shedding of most of the cytoplasm. It takes approximately 64 days for a spermatogonium to become a mature spermatozoon.

Infertility Infertility is defined as the inability to conceive after 1 year of regular, unprotected intercourse. The incidence of infertility is approximately 15%. Common causes of infertility include male factor (40%), female factor (40%), and unidentifiable causes (20%). Female factor infertility can be further subdivided into the following causes: ovulatory factors (e.g., intracranial tumors, premature ovarian failure, polycystic ovarian syndrome, endocrine diseases), uterine or tubal factors (e.g., fibroids, PID, synechiae), cervical factors (e.g., cervical stenosis, abnormal mucous production), and peritoneal factors (e.g., endometriosis, pelvic adhesions). In approximately 20% of cases, multiple factors are identified.

Because the causes of infertility are myriad, the evaluation of infertility should be systematic and include detailed history and physical exams on both partners, with specific emphasis on history of prior pregnancies, surgeries, medical

Mitosis

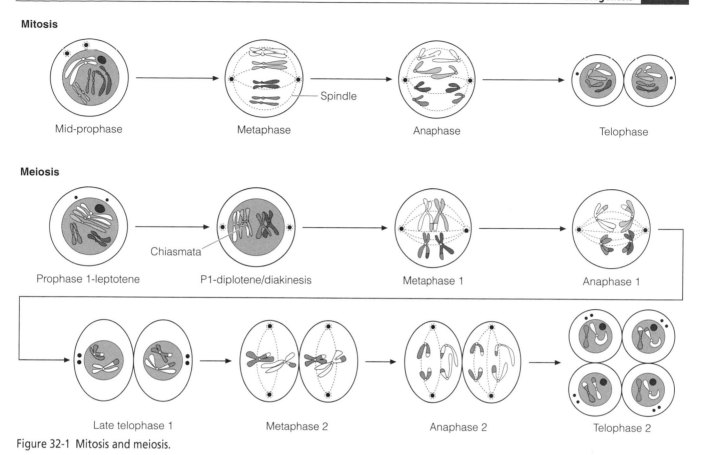

Figure 32-1 Mitosis and meiosis.

problems, genitourinary infections, and exposure to toxins or radiation. Additionally, male partners should be asked about history of postpubertal mumps or varicocele, impotence, and hernia repair. Female partners should be asked specifically about menstrual history, history of abnormal Pap smears, endometriosis, galactorrhea, and prior IUD use.

Case Conclusion Further history of the male partner reveals that he is in good health and denies history of surgery or testicular trauma. Although he reports intermittent condom usage with past partners, he has not had prior pregnancies with other partners. He reports a history of mumps infection at age 14. Your continued evaluation of the female partner is as follows:

Labs: FSH 12 mIU/mL, TSH 2.1 μU/mL, LH 10 mIU/mL, PRL 15 ng/mL. Endometrial biopsy (luteal phase) = WNL.

Semen Analysis: pH 7.3, 2 mL volume (normal 2–5 mL), 10% motile (normal >50%), 5 million per mL (normal >20 million/mL), 95% abnormal forms (normal <70%).

Given the patient's normal endocrine profile and her partner's abnormal semen analysis, the couple is diagnosed with male factor infertility, likely secondary to mumps orchitis, which can impair spermatogenesis. They subsequently undergo intracytoplasmic sperm injection (ICSI) and in vitro fertilization (IVF) to achieve pregnancy.

Thumbnail: Spermatogenesis and Oogenesis

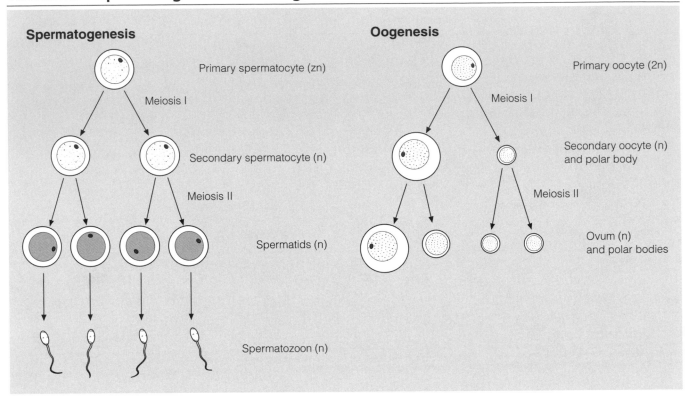

Spermatogenesis

Primary spermatocyte (zn)

Meiosis I

Secondary spermatocyte (n)

Meiosis II

Spermatids (n)

Spermatozoon (n)

Oogenesis

Primary oocyte (2n)

Meiosis I

Secondary oocyte (n) and polar body

Meiosis II

Ovum (n) and polar bodies

Key Points

- In mitosis the entire chromosome content of a cell is duplicated.
- In meiosis the genetic material undergoes crossover and the number of chromosomes is reduced from diploid (46) to haploid (23) to produce gametes.
- Females are born with all the germ cells they will ever have, and these are arrested in prophase I of meiosis until ovulation initiates metaphase I. The second meiotic division is only completed if the oocyte is fertilized.

- Males have a reserve of spermatogonia, which provides stem cells from which primary spermatocytes are created. These primary spermatocytes then undergo meiosis to ultimately produce four spermatids that then undergo spermiogenesis to generate mature spermatozoa.
- Infertility is the inability of a couple to conceive after 1 year of regular, unprotected intercourse. The incidence is approximately 15% and the etiologies include male factors, female factors, and multifactorial.

Questions

1. A 26-year-old woman with regular menses comes to your office requesting an infertility evaluation because she and her husband have been unable to conceive despite regular, unprotected intercourse for the past 3 years. Which aspect of her history is a potential cause of female factor infertility?

   A. History of one prior therapeutic abortion
   B. Early age of menarche
   C. Diethylstilbestrol (DES) exposure in utero
   D. Use of oral contraceptive pills
   E. Her age

2. A 38-year-old man in good health presents to your office concerned about his inability to conceive with his new wife, who has two children from a previous marriage. Of note, he is quite muscular and regularly competes in body-building competitions. Which of the following would be the most likely cause of infertility in this patient?

   A. Absence of spermatogonia
   B. Immotile spermatozoa
   C. Retrograde ejaculation
   D. Chromosomal abnormalities
   E. Failure of spermatogenesis

3. A 39-year-old woman presents to your office for the results of her amniocentesis, which reveals that she has an infant with trisomy 21. During which step of meiosis is nondisjunction likely to have occurred in this patient?

   A. Prophase I
   B. Prophase II
   C. Metaphase I
   D. Telophase I
   E. Telophase II

HPI: PP is a 5-year-old girl who is brought to your office by her mother who is concerned that her daughter has begun developing breasts and pubic hair. Her prenatal and birth histories were significant only for neonatal jaundice, and to date she has been healthy.

PE: On physical exam, you confirm that the child has indeed undergone thelarche (onset of breast development) and pubarche (onset of pubic hair growth) and also note multiple brown skin patches on the child's buttocks, back, and extremities, which her mother states have been there since birth.

Labs: Concerned for McCune-Albright syndrome, you order plain x-rays of the femur and pelvis as well as check estrogen, FSH, and LH levels.

Thought Questions

- What are the key changes observed in female puberty?
- What are the key changes observed in male puberty?
- Discuss precocious puberty.

Basic Science Review and Discussion

Puberty is the series of events leading to sexual maturity. This process includes the development of behavioral and physical characteristics that ultimately lead to adult reproductive function. While there is some variance in mean age of each stage of puberty, age 5 is certainly far outside the norm of age ranges of puberty.

Puberty in Girls In girls, the stages of puberty include adrenarche, gonadarche, thelarche, pubarche, and menarche. **Adrenarche,** which is the increase in adrenal hormone synthesis as a result of regeneration of the zona reticularis, occurs between the ages of 6 and 8 before any visible signs of puberty are evident. Dehydroepiandrosterone (DHEA), dehydroepiandrosterone sulfate (DHEAS), and androstenedione are the adrenal androgens responsible for initial development of pubic and axillary hair.

Pulsatile secretion of GnRH from the hypothalamus around the age of 8 marks the beginning of **gonadarche.** The gonadotrophs in the anterior pituitary are stimulated to secrete LH and FSH, which eventually lead to stimulation of the ovary and estrogen secretion.

The first visible sign of puberty occurs with **thelarche,** the development of breasts. This typically occurs around age 11 in response to rising estrogen levels and continues throughout adolescence, as described by Tanner (Figure 33-1). The vaginal mucosa, uterus, and labia minora and majora also grow in response to estrogen.

Pubarche is the growth of pubic hair in response to circulating androgens and usually occurs in conjunction with

axillary hair growth around age 12. The onset of menstruation, **menarche,** typically occurs 1 to 3 years after thelarche, around age 12 to 13. Menstrual cycles are irregular and

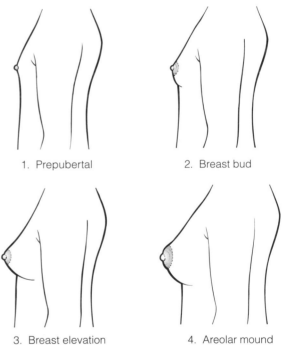

1. Prepubertal   2. Breast bud

3. Breast elevation   4. Areolar mound

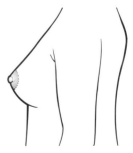

5. Adult contour

Figure 33-1 Tanner stages of thelarche. (Reprinted from *Blueprints Obstetrics and Gynecology,* 3rd ed. Malden, MA: Blackwell Publishing, 2004.)

anovulatory for the first 6 months to 2 years, and can take up to 5 years to develop regular, ovulatory cycles.

Somatic growth is most noticeable during the growth spurt, which is an acceleration in growth rate around age 9 or 10 in response to growth hormone (GH) and insulin-like growth factor-1 (IGF-1). Excess levels of estrogen, as seen in precocious puberty, can lead to short stature via decreased secretion of GH and IGF-1, as well as premature fusion of the epiphyseal plate in long bones.

Despite the orderly fashion described above, it is not unusual for some girls to experience a different order of the presenting signs and symptoms of puberty. The ages at which some girls go through the different stages can vary quite a lot as well.

Puberty in Boys   The stages of puberty in boys include adrenarche, pubarche, testicular maturation, and further development of secondary sexual characteristics. Adrenarche occurs similarly to girls except that the adrenal steroids DHEA, DHEAS, and androstenedione are converted peripherally to the more potent androgens, testosterone, and DHT. These, in turn, promote pubic and axillary hair development. Along with enlargement of the testes, these are the first visible signs of puberty and usually begin between ages 9 and 14.

Testicular maturation is mediated by the pulsatile release of GnRH, which stimulates the diurnal secretion of FSH and LH approximately 1 year prior to testicular enlargement. These gonadotropins initiate androgen production by Leydig cells, growth of the seminiferous tubules, and spermatogenesis.

Although the growth spurt typically occurs 2 years after girls, the mechanism of somatic growth and eventual epiphyseal plate closure is similar. Other somatic changes that occur during puberty include deepening of the voice, increase in bone and muscle mass, increase in laryngeal size, and the development of facial and trunk hair.

Precocious Puberty   True precocious puberty involves the premature maturation of the hypothalamic-pituitary-gonadal axis and is considered when puberty occurs before age 8. Precocity is five times more frequent in girls than boys, with over 70% of cases being idiopathic. In addition to nonorganic causes of precocity such as drug ingestion, neoplastic etiologies such as intracranial, gonadal, and adrenal tumors should be ruled out. Finally, hypothyroidism can rarely cause precocious puberty possibly via stimulation of the FSH receptor by elevated levels of TSH.

McCune-Albright syndrome, also known as polyostotic fibrous dysplasia, is considered precocious pseudopuberty since sexual maturation occurs via early production of estrogen by the ovaries rather than maturation of the hypothalamic-pituitary-gonadal axis. It accounts for 5% of female precocity and manifests as multiple cystic bone lesions prone to fracture, café au lait skin spots, and sexual precocity. It is caused by a mutation during embryogenesis and is not hereditary. While there is no cure for McCune-Albright syndrome, management of endocrine and metabolic abnormalities can result in achievement of normal stature, fertility, and life span.

Case Conclusion   The labs reveal an elevated estrogen level and decreased levels of gonadotropins. The x-rays reveal multiple lytic lesions with scalloped borders in the cortex and ground-glass pattern centrally. You diagnose PP with McCune-Albright syndrome and send her for immediate endocrinology consultation.

Thumbnail: Puberty

Stage	Age of onset (yr)	Description
Girls		
Adrenarche	6–8	Adrenal gland secretion of adrenal androgens
Gonadarche	8	Gonadotropin stimulation of ovarian hormone secretion
Thelarche	11	Breast development
Pubarche	12	Pubic hair development
Menarche	12–13	Onset of menses
Somatic growth	9–10	Growth spurt
Boys		
Adrenarche	8	Adrenal gland secretion of adrenal androgens
Pubarche	9–14	Pubic hair development
Gonadarche	9–14	Gonadotropin stimulation of testicular maturation, testosterone secretion, spermatogenesis
Somatic growth	11–16	Growth spurt, deepening of voice, facial/trunk hair, increased bone and muscle mass

Key Points

▶ Gonadarche is initiated by pulsatile GnRH released from the hypothalamus in both sexes.

▶ The effects of GnRH are mediated by FSH and LH and their actions on the gonads.

▶ The range in timing of the stages of puberty is more varied in males than females.

▶ McCune-Albright syndrome is considered precocious pseudopuberty because rather than early maturation of the hypothalamic-pituitary axis, it involves early estrogen secretion from the ovaries, leading to acceleration of many of the phenotypic changes of puberty.

Questions

1. It is still unclear exactly what occurs on the molecular level to initiate puberty. However, we do know how a variety of the changes are mediated. Which of the following hormones is correctly paired with its role in puberty?

   A. Increased estrogen—increased hepatic enzyme activity.
   B. DHEAS—primarily responsible for pubic and axillary hair in males and females.
   C. LH—stimulation and maturation of breast tissue.
   D. FSH—maturation of secondary sexual characteristics.
   E. GnRH—constant release of this hormone increases its effects.

2. LB is a 13-year-old girl who presents to your office. She has had breast development for over 2 years, but has not begun menstruating and is quite concerned. You discuss that the typical order of the stages of puberty in a female are:

   A. Gonadarche, adrenarche, pubarche, thelarche, menarche
   B. Adrenarche, gonadarche, thelarche, pubarche, menarche
   C. Gonadarche, adrenarche, menarche, thelarche, pubarche
   D. Adrenarche, gonadarche, menarche, thelarche, pubarche
   E. Pubarche, adrenarche, gonadarche, thelarche, menarche

HPI: NM is a 17-year-old gravida 0 competitive gymnast who comes to your office because she has not had her period for approximately 2 years. She began menstruating at age 13 but never had regular periods. She has always been thin and physically active but increased her level of activity at age 14 when she left school to train as a professional gymnast. Approximately 6 months later, her periods stopped entirely. She denies current sexual activity or galactorrhea and does not take any medications.

PE: On physical exam, she is slim but muscular. Her exam is entirely within normal limits, and there are no signs of pregnancy.

Thought Questions

- What are the steps of the menstrual cycle?

- What are the causes of amenorrhea?

- How is amenorrhea evaluated?

Basic Science Review and Discussion

Most women of childbearing age experience ovulatory menstrual cycles every 24 to 35 days (average 28 days). The menstrual cycle involves the hypothalamus, pituitary, ovaries, and endometrium all working in concert to coordinate ovulation and prepare the endometrium for implantation should fertilization occur. It is divided into four phases: menstrual, follicular, ovulatory, and luteal (Figure 34-1).

Menstrual Phase   The first day of menstruation is considered day 1 of the menstrual cycle. The endometrium that was built up from the previous cycle is shed in response to the loss of progesterone support from the corpus luteum. While bleeding typically lasts 3 to 7 days, the start of the follicular phase begins prior to the cessation of menses.

Follicular/Proliferative Phase   The **follicular phase** starts around day 4 of the cycle and lasts until ovulation occurs approximately at mid-cycle (day 14 of an average 28-day cycle). Differences in cycle length can generally be attributed to variations in this phase of the menstrual cycle. Levels of **FSH** from the anterior pituitary begin to rise in response to hypothalamic **GnRH,** which is stimulated by the decrease in estrogen and progesterone during the luteal phase of the prior cycle. FSH stimulates the growth of 5 to 15 primordial follicles that continue to develop until one becomes a dominant follicle that will be ovulated. The dominant follicle produces estrogens that enhance its own maturation as well as increase the production of FSH and **LH** receptors. In response to the rising estrogen levels, the endometrium begins to proliferate and thicken. LH begins to rise late in the follicular phase, stimulating the synthesis of androgens that are converted to estrogen.

Ovulation   When the dominant follicle secretes a sustained critical level of estrogen, this positively feeds back to the anterior pituitary, which responds by secreting a surge of LH, causing the dominant follicle to rupture and release the mature **ovum** approximately 24 to 36 hours later. The ovum is then swept into the fallopian tube and makes its way toward the uterus.

Luteal/Secretory Phase   The **luteal phase** begins after ovulation. Under stimulation by LH, the **corpus luteum** forms from the granulosa and theca interna cells lining the wall of the empty follicle. The corpus luteum then synthesizes progesterone to both stabilize the endometrium and make it more glandular and secretory to prepare it for possible implantation. If implantation does not occur, the corpus luteum degenerates, leading to a rapid decline in progesterone and onset of menses (as described above). The decreasing levels of estrogen and progesterone release the negative feedback mechanism, and the pituitary begins to secrete FSH again to start a new cycle.

If fertilization does occur, the trophoblast produces **human chorionic gonadotropin** (hCG), which is very similar to LH, to maintain the corpus luteum. Endometrial support via progesterone production shifts from the corpus luteum to the placenta by 7 to 9 weeks gestational age.

Evaluation of Amenorrhea   **Amenorrhea** is the absence or cessation of menses. It is generally categorized as either primary or secondary amenorrhea to guide the evaluation process. **Primary amenorrhea** is the absence of **menarche** (onset of menses) by age 16 and can be caused by anatomic abnormalities resulting in outflow tract obstruction, hypothalamic dysfunction, gonadal failure, chromosomal abnormalities, enzyme or hormonal deficiencies, and other rare causes. **Secondary amenorrhea** is the absence of menses for 6 months or three menstrual cycles in a previously menstruating woman and can be caused by hypothalamic dysfunction, polycystic ovarian syndrome (PCOS), pituitary or thyroid disease, abnormal prolactin secretion, premature ovarian failure, or anatomic abnormalities.

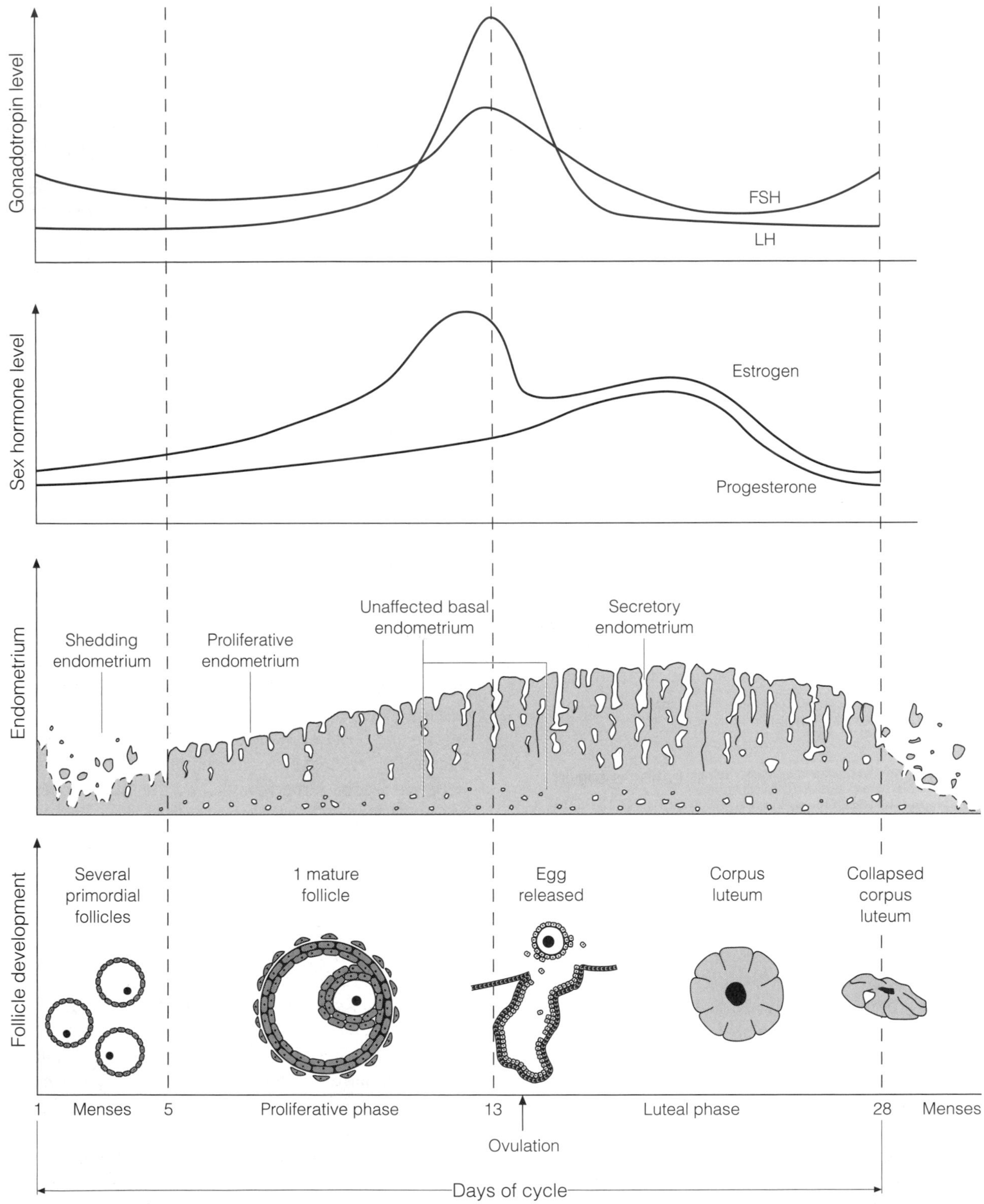

Figure 34-1 Normal menstrual cycle. (Adapted with permission from Impey, L. *Obstetrics and Gynaecology.* Oxford: Blackwell Science, Ltd., 1999.)

The evaluation of primary amenorrhea is guided by the absence or presence of the uterus and breasts (see Thumbnail). If both uterus and breasts are absent, the karyotype is usually 46,XY. When the uterus is present but the breasts absent, **hypergonadotropic hypogonadism** (e.g., gonadal dysgenesis) must be differentiated from **hypogonadotropic hypogonadism** (e.g., hypothalamic dysfunction) by checking serum FSH levels, which will be low in the latter situation.

Additionally, a karyotype may be necessary to rule out gonadal agenesis in a 46,XY individual. If breasts are present but uterus absent, a karyotype is necessary to differentiate between testicular feminization and müllerian agenesis. Finally, patients with both uterus and breasts should be evaluated as patients with secondary amenorrhea.

The most common cause of secondary amenorrhea is pregnancy. When this has been ruled out, anatomic abnormalities that can disrupt the patency of the outflow tract such as cervical stenosis and Asherman's syndrome (intrauterine synechiae or adhesions) should be investigated.

Several endocrine abnormalities can lead to secondary amenorrhea, either via hypogonadotropic hypogonadism or hypergonadotropic hypogonadism. High levels of prolactin are known to cause galactorrhea and amenorrhea via interference in gonadotropin secretion, resulting in hypogonadotropic hypogonadism. Treatment of **hyperprolactinemia** ranges from medication to surgery depending on the etiology. Hypothyroidism can cause amenorrhea via elevated levels of TSH and TRH that in turn can cause hyperprolactinemia. Treatment of the hypothyroidism usually corrects the amenorrhea. Nonendocrine factors that lead to hypothalamic dysfunction and hypogonadotropic hypogonadism include anorexia nervosa and extreme levels of stress and exercise. Hypergonadotropic hypogonadism etiologies of secondary amenorrhea include menopause and premature ovarian failure. In these two conditions, the ovaries no longer produce estrogen and progesterone. In addition to clinical signs and symptoms consistent with menopause, diagnosis is confirmed by an abnormally elevated FSH level.

Secondary amenorrhea can be seen in patients with obesity and PCOS. In these patients, chronically elevated estrogen levels secondary to peripheral aromatization of adrenal androgens to estrogens by adipose cells leads to a disruption in the feedback loop and anovulation. Patients may have only several menses per year and can present with amenorrhea. This can be differentiated from hypogonadism by performing a **progesterone challenge.** If a withdrawal bleed occurs after administration of progesterone for 10 days, anovulation with normal gonadal estrogen production is the likely cause of amenorrhea. These patients can be placed on oral contraceptives to regulate their cycles.

Case Conclusion A pregnancy test is negative, and prolactin and TSH levels both return within normal limits. You prescribe a progesterone challenge and the patient subsequently reports a withdrawal bleed, indicating that she has an intact, estrogen-primed uterus and is likely experiencing amenorrhea as a result of hypothalamic dysfunction due to excessive exercise. You place her on oral contraceptives and schedule a follow-up appointment in several months.

Thumbnail: Etiology of Primary Amenorrhea

	Uterus absent	Uterus present
Breasts absent	Gonadal agenesis in 46,XY Enzyme deficiencies in testosterone synthesis	Gonadal failure/agenesis in 46,XX Disruption of hypothalamic-pituitary axis
Breasts present	Testicular feminization Müllerian agenesis or Mayer-Rokitansky-Küster-Hauser syndrome (MRKH)	Hypothalamic, pituitary, or ovarian pathogenesis similar to that of secondary amenorrhea Congenital abnormalities of the genital tract

Key Points

▶ Menstruation is the cyclical shedding of the endometrium experienced by women of reproductive age.

▶ The menstrual cycle is driven by a feedback loop between the hypothalamus (GnRH), pituitary gland (FSH and LH), and ovaries (estrogen and progesterone).

▶ Primary amenorrhea is the absence of menarche by age 16 or 4 years after thelarche.

▶ Evaluation of primary amenorrhea is guided by the presence or absence of the breasts and uterus.

▶ Secondary amenorrhea is the absence of menses for more than 6 months or the equivalent of three menstrual cycles in a previously menstruating woman.

Questions

1. A 16 year-old girl presents to your office complaining of primary amenorrhea. On physical exam, she has both breasts and a uterus. A pregnancy test returns positive and explains the patient's amenorrhea. Which of the following does not lead to primary amenorrhea?

   A. Testicular feminization
   B. Imperforate hymen
   C. Transverse vaginal septum
   D. Intense physical activity since age 8
   E. Removal of left ovary secondary to torsion at age 8

2. A 24-year-old woman presents to your office with complaints of secondary amenorrhea since age 22. She had regular menses from age 13 to age 21, but only four periods during her last year of college. She reports no sexual intercourse since age 18. She gained 110 pounds during college, increasing from 140 to 250 pounds. Since age 22, she has lost 40 pounds, back down to 210 pounds. During this time she has increased her exercise to five times per week, 1 to 1½ hours each time. Which of the following is the most likely cause of her secondary amenorrhea?

   A. Elevated hCG leading to maintenance of her corpus luteum
   B. Elevated circulating estrogen leading to a disruption in FSH/LH production by the pituitary
   C. Sudden weight loss leading to hypogonadotropic hypogonadism
   D. Excessive exercise leading to hypogonadotropic hypogonadism
   E. Testicular feminization

3. A 34-year-old woman is undergoing evaluation for secondary amenorrhea of 8 months' duration. She also reports occasional hot flushes. She has never been pregnant before. Her physical exam is within normal limits and a pregnancy test is negative. PRL and TSH values are also within normal limits. You schedule her for a progestin challenge. Which of the following results is correctly matched to a plausible etiology of her secondary amenorrhea?

   A. Withdrawal bleed seen with progestin challenge—Asherman's syndrome
   B. Withdrawal bleed seen with progestin challenge—premature ovarian failure
   C. Withdrawal bleed seen only with estrogen/progestin challenge and FSH abnormally low—PCOS
   D. Withdrawal bleed seen only with estrogen/progestin challenge and FSH abnormally elevated—premature ovarian failure
   E. Withdrawal bleed seen only with estrogen/progestin challenge and FSH abnormally elevated—testicular feminization

HPI: A 17-year-old girl presents to your office reporting amenorrhea for 1½ months. She recently became sexually active with her boyfriend and uses condoms "sometimes." She thinks she may be pregnant and requests a pregnancy test.

Thought Questions

- What are common methods for contraception?
- Which methods are considered most effective?
- What are contraindications to these methods of contraception?

Basic Science Review and Discussion

Over the course of 1 year, the pregnancy rate for women not using any form of contraception is 85%. **Contraception** is the intentional prevention of pregnancy by utilizing one or more of the various methods available. There are several categories of contraception including natural methods, IUDs, spermicides, barrier methods, hormonal methods, and surgical sterilization. Within each of these categories, there exist a number of alternatives. Since no single contraceptive method is 100% effective, easy to use, or free of side effects, the choice of contraception depends on individual preferences.

Natural Methods **Periodic abstinence,** also known as the **rhythm method,** is a form of natural contraception that requires a highly motivated user since it relies on accurate prediction of ovulation and subsequent abstinence surrounding the estimated time of ovulation. Another natural form of contraception is **coitus interruptus,** which involves withdrawal of the penis from the vagina prior to ejaculation. This method can be unreliable because semen can be deposited in the vagina even prior to ejaculation. Not surprisingly, natural methods of contraception have a high failure rate of approximately 20% compared with other forms of contraception. While there are no true contraindications to these natural forms of contraception, the high failure rate and necessity for self-control and regular menses make them a less desirable option for many couples.

Intrauterine Device The **IUD** is the most widely used form of reversible contraception worldwide. It is a T-shaped device composed of plastic that is inserted into the uterus by a physician, where it can remain effective for 5 to 10 years. The addition of copper or progestin affects the mechanism by which IUDs prevent pregnancy, which is primarily via prevention of implantation. Copper IUDs function primarily by generating a local sterile spermicidal inflam-

matory response, while progestin-containing IUDs disrupt normal endometrial development that is necessary for implantation. The side effects associated with IUDs include increased risk of pelvic inflammatory disease **(PID)**, ectopic pregnancy, and excessive or painful menstrual bleeding. As such, IUDs are contraindicated in women who are currently pregnant, are at high risk for sexually transmitted diseases, or have undiagnosed vaginal bleeding. Additionally, they are relatively contraindicated in women who have not had children because insertion can be more difficult and painful. The IUD is considered a very effective form of contraception, with a failure rate of 1–2%, which is comparable with that of sterilization.

Barrier Methods Barrier methods of contraception are available for both sexes and function by inhibiting sperm entry into the uterus. The **male condom** is a sheath composed of latex, polyurethane, or animal intestine that is placed over the erect penis to prevent the deposition of sperm or infectious agents into the vagina. While they are ideal for some individuals because they can prevent the transmission of STDs, are inexpensive, and are readily available, male condoms can also be inconvenient and unreliable if used incorrectly, reducing the ideal efficacy rate of 98% to an actual efficacy rate of 85% to 90%.

The **female condom** is composed of polyurethane and has two flexible rings, with one fitting loosely inside the vagina near the cervix and the other remaining outside the vagina at the perineum. Initial studies indicate that the female condom is slightly less effective as well as less popular than the male condom. The only absolute contraindication to male or female condom usage is allergy to the material.

The **diaphragm** is a dome composed of soft latex or plastic that is fitted over the cervix and used with spermicides. It must be placed in the vagina before intercourse and left in place for 6 to 8 hours afterward. When used in conjunction with spermicides, the failure rate is 15% to 20%. It is contraindicated in women who are allergic to the material, cannot be properly fitted, or are not comfortable inserting the diaphragm. The **cervical cap** is similar to the diaphragm but is smaller and can be left in for 1 to 2 days. Because it is more difficult to place than the diaphragm, it has a slightly higher failure rate.

Spermicides are commonly used in conjunction with barrier methods of contraception and function by killing sperm via destruction of the cell membrane. Common spermicidal formulations include nonoxynol-9 and octoxynal-9, which are available as foam, jelly, or wax suppositories. The only absolute contraindication to spermicides is allergy to the ingredients. When used alone, the failure rate of spermicides is 5% to 15%.

Hormonal Contraception   **Hormonal methods** of contraception are quite varied and include oral, injectable, implantable, and emergency forms. **Oral contraceptive pills** (OCPs) are one of the most popular methods of reversible contraception in the United States. They are available in combination estrogen and progestin formulations as well as progestin-only pills. Combination OCPs function by preventing ovulation, thickening the cervical mucus, and altering the endometrium to make implantation unfavorable. Progestin-only pills function similarly, although they will only inhibit ovulation in some women. They are used in situations where estrogen is contraindicated, such as in breast-feeding women. Typical dosing of OCPs involves a 28-day regimen that includes 21 days of hormone-containing pills followed by 7 days of placebo pills, during which time the woman should experience a withdrawal bleed. Because OCPs are associated with increased risk for thromboembolic disease, nausea, elevated BP, and irregular breakthrough bleeding, they are absolutely contraindicated in women with a history or tendency toward thromboembolic disease, chronic liver disease, pregnancy, estrogen-dependent neoplasia, and undiagnosed vaginal bleeding. Relative contraindications include women over the age of 35 years who smoke or have cardiac disease or migraine headaches. OCPs are 95% to 99% effective in preventing pregnancy.

There are currently two **injectable contraceptives** available in the United States, Depo-Provera and Lunelle. **Depo-Provera** (medroxyprogesterone acetate, or DMPA) is an intramuscular injection of progestin that is dosed every 3 months and works by inhibiting ovulation, thickening cervical mucus, and altering the endometrium. Side effects include irregular bleeding, weight gain, hair loss, and mood changes. The failure rate is less than 1%. The other injectable contraceptive is **Lunelle** (medroxyprogesterone acetate and estradiol cypionate), which is very similar to DMPA except that it is dosed once a month, providing more

flexibility for women desiring more rapid return of fertility following cessation of usage. In addition, the estrogen component stabilizes the endometrium to reduce the side effect of irregular bleeding.

Norplant is a subdermal implant system consisting of six rod-shaped capsules containing progestin (levonorgestrel) that is slowly released over 5 years. The rods must be placed and eventually removed by a physician. A single-rod system effective for 3 years is under investigation. The mechanism of action and efficacy are similar to that of DMPA. Side effects are also similar to those of DMPA but are generally considered to be milder. These progestin-only contraceptives are absolutely contraindicated in pregnant women and in women with undiagnosed vaginal bleeding and breast cancer. Relative contraindications include active liver disease, coronary artery disease, HTN, and diabetes with complications.

Emergency contraception, also called the "morning after pill," comes in combination estrogen and progestin as well as progestin-only formulations. It can be used to prevent pregnancy if taken within 72 hours from the time of unprotected intercourse. The mechanism of action as well as side effects are similar to that of combination or progestin-only contraceptives, with the exact mechanism of action depending on where the woman is in her menstrual cycle. Used properly, emergency contraception is 75% effective in preventing pregnancy.

Sterilization   **Sterilization** is a permanent form of contraception that can be implemented in males or females. Although the methods vary, the goal of surgical sterilization is to prevent gametes from reaching one another. Male sterilization can be performed in an outpatient setting and is called **vasectomy.** It involves cutting and tying the vas deferens to prevent sperm from leaving the testes. The failure rate is less than 1% after confirmation of azoospermia. Female sterilization involves occluding both fallopian tubes and can be achieved by ligation, banding, clipping, or coagulation. It can be performed on an inpatient or outpatient basis and has a failure rate of 0.2% to 1.0%. Although reversal of sterilization is possible, success rates vary. As such, sterilization is contraindicated in individuals who wish to preserve future fertility.

Case Conclusion   A urine pregnancy test returns negative. You counsel the patient regarding safe sexual practices as well as contraceptive alternatives. After your discussion, she elects to get a Depo-Provera shot.

Thumbnail: Methods of Contraception

Method	Mode of action	Contraindications
Natural		
Rhythm method	Abstinence during periods of predicted ovulation	Individuals in whom contraception is important since it has a high failure rate
Coitus interruptus	Withdrawal of penis from vagina prior to ejaculation	Individuals in whom contraception is important since it has a high failure rate
Barrier		
Male condom	Sheath placed over penis to prevent deposition of semen into vagina	Allergic reaction
Female condom	Sheath placed within vagina and covering perineum to prevent deposition of semen into vagina	Allergic reaction
Diaphragm	Latex/plastic dome that covers cervix—prevents semen entry into uterus	Anatomic condition prohibiting proper fitting of diaphragm; discomfort
Cervical cap	Latex/plastic cap that covers cervix—prevents semen entry into uterus	Anatomic condition prohibiting proper fitting of cervical cap; discomfort
Hormonal		
Oral contraceptive pills	Combination pills: suppression of ovulation, thickening of cervical mucus, alteration of endometrium to make implantation unsuitable Progestin-only pills: thickening of cervical mucus, alteration of endometrium to make implantation unsuitable	Absolute: pregnancy thromboembolic disease, CVA, breast or endometrial cancer, hepatic tumor or abnormal function Relative: DM, HTN, smokers > 35 yr, age > 40 yr with high risk for vascular disease
Injectable	Depo-Provera: suppression of ovulation, thickening of cervical mucus, alteration of endometrium to make implantation unsuitable; dosed every 3 mo Lunelle: similar to Depo-Provera but dosed every month	Absolute: pregnancy, undiagnosed vaginal bleeding, breast cancer Relative: liver tumor, disease or decreased function; hypertension with or without vascular disease; history of CVA; diabetes with complications
Implantable	Norplant: subdermal implant system of slow-release progestin to prevent suppression of ovulation, thickening of cervical mucus, alteration of endometrium to make implantation unsuitable; dosed every 5 yr	See Injectable contraceptive contraindications
Emergency	Combination estrogen/progestin or progestin-only formulations: depending on woman's cycle phase, suppression of ovulation, thickening of cervical mucus, and/or alteration of endometrium to make implantation unsuitable; taken within 72 h of unprotected intercourse	Similar to oral contraceptive pills
Sterilization		
Vasectomy	Occlusion of the vas deferens via ligation to prevent sperm from leaving testes	Couples desiring future fertility
Tubal occlusion	Occlusion of the fallopian tubes via ligation, cautery, clipping, or banding	Couples desiring future fertility
Other		
IUD	Sterile spermicidal inflammatory response, alteration of tubal motility, inhibition of implantation	Absolute: suspected gynecologic malignancy; acute cervical, uterine, or salpingeal infection; history of PID; pregnancy Relative: multiple sexual partners; nulliparity
Spermicide	Sperm destruction via degradation of sperm cell wall	Allergic reaction

Key Points

- Although natural methods of contraception have no true contraindications, they have high failure rates and should therefore not be used by couples for whom pregnancy prevention is a high priority.
- IUDs function primarily by preventing implantation and are a highly effective method of contraception.
- Barrier methods such as condoms, diaphragms, and cervical caps function by forming physical barriers that prevent gametes from meeting.
- The diaphragm and cervical cap require motivated users because they must be fitted by a physician, they must be used in conjunction with spermicides, and the user must be comfortable with proper insertion.

- Combination estrogen and progestin hormonal contraceptives are very effective when used properly and function by suppression of ovulation, thickening of cervical mucus, and alteration of the endometrial lining to make implantation unfavorable.
- Progestin-only OCPs function similarly to combination oral contraceptives except that they only suppress ovulation in some women. Although they are not as effective as combination hormonal contraceptives, they are useful for women in whom estrogen usage is contraindicated (e.g., lactation, HTN, severe headaches).
- Injectable contraceptives (Depo-Provera and Lunelle) are progestin-only contraceptives that function similarly to the progestin-only pills.

Questions

1. A 36-year-old G3 P2 smoker with a history of depression presents to your office to discuss birth control options. Which of the following is the most appropriate contraceptive for her?
   - **A.** Copper IUD
   - **B.** Norplant
   - **C.** Depo-Provera
   - **D.** Combination OCPs
   - **E.** Progestin-only OCPs

2. You are discharging a 20-year-old G3 P1 from the hospital after treating her for PID. She is currently in a monogamous relationship but has had two partners in the past few months. Which of the following forms of contraception would be most effective in preventing future similar hospitalizations?
   - **A.** Diaphragm
   - **B.** Condoms
   - **C.** IUD
   - **D.** OCPs
   - **E.** Depo-Provera

3. Which of the following is correctly matched to its primary mechanism of action?
   - **A.** Diaphragm—makes endometrium unsuitable for implantation
   - **B.** Depo-Provera—kills sperm by degrading cell walls
   - **C.** IUD—acts as a barrier between sperm and egg
   - **D.** Combination OCPs—prevent ovulation, thicken cervical mucus, make endometrium unsuitable for implantation
   - **E.** Norplant—kills sperm by generating a foreign body reaction

> **HPI:** A 27-year-old G1P0 woman presents to your office stating that her period is almost 1 week late and that she has been experiencing bilateral breast tenderness. She is sexually active with her boyfriend and reports 100% condom usage. However, she reports that approximately 3 weeks ago, the condom slipped off during intercourse. Since her periods are normally quite regular, she is worried that she may be pregnant.
>
> **PE:** On physical exam, her blood pressure is 100/60 mm Hg, and her heart, lung, and abdominal exams are normal. Upon inspection of the cervix, there is a slight bluish hue, and on palpation her cervix is soft with a slightly enlarged uterus to 5- to 6-week size. You send off several lab tests.

Thought Questions

- What medical methods are available for pregnancy termination?

- What are the physiologic principles behind medical abortion?

- What are common surgical methods used to terminate pregnancies?

Basic Science Review and Discussion

Approximately 5 million women become pregnant in the United States every year, with 55% of these pregnancies being unintended. The landmark case, *Roe v. Wade,* legalized abortion throughout the United States in 1973. Approximately 1.2 million elective pregnancy terminations are performed each year, and it is estimated that by age 45, nearly half of all women in the United States will have an abortion.

Several methods exist for elective pregnancy termination, the choice of which is usually dictated by the duration of the pregnancy. In the first trimester (less than 12 weeks of gestation), the options include suction curettage and medical abortion. The available options in the second trimester (12–24 weeks of gestation) are induction of labor or dilatation and evacuation (D&E). After the fetus reaches viability at 24 weeks of gestation (i.e., it is theoretically capable of independent survival), abortions are only allowed in situations where maternal life is at risk.

First-Trimester Terminations **Medical abortion** involves the usage of **mifepristone** (RU-486) in combination with a prostaglandin to induce pregnancy termination. Mifepristone is a progesterone receptor antagonist that blocks progesterone action, which results in alteration of endometrial growth and detachment of the embryo. It is given in a single oral dose followed 36 to 48 hours later by a prostaglandin (usually **misoprostol**) to induce cervical dilatation and uterine contractions in order to expel the uterine contents. Mifepristone in conjunction with miso-

prostol is over 90% effective for inducing pregnancy termination.

Another regimen for medical abortion employs **methotrexate,** a folic acid antagonist that is used in cancer therapies, in conjunction with a prostaglandin. Methotrexate will stop embryonic cells from dividing and is given as an intramuscular injection, followed several days later by intravaginal misoprostol. Other medical abortion regimens are under investigation and include the usage of intravaginal prostaglandin alone to induce cervical dilatation and uterine contractions.

Medical abortion is only approved for pregnancies of up to 7 weeks of gestation due to the lower efficacy rate for pregnancies beyond this gestational age. Although medical abortion is restricted to early gestation pregnancies, it provides a safe, private, and effective alternative for women who wish to avoid uterine instrumentation. The disadvantages of medical abortion include the possibility of failed abortion, which would eventually require suction curettage, and the risk of heavy uterine cramping and bleeding, which some women may wish to avoid by electing to undergo suction curettage.

Dilatation and curettage (D&C) is another first-trimester alternative for pregnancy termination. Currently, the majority of abortions in the United States employ suction curettage. The procedure is often performed in an outpatient setting under local anesthesia and conscious sedation but can also be performed under general anesthesia when necessary. Dilatation of the cervix is achieved via placement of laminaria prior to the procedure or mechanical dilation using metal dilators. A suction cannula attached to a vacuum aspirator is then introduced into the uterus and rotated as well as moved in and out of the uterus to evacuate the contents. Suction curettage is highly effective, and complications are rare, but include infection (1%), excessive bleeding (2%), and uterine perforation (1%). The mortality rate associated with D&C is less than that of a term delivery.

Second-Trimester Terminations For pregnancies beyond 12 weeks of gestation, pregnancy termination can be achieved via dilatation and evacuation (D&E) or labor induction. **D&E** can be performed on pregnancies up to 24 weeks of gestational age. It is similar to D&C except that greater cervical dilatation must be achieved so that large suction cannulas and specialized instruments may be introduced to remove fetal parts and the placenta. Complications of D&E are similar to that of D&C, but the former has a higher mortality rate that is comparable with that of term delivery. One advantage of D&E over labor induction is that D&E can be performed in an outpatient setting.

Pregnancy termination by **labor induction** can be performed for pregnancies up to 24 weeks of gestation and is achieved by a number of methods, including cervical ripening with prostaglandins, amniotomy, oxytocin, and intra-amniotic instillation of prostaglandin $F_{2\alpha}$, hyperosmolar urea, or hypertonic saline, of which the latter agent is now rarely used due to the increased risk for complications. Overall, complications are more common in comparison with other methods and include hemorrhage, retained placenta, or incomplete abortion, in addition to the side effects of nausea, vomiting, fever, and diarrhea. Additionally, prostaglandin use has been associated with a higher incidence of live births and gastrointestinal side effects. One disadvantage of labor induction as opposed to D&E is the fact that inductions can be quite lengthy and emotionally exhausting for the patient and her partner.

Case Conclusion   A serum pregnancy test confirms that the patient is pregnant and ultrasonography confirms that the pregnancy is intrauterine and approximately 5 weeks of gestation, which is consistent with dating as calculated by her last menstrual period. After discussing various options with the patient, she elects to undergo medical abortion. She receives mifepristone, and 48 hours later a single dose of vaginal misoprostol. The next day she has cramping and self-limited vaginal bleeding for several hours. Her one week follow-up visit confirms that her uterus is now empty.

Thumbnail: Abortion

Methods of Abortion

Method	Weeks of gestational age available	Mode of action
Medical		
Mifepristone (RU-486)	Up to 7	Asynchronization of endometrium leading to embryo detachment
Methotrexate	Up to 7	Cessation of cell division, leading to embryonic death
Labor induction	16–24	Delivery of fetus from vagina using prostaglandins, amniotomy, oxytocin, or intra-amniotic infusion
Surgical		
D&C	Up to 12	Dilation of cervix followed by suction curettage of uterine contents
D&E	13 -24	Dilation of cervix followed by suction curettage as well as manual extraction of fetal parts and placenta

---

Key Points

▶ Elective pregnancy termination, or therapeutic abortion, is a common procedure in the United States and can be achieved by medical or surgical methods.

▶ Medical abortion can be safely and effectively performed up to 7 weeks gestational age and involves the usage of mifepristone (RU-486), methotrexate, or prostaglandins.

▶ Surgical methods of abortion can be utilized up to 24 weeks of gestation and involve cervical dilatation followed by evacuation of uterine contents either by vacuum aspiration or manual extraction of fetal parts via specialized tools.

▶ Labor induction can be utilized for pregnancy termination in the late second trimester and utilizes various agents and interventions to accelerate the labor process and facilitate expulsion of the fetus and placenta.

Questions

1. A 22-year-old woman is referred to your office for termination of pregnancy at 6 weeks of gestation. Which of the following correctly matches the method with the mechanism of action?

   A. Mifepristone—folic acid antagonist that stops cell division

   B. Methotrexate—induces contractions to expel uterine contents

   C. Misoprostol—progesterone antagonist

   D. Misoprostol—folic acid antagonist

   E. Mifepristone—progesterone antagonist

2. Statistical record keeping about abortion has improved since its legalization. Which of the following is true about the practice of abortion in the United States?

   A. Approximately 15% of all women will have an abortion in their lifetime.

   B. To this day, abortion remains illegal in Utah.

   C. Abortion was illegal in all 50 states prior to 1973.

   D. Over 1 million abortions are performed each year in the United States.

   E. Over 50% of abortions are performed on women under the age of 20.

HPI: A 22-year-old G3P0 recent immigrant from Mexico presents to the emergency room complaining of shortness of breath, fatigue, palpitations, and cough, especially at night, for the past 2 weeks. She denies night sweats, weight loss, or exposure to tuberculosis. She also reports that she is approximately 25 weeks pregnant and has not received any prenatal care during this pregnancy. Her past medical history is significant for recurrent strep throat infections as a child. She works as a nanny and does not smoke.

PE: On physical exam, she is tachycardic and appears to be in moderate distress. Her neck veins are distended and she has a diastolic rumble heard best in the left lateral decubitus position, an opening snap (OS), and an S_3 gallop. Her fundal height is 26 cm, and she has 2+ bilateral lower extremity edema. CXR shows bilateral pulmonary edema.

Thought Questions

- What pathophysiologic process is most consistent with this patient's symptoms?

- What are the key changes of maternal physiology in pregnancy?

- How would these changes affect cardiac valvular disease?

Basic Science Review and Discussion

The findings of distended neck veins (JVD), 2+ bilateral edema, pulmonary edema, and a diastolic murmur are most consistent with congestive heart failure (CHF), particularly in the setting of mitral stenosis. There are other etiologies of CHF, and certainly an echocardiogram to determine cardiac function should be done. Although unlikely, the patient should also be evaluated for recent MI. This patient with no known prior disease may have a history of a valvular heart disease that is now exacerbated by the physiologic changes of pregnancy. Pregnancy places new demands on the mother that require physiologic adaptations in almost every organ system in order to meet these demands. These changes are reviewed by organ systems below.

Cardiovascular Elevated progesterone levels during pregnancy lead to smooth muscle relaxation, which results in decreased SVR and BP. The decrease in BP nadirs at 24 weeks of gestation and slowly returns to prepregnancy levels by term. Any further increases in BP are abnormal and should be evaluated. Because preload increases via the increase in blood volume, cardiac output increases by 30% to 50%.

Pulmonary Because the enlarging uterus elevates the diaphragm, the total lung capacity is decreased by 5% during pregnancy. Nevertheless, the tidal volume increases by 30% to 40% and the RR stays the same, which leads to a 30% to 40% increase in the minute ventilation and a con-

comitant decrease in arterial P_{CO_2}. However, bicarbonate decreases to maintain the pH and results in a compensated respiratory alkalosis.

Renal The GFR increases by 50% during pregnancy, resulting in 25% decreases in both serum creatinine and BUN. The increased GFR also leads to decreased resorption of glucose, leading to glycosuria in approximately 15% of normal pregnancies. High progesterone levels lead to dilatation of the ureters and mild hydronephrosis, which can be further exacerbated by mechanical compression by the enlarging uterus. Increased sodium filtration also occurs due to the increased GFR, but plasma levels of sodium do not increase because of a concomitant increase in aldosterone to resorb this sodium.

GI Progesterone relaxation of gastrointestinal smooth muscle leads to delayed gastric emptying, decreased tone of the gastroesophageal sphincter, and decreased large bowel motility. These changes lead to the symptoms of increased reflux and constipation. Nausea occurs in more than 70% of pregnancies and tends to resolve by 17 weeks of gestation. While this phenomenon has been termed "morning sickness," it can occur at any time of the day.

Heme The red cell mass also increases during pregnancy (20%–30%), although proportionally less than the increase in blood volume (50%). Thus, a mild dilutional anemia results. A leukocytosis also occurs, but should not affect the differential count. Approximately 10% of women experience a mild thrombocytopenia (<150,000 platelets/mL) but this is rarely of clinical significance. Increased levels of factors I (fibrinogen), VII, VIII, IX, and X, as well as increased stasis, make pregnancy a hypercoagulable state.

Endocrine Elevated levels of estrogen in pregnancy stimulate production of thyroid-binding globulin by the liver. However, levels of free T_3, T_4, and TSH remain unchanged in pregnancy due to increased production of T_3 and T_4 via the thyroid-stimulating properties of placental hormones such as hCG. While PRL levels increase during pregnancy, they paradoxically decrease after delivery and then rise again in response to suckling.

Cardiac Valvular Disease in Pregnancy Preexisting maternal heart disease that does not compromise function in the non-pregnant state can worsen during pregnancy as a result of its associated cardiovascular changes. Specifically, cardiac output is relatively fixed in cases of tight mitral stenosis. Elevation of

preload and cardiac output in normal pregnancy can lead to ventricular failure and pulmonary HTN. Additionally, worsening left atrial (LA) enlargement can lead to arrhythmias and thrombus formation. As such, tachycardia and heart failure from fluid overload can be seen in mitral stenosis during pregnancy. Since 25% of women with mitral stenosis have cardiac failure for the first time in pregnancy, mitral stenosis can be confused with idiopathic peripartum cardiomyopathy.

Case Conclusion The patient has heart failure likely from undiagnosed rheumatic heart disease resulting in mitral stenosis. You admit her to the hospital for diuresis, bedrest, and start her on a low-dose beta-blocker to control her heart rate (HR) and prevent rate-related heart failure. Echocardiography confirms mitral stenosis. She responds well to this regimen and is eventually discharged home on a diuretic and beta-blocker with instructions to limit her activity and adhere to a low-salt diet.

Thumbnail: Maternal Adaptations in Pregnancy

Maternal Adaptations to Pregnancy

Organ system	Changes
Hematologic	Red cell mass increases 20%–30% Plasma volume increases 50% Leukocytosis Thrombocytopenia (mild) Elevated factors I, VII-X
Endocrine	Estrogen increases Progesterone increases Thyroid-binding globulin increases Prolactin increases
Renal	GFR increases 50% BUN and creatinine decrease 25% Mild hydronephrosis and hydroureter
Gastrointestinal	Gastric emptying times prolonged Gastroesophageal sphincter tone decreases Large bowel motility decreases
Pulmonary	Total lung capacity decreases 5% Respiratory rate stays the same Tidal volume increases 30%–40% Expiratory reserve volume decreases 20% Minute ventilation increases 30%–40%
Cardiovascular	SVR and BP decrease Cardiac output increases 30%–50%

Key Points

- ▶ Pregnancy induces maternal physiologic adaptations in almost every organ system.

- ▶ Blood volume increases by approximately 50%, leading to an increase in cardiac output of approximately 30% to 50%.

- ▶ While total lung capacity is decreased by the enlarging uterus, tidal volume and minute ventilation both increase by 30% to 40%.

- ▶ GFR increases by 50%, resulting in decreased levels of both serum creatinine and BUN.

- ▶ Elevated progesterone levels in pregnancy cause decreased esophageal sphincter tone, leading to increased gastroesophageal reflux.

Questions

1. A 28-year-old woman presents for a routine prenatal appointment at 24 weeks of gestation. Which of the following cardiovascular and/or hematologic indices are elevated?

   A. Systemic vascular resistance
   B. Cardiac output
   C. Platelets
   D. BP
   E. Hematocrit

2. A 30-year-old woman presents for a routine prenatal appointment at 22 weeks of gestation. Which of the following pulmonary and/or renal indices are decreased?

   A. Tidal volume
   B. GFR
   C. RR
   D. BUN and serum creatinine
   E. Minute ventilation

HPI: HF is a 32-year-old G2P1 pregnant woman at 10 2/7 weeks of gestation who presents for her initial prenatal visit. On review of her prenatal labs, you notice that her blood type is A-negative and that her antibody screen for rhesus factor (Rh) is positive with a titer of 1:16. Her past obstetric history is significant for an uncomplicated spontaneous vaginal delivery of a term infant 2 years ago in South America. She recalls getting one dose of RhoGAM mid-pregnancy but not at delivery. The blood type of the father of the baby is A-positive and the first child's blood type is also A-positive. Her past medical history is otherwise noncontributory.
You repeat the antibody screen and confirm that the titer is correct. You advise the patient that she has been alloimmunized to fetal D antigen and that this pregnancy is at risk for hydrops fetalis if the blood type of the fetus is confirmed to be Rh-positive. You schedule her for serial antibody titers and amniocentesis to determine fetal blood type.

Thought Questions

- Discuss maternal-fetal circulation and the fetal adaptations that facilitate fetal oxygenation.

- What is Rh D alloimmunization?

- What is the management of a pregnant Rh-negative woman who has been sensitized to Rh antigen?

- What is RhoGAM and how is it used?

Basic Science Review and Discussion

Fetal circulation is designed to maximize fetal oxygenation. Because the fetal lungs are functionally inactive until birth, the fetus is dependent on the placenta for oxygen and nutrition. The placenta also facilitates clearance of fetal waste. It consists of fetal villi that are bathed in maternal blood contained in the intervillous spaces and have a large surface area for exchange.

Oxygenated blood reaches the fetus from the placenta via the umbilical cord, which consists of one **umbilical vein** and two **umbilical arteries.** The umbilical vein transports maternally oxygenated blood, half of which passes through the fetal liver and the remainder of which bypasses the liver to the IVC via the **ductus venosus.** In the vena cava, blood from the ductus venosus, hepatic veins, and lower trunk and extremities combines. This blood then travels to the RA,

where the majority is shunted to the LA via the **foramen ovale,** which separates the two atria and allows oxygenated blood to bypass the pulmonary system. In fact, only one tenth of RV output goes to the lungs because of the large pulmonary resistance. The remainder of the blood bypasses the pulmonary system by traveling from the pulmonary artery through the **ductus arteriosus** to the aorta. Blood returns from the lungs to the LA and is subsequently pumped to the aorta and the rest of the body via the LV. Deoxygenated blood and fetal waste then return to the placenta via the umbilical arteries (Table 38-1).

Fetal blood is also designed to maximize fetal oxygenation. Fetal hemoglobin (**hemoglobin F**) has a higher affinity for oxygen than adult hemoglobin (hemoglobin A). Additionally, the fetal oxyhemoglobin dissociation curve is shifted to the left to favor fetal over maternal oxygenation. Sites of fetal hematopoiesis change with gestational age (GA), starting with the yolk sac and transitioning to the fetal liver, spleen, lymph nodes, and finally bone marrow.

At birth, the umbilical vessels are clamped and ligated, resulting in increased total peripheral resistance and BP. Additionally, the umbilical vessels, ductus arteriosus, and ductus venosus constrict. With the infant's first breath, pulmonary vascular resistance decreases to about one tenth of its previous level. This reverses the pressure gradient between the left and right atria and causes the foramen ovale to close and eventually fuse. Additionally, the pressure in the pulmonary artery falls to about half its previous

Table 38-1 Fetal circulatory adaptations

Structure	Purpose	Adult structure
Umbilical vein	Transport oxygenated blood to fetus	Ligamentum teres
Umbilical arteries	Return deoxygenated blood from fetus to placenta	Umbilical ligaments
Ductus venosus	Bypass oxygenated blood from liver to inferior vena cava	Ligamentum venosum
Foramen ovale	Bypass pulmonary system (RA to LA)	Closed foramen ovale
Ductus arteriosus	Bypass pulmonary system (pulmonary artery to aorta)	Ligamentum arteriosum

level, facilitating the reversal of flow through the ductus arteriosus, which proceeds to constrict and close over the course of 1 or 2 days.

Rh D Alloimmunization   The **D antigen,** also known as **rhesus factor** (Rh), is the most antigenic protein on the surface of erythrocytes. Rh incompatibility occurs when an Rh-negative woman (i.e., a woman who does not possess the D antigen on her erythrocytes) carries an Rh-positive fetus and is exposed to Rh-positive fetal blood during the pregnancy or labor. If the exposure is significant, she can form antibodies to D antigen and become alloimmunized. These antibodies can then cross the placenta and attack fetal erythrocytes that possess the D antigen in subsequent pregnancies, resulting in hemolysis, anemia, and possible **hydrops fetalis.** Aside from death, fetal hydrops is the most severe sequela of Rh D alloimmunization and consists of a hyperdynamic state resulting in fetal heart failure, diffuse edema, and ascites. Alternatively, if the fetus is Rh-negative, it will not be affected by circulating anti-D antibodies. In general, the pregnancy that causes the sensitization is not affected because the initial immune response is IgM, which does not cross the placenta. It is only with subsequent pregnancies that an IgG response is triggered.

Rh D alloimmunization can be prevented in unsensitized Rh-negative women by administration of **RhoGAM,** which is anti-D immunoglobulin that destroys fetal erythrocytes before a maternal immune response can be mounted. To be effective, RhoGAM must be administered any time fetal-maternal hemorrhage is a potential, including pregnancy, miscarriage, invasive procedures (e.g., amniocentesis), delivery, and abortion. Additionally, mismatched blood transfusion can also cause alloimmunization. Prior to administration of RhoGAM to an Rh-negative woman, an antibody screen and titer if appropriate should be performed to confirm that she has not already been sensitized. Once this is confirmed, routine prophylaxis includes administration of RhoGAM at 28 weeks of GA and again within 72 hours of delivery if the infant's blood type is undetermined or found to be Rh-positive. A standard dose of RhoGAM is 300 µg, which should cover maternal exposure to 30 mL of fetal blood. However, if maternal-fetal hemorrhage is suspected to exceed this amount, a **Kleihauer-Betke test** can be performed to quantitate the amount of fetal erythrocytes in the maternal circulation and allow for adjustment of RhoGAM dosing.

Management of the Rh D alloimmunized woman during pregnancy depends on the blood type of the fetus, which can be determined by amniocentesis. Alternatively, if paternity is certain and paternal blood type is Rh-negative, the fetus must therefore be Rh-negative as well and will not be affected. If fetal blood type is unknown or confirmed to be Rh-positive, maternal antibody titers should be followed serially. Pregnancies with titers less than 1:16 can be

managed expectantly. However, because titers of 1:16 or greater have been associated with fetal hydrops, serial amniocentesis should be performed in these pregnancies starting at 16 to 20 weeks to obtain amniotic fluid samples. Fetal hemolysis releases bilirubin into the amniotic fluid, which can then be analyzed by a spectrophotometer to measure the light absorption by bilirubin (ΔOD_{450}). These serial values are then plotted on the **Liley curve** (Figure 38-1), which is used to estimate the extent of fetal disease and guide management. The Liley curve is divided into three zones. Zone 1 indicates a mildly affected fetus, allowing the interval of amniocentesis to be every 2 to 3 weeks. Zone 2 indicates a moderately affected fetus that should undergo amniocentesis every 1 to 2 weeks. When ΔOD_{450} values enter zone 3, the fetus is assumed to be severely affected and should undergo weekly amniocentesis as well as detailed ultrasound examination to assess for signs of hydrops. Additional invasive therapeutic procedures can be performed if the fetus is severely affected. These procedures include intraperitoneal transfusion and **percutaneous umbilical cord sampling** (PUBS) during which time the PUBS needle can be used to transfuse the fetus if necessary. Premature delivery may be indicated in cases where the risk of remaining *in utero* exceeds that of prematurity. If premature delivery is likely and the fetus is beyond 24 weeks GA, a course of antenatal corticosteroids can be administered to promote fetal lung maturity.

Of note, several other erythrocyte antigens can also cause alloimmunization. These include ABO blood type, C, E, Kell,

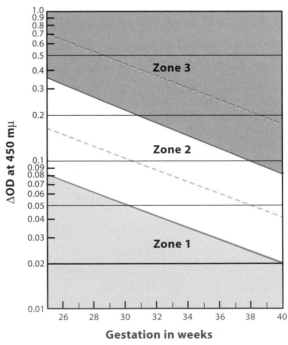

Figure 38-1 Liley curve used to depict severity of fetal hemolysis with red cell isoimmunization.

Duffy, and Lewis. The sequelae range from immune hydrops to mild hemolysis and anemia. These antigens are managed in a similar fashion to Rh D alloimmunization with the exception of RhoGAM administration.

Case Conclusion   At 16 weeks GA, the patient undergoes amniocentesis, which unfortunately confirms a fetal blood type of A-positive. During the amniocentesis, amniotic fluid is sampled to test for ΔOD_{450}. This returns a result in zone 1 of the Liley curve. The patient subsequently undergoes serial amniocentesis every 2 weeks. At 26 weeks GA, the ΔOD_{450} level enters zone 3 and fetal ultrasonography shows ascites. The patient is given a course of corticosteroids in anticipation of premature delivery and starts undergoing weekly PUBS transfusions. At 28 weeks GA, fetal ultrasound indicates worsening ascites as well as the presence of a pericardial effusion. The risk of fetal harm is determined to exceed that of maintaining the pregnancy and the patient undergoes delivery via cesarean section.

Thumbnail: Maternal-Fetal Circulation

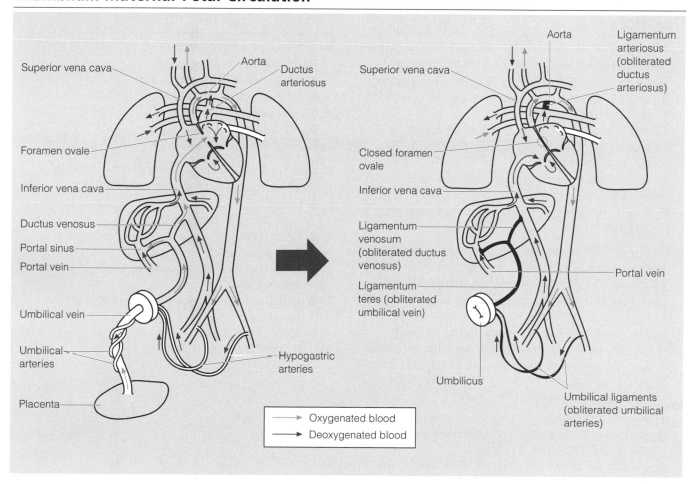

Key Points

▸ Fetal adaptations such as the foramen ovale, ductus arteriosus, and ductus venosus allow maximal fetal oxygenation by bypassing functionally inactive structures.

▸ The decrease in pulmonary vascular resistance caused by lung inflation at birth reverses the pressure gradient between the atria and causes the foramen ovale to close.

▸ The umbilical vessels, ductus arteriosus, and ductus venosus constrict at birth.

▸ Fetal hemoglobin and the fetal oxyhemoglobin dissociation curve favor fetal over maternal oxygenation.

▸ D antigen, or rhesus factor, is the most antigenic protein found on erythrocytes and can cause immune fetal hydrops when maternal antibodies cross the placenta and cause fetal hemolysis and anemia.

Questions

1. Which of the following is not an absolute indication for RhoGAM administration in an Rh D-negative woman?

   A. An Rh D-negative woman at 28 weeks of gestation
   B. An Rh D-negative woman who has just delivered at 37 weeks GA
   C. An Rh D-negative woman who has just experienced a spontaneous abortion at 10 weeks of gestation
   D. An Rh D-negative woman undergoing an amniocentesis
   E. An Rh D-negative woman with a ruptured ectopic pregnancy

2. You have been following an Rh D-negative woman with antibody titers of 1:32 at her intake obstetric visit and a prior history of a mildly affected infant requiring no interventions by performing serial amniocenteses for ΔOD_{450} values. Her prior ΔOD_{450} values have resided within Liley zone 1 but have slowly been increasing. Today at her 29-week prenatal visit, she is found to have a ΔOD_{450} value within Liley zone 3. However, ultrasonography shows no signs of fetal hydrops. What is the next step in the management of this patient?

   A. Immediate delivery.
   B. PUBS to determine severity of fetal disease and possible IV transfusion if indicated.
   C. Confirm presence of fetal lung maturity and deliver as soon as it is achieved.
   D. Short course of antenatal corticosteroids followed by immediate delivery.
   E. Continued serial amniocenteses to assess ΔOD_{450} value trends and PUBS and transfusion as indicated.

3. Which of the following can be an indication of severe fetal disease?

   A. ΔOD_{450} value in Liley curve zone 3
   B. Fetal ascites
   C. Fetal pericardial effusion
   D. Fetal pleural effusion
   E. All of the above

4. Which of the following fetal structures is correctly matched to its purpose in fetal circulation?

   A. Ductus arteriosus—bypass liver by shunting blood from umbilical vein to IVC
   B. Ductus venosus—bypass lungs by shunting blood from pulmonary artery to aorta
   C. Foramen ovale—Bypass lungs by shunting blood from RA to LA
   D. Umbilical vein—transport deoxygenated fetal blood back to placenta
   E. None of the above

HPI: BD is a 53-year-old man who presents complaining of inability to maintain an erection for the past month despite normal libido. His past medical history is significant for HTN and mild acid reflux. He denies tobacco usage but reports a glass of wine with dinner each night. His medications include cimetidine and metoprolol.

PE: On physical exam, his BP is within normal limits and he is mildly obese.

Thought Questions

- Discuss the sexual response cycle.

- Compare and contrast male and female sexual response.

- Discuss the various etiologies for erectile dysfunction.

Basic Science Review and Discussion

Human sexuality differs from that of most animals in that procreation is not the only purpose for sexual interaction. Rather, pleasure and recreation also drive human sexual behavior. Masters and Johnson first described the human sexual response cycle in the 1960s. Their description included four major phases: excitement, plateau, orgasm, and resolution. In addition to these four phases, sexual attraction or arousal can be included in the human sexual response cycle.

Sexual attraction and arousal vary immensely from individual to individual as well as between different cultures. While groups may place value on different external features such as breast size, the factors that appear to be universally considered attractive are health and youth. The **excitement phase** occurs when stimuli from the preceding stage initiate physiologic changes. This manifests as penile erection in males when the corpora cavernosa and corpus spongiosum become engorged, which is mediated by the parasympathetic system and blood supply of the penis. Vaginal lubrication, lengthening of the vagina, vasocongestion of the clitoris, and engorgement of the labia minora occur in females. These changes intensify in the **plateau phase.** In males, the testes increase in size due to vasocongestion, the scrotum is drawn toward the perineum, and HR, BP, and muscle tension increase. Plateau phase in the female is marked by intense red coloration of the labia minora from vasocongestion, clitoral retraction behind the clitoral hood, and increased HR and BP. If stimulation continues to a sufficient degree, release of sexual tension via **orgasm** occurs. In males, this is mediated by the sympathetic system and is characterized by ejaculation of semen from the penis via rhythmic contractions of smooth muscles in the urethra, and bulbocavernosus and ischiocavernosus muscles. Female orgasm also involves rhythmic contractions of smooth muscles, but there is no ejaculation. Unlike males, females do not have a refractory period during which further stimulation cannot elicit further sexual response; as such, females are capable of prolonged and multiple orgasms. **Resolution** occurs as vascular congestion and muscle tension resolve. The penis becomes flaccid and refractory to further stimulation, while in females, the labia and clitoris decongest.

Erectile dysfunction is the inability to attain or maintain an erection satisfactory for intercourse. Data from the Massachusetts Male Aging study suggest that it affects approximately 50% of men. Although the etiology is often multifactorial in aging men, the most common cause is vascular, as would be suggested by the strikingly high incidence in men with diabetes, HTN, and cardiovascular disease. Atherosclerosis causes arterial flow abnormalities, while venous leakage can cause cavernosal problems. In addition to vascular abnormalities, other etiologies include medications, neurologic and psychiatric factors, and endocrine abnormalities. Several classes of medications can cause erectile dysfunction, including beta-blockers, thiazide diuretics, antidepressants, NSAIDs, and H2 blockers. Additionally, tobacco, alcohol, and opiates also contribute to erectile dysfunction. Neurologic and psychiatric etiologies consist of autonomic and peripheral neuropathies, multiple sclerosis, stroke, temporal lobe epilepsy, spinal cord injuries, depression, and anxiety. Several endocrine abnormalities can lead to erectile dysfunction. In particular, diabetes causes vascular changes, accelerated atherosclerosis, and autonomic and peripheral neuropathies. Erectile dysfunction has also been seen with Cushing's syndrome, hypothyroidism, hyperthyroidism, and hyperprolactinemia. Because the etiologies of erectile dysfunction are so varied and multifactorial, evaluation and determination of treatment options must be methodical and include a thorough social and medication history and physical exam (Figure 39-1).

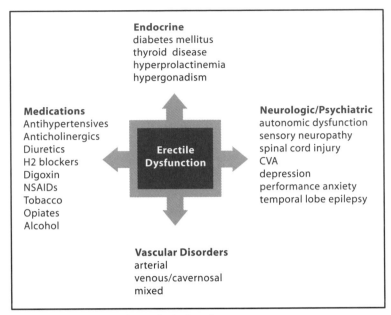

Figure 39-1 Etiologies of erectile dysfunction.

Case Conclusion After careful review of the patient's medications, you discover that he was recently started on metoprolol. Although the patient has several risk factors for erectile dysfunction, including his other medication (an H2 blocker) and HTN, you decide to change his medication to an ACE inhibitor, which has been associated with fewer cases of erectile dysfunction.

Thumbnail: Human Sexual Response Cycle

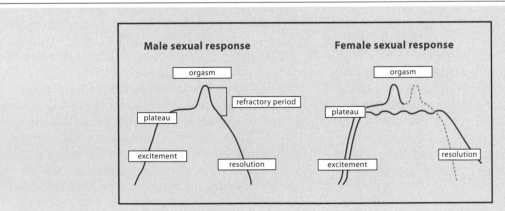

Key Points

▶ Unlike most animals, the purposes of human sexual interaction include procreation as well as pleasure and recreation.

▶ There are five phases of the human sexual response cycle: sexual attraction and arousal, excitement, plateau, orgasm, and resolution.

▶ Male sexual response differs primarily from that of females because males must undergo a refractory period during which time the penis is incapable of responding to further stimulation, whereas females are capable of experiencing multiple orgasms in rapid succession; additionally, unlike females, male orgasm involves ejaculation of semen.

▶ Erectile dysfunction is the inability to attain or maintain an erection satisfactory for intercourse.

▶ Etiologies of erectile dysfunction are varied and often multifactorial, including vascular, neurologic, psychiatric, endocrine, and medication-induced.

Questions

1. Which of the following correctly orders the phases of the human sexual response cycle?
   A. Excitement, sexual arousal, plateau, orgasm, resolution
   B. Excitement, sexual arousal, orgasm, plateau, resolution
   C. Sexual arousal, plateau, excitement, orgasm, resolution
   D. Sexual arousal, excitement, plateau, orgasm, resolution
   E. Sexual arousal, excitement, orgasm, plateau, resolution

2. A 48-year-old man presents to your office complaining of impotence and requesting Viagra. On further history, you discover that the patient is not taking any medications, and he denies any significant medical or social history. Physical exam is essentially within normal limits with the exception of moderate obesity. You run several lab tests and discover that the patient has a fasting glucose of 182 mg/dL. The patient is diagnosed with DM and subsequent evaluation suggests possible long-standing disease that is the likely cause of the patient's erectile dysfunction. Which of the following is not a cause of erectile dysfunction?
   A. Stroke
   B. Depression
   C. Acid reflux
   D. Hyperthyroidism
   E. Atherosclerosis

HPI: MP is a 50-year-old G3P3 woman who presents complaining of having hot flushes and night sweats for approximately 2 months. In addition, her periods have been irregular for the past several months. She thinks she has entered menopause but would like to make sure and see if there is any treatment for her hot flushes, which are disrupting and embarrassing.

Her past gynecologic history is significant for previously regular menses, three vaginal deliveries, and a tubal ligation at age 37. She reports mildly elevated cholesterol but is otherwise in good health. She denies a family history of osteoporosis or gynecologic cancers.

PE: On physical exam, she is slim and appears her stated age. A rectovaginal exam is within normal limits. An FSH level is sent.

Thought Questions

- Define menopause.
- How is menopause diagnosed?
- What is the physiology of menopause?
- Discuss the changes associated with menopause.
- Discuss hormone replacement therapy (HRT).

Basic Science Review and Discussion

Menopause is the permanent cessation of menstruation and marks the end of ovarian, and hence reproductive, function in women. It is preceded by the **climacteric** or perimenopause, which is the time period during which a woman transitions into menopause and undergoes characteristic physiologic changes. The mean age of menopause in the United States is 51 but ranges from ages 45 to 55. Additionally, smoking has been shown to hasten the onset of menopause.

Menopause is typically diagnosed by clinical history and supportive physical findings. Patients will often present in their late forties to early fifties with complaints of vasomotor instability, irregular or absent menses, and mood changes. While these symptoms typically resolve within a year, some women can remain symptomatic for several years. Physical findings consistent with menopause include decrease in breast size, and vaginal atrophy and dryness. If a woman presents with menopausal symptoms and signs before the age of 40, premature ovarian failure should be investigated.

The ovarian failure that precedes menopause develops as a result of ovarian follicle atresia and eventual disappearance, leading to reduced estrogen production. The ovary subsequently becomes shriveled. However, postmenopausal women have alternate sources of estrogen, which are derived primarily from peripheral conversion of ovarian and adrenal androgens. Of note, obese women have higher circulating estrogen levels due to increased peripheral conversion in adipose cells. In response to decreased estrogen production, the gonadotropins increase. In particular, FSH levels increase 10- to 20-fold. As such, an elevated FSH level is often used to confirm menopause. Additionally, LH levels triple. Gonadotropin levels peak 1 to 3 years after menopause and then decline gradually over time.

The diminished ovarian estrogen production that defines menopause results in most of the characteristic changes of menopause. **Vasomotor instability** affects approximately 70% of perimenopausal women, causing the characteristic **hot flushes** or flashes, which are described as the sensation of intense warmth, ascending flushing, and diaphoresis, lasting approximately 1 to 5 minutes. They are due to acute estrogen withdrawal rather than decreased estrogen levels. As such, they should decline with time. Additionally, obese women tend to be less symptomatic due to higher circulating levels of estrogen. If vasomotor instability symptoms are unbearable, estrogen replacement can be prescribed to assist the patient through the perimenopausal period. If the patient has not undergone hysterectomy in the past, progesterone should be given in conjunction with estrogen to protect the endometrium from unopposed estrogen exposure. Nonhormonal treatments for vasomotor instability include clonidine, some selective serotonin reuptake inhibitors (SSRIs), behavioral therapy, and herbal medications.

Because estrogen inhibits bone resorption by osteoclasts, the risk of osteoporosis increases with menopause when increased bone resorption coupled with decreased bone formation leads to net bone loss. A **bone mineral density** scan can be used to diagnose bone loss as either **osteoporosis** (2.5 standard deviations or more below the adult peak mean) or **osteopenia** (1.0–2.5 standard deviations below the mean). Risk factors for osteoporosis include white or Asian ethnicity, low body mass index, family history of osteoporosis, and smoking. Osteoporosis predisposes women to bone fractures that can result in disability and death. As with the treatment of vasomotor instability, estrogen replacement is a treatment option, but due to recent evidence linking estrogen replacement with increased risks of cancer, heart attack, and stroke, alternative treatments such as calcitonin and bisphosphonates may be more appropriate. Additionally, selective estrogen receptor modulators (SERMs) such as raloxifene have been shown to have estrogen-agonist effects on bone but estrogen-antagonist effects on breast and endometrial tissues.

Atrophy of the genital tract due to estrogen loss can lead to dyspareunia, vaginismus, dysuria, and other urinary symptoms. These can be treated with estrogen replacement as well as local estrogen creams.

Until recently, hormone replacement therapy (HRT) was prescribed on a long-term basis for almost all perimenopausal women for the treatment of symptoms as well as prevention of osteoporosis and cardiovascular disease. Although HRT has been associated with increased risks for breast cancer as well as endometrial hyperplasia and cancer, the benefits of HRT were previously believed to outweigh these risks in most women, and thus it was widely prescribed. However, recent evidence challenges this practice, particularly with regard to cardiovascular disease. The Women's Health Initiative (WHI), a long-term study by the National Institutes of Health (NIH), was designed to study the relationship between HRT and its effects on heart disease, hip fractures, breast cancer, endometrial cancer, and blood clots. However, after 5 years, the study was prematurely terminated in July 2002 when preliminary analyses revealed increased risks for breast cancer, heart disease, stroke, and blood clots. While the individual risks were small, they were considered significant given that HRT is taken by millions of women over many years, which could result in a large number of women developing the above conditions. Additionally, the small increase in individual risk appears to be cumulative for certain conditions, such as breast cancer.

To be complete, the WHI also showed some benefits of HRT. Specifically, the risks for colon cancer and bone fracture were both reduced. Given all these findings, it is currently recommended that HRT be prescribed to a perimenopausal woman who is affected by menopausal symptoms only after careful discussion and consideration of her potential risks and benefits from HRT; and even in such situations, a limited trial of HRT is often prescribed. Additionally, women currently on HRT have been encouraged to discuss possible cessation of HRT with their health-care providers. Of note, a separate WHI trial looking at estrogen use in women with a prior hysterectomy is ongoing because similar adverse effects have not been seen. Until further evidence is provided, use of HRT must be considered on a case-by-case basis.

Case Conclusion After careful review of the patient's history as well as a discussion of possible risks and benefits of HRT, the patient elects to implement a new exercise and diet regimen that includes calcium supplementation to counteract her risks of heart disease and osteoporosis rather than start HRT.

Thumbnail: Menopause

Change	Treatment options
Vasomotor instability	Clonidine SSRIs Behavioral therapy Herbal medications Hormone replacement
Osteoporosis	Calcitonin Bisphosphonates SERMs Hormone replacement
Genital atrophy	Local estrogen replacement Vaginal lubricants

Key Points

▶ Menopause is the permanent cessation of menses due to diminished ovarian estrogen production and marks the end of a woman's reproductive life.

▶ The mean age of menopause is 51 years.

▶ The characteristic signs and symptoms of menopause include hot flushes, vaginal atrophy and dryness, and osteoporosis.

▶ Menopause is diagnosed clinically by history and physical exam but can be confirmed by elevated levels of FSH.

▶ Osteoporosis is one of the major sequelae of diminished estrogen and can be treated with calcitonin, bisphosphonates, SERMs, and hormone replacement in select individuals.

▶ Treatments for menopausal symptoms include herbal medications, behavioral therapy, clonidine, SSRIs, and hormone replacement in select individuals.

▶ Hormone replacement has been associated with increased risks of heart disease, hip fractures, breast cancer, endometrial cancer, and blood clots and is therefore only indicated in individuals in whom the benefits outweigh these risks.

Questions

1. A 54-year-old G4P4 presents complaining of amenorrhea for approximately 1 year but continues to have persistent vasomotor symptoms. She has weighed the risks and benefits of HRT and feels strongly that she would like a trial of HRT. Which of the following is associated with HRT?
   A. Decreased risk for colon cancer
   B. Decreased risk for uterine cancer
   C. Decreased risk for heart disease
   D. Decreased risk for breast cancer
   E. All of the above

2. Which of the following signs and symptoms are seen in menopause?
   A. Decreased breast size
   B. Night sweats
   C. Vaginal atrophy
   D. Hot flushes
   E. All of the above

3. A 49-year-old Asian woman who is perimenopausal and does not wish to take HRT comes to your office to discuss potential treatments and lifestyle changes that she can take to prevent osteoporosis. Her mother passed away after a prolonged hospitalization that began when she fell and broke her hip. On exam, the patient is 5 feet tall and 100 pounds. Her exam is within normal limits. Which of the following are risk factors for osteoporosis?
   A. White or Asian ethnicity
   B. Low body mass index
   C. Smoking
   D. Family history of osteoporosis
   E. All of the above

HPI: PB is a 47-year-old G5P2 woman who recently immigrated from China and presents to your office for her first pelvic exam. She reports recurrent postcoital bleeding for several months and now has irregular menses. She is sexually active with her husband only, and her gynecologic history includes two spontaneous vaginal deliveries, three therapeutic abortions, and regular menses until 5 months ago. Her past medical history is significant for hepatitis B infection and tubal ligation at age 37.

PE: On physical exam, she is found to have a large, friable lesion involving the right side of her cervix. No adnexal masses are palpated, and rectovaginal exam reveals that the mass does not involve the parametria or cul de sac. You suspect cervical cancer and refer the patient to gynecologic oncology for further evaluation and treatment.

Thought Questions

- What is the incidence of cervical cancer, and what are the associated risk factors?
- How can we screen for cervical cancer?
- Discuss cervical dysplasia.
- How is cervical cancer staged?
- Discuss the treatment of cervical cancer.

Basic Science Review and Discussion

An estimated 15,000 women are diagnosed with cervical cancer in the United States every year. With approximately 4,600 deaths per year, cervical cancer is the sixth leading cause of death from cancer in women in the United States. In undeveloped countries where screening is unavailable, cervical cancer is the leading cause of cancer deaths in women.

Infection with **human papilloma virus (HPV)** causes over 90% of cervical cancer cases, especially infections due to genotypes 16, 18, and 31. Other risk factors for cervical cancer include cigarette smoking, early onset of sexual activity, large number of sexual partners, and history of sexually transmitted diseases, especially human immunodeficiency virus (HIV).

Because the natural history of cervical cancer is typically slow and predictable, starting with dysplasia and moving to **cervical intraepithelial neoplasia (CIN)** and finally invasive disease, early detection can lead to improved outcomes. The **Papanicolaou smear,** or Pap smear, was implemented in the 1950s to screen for cervical dysplasia and cancer. It involves scraping cells from the cervix to sample the squamocolumnar junction, or transformation zone. Pap smears should be performed annually in all sexually active women and those over the age of 18. Screening frequency can be adjusted depending on risk factors and presence of dysplasia.

Cervical cytology is evaluated using the Bethesda System, which classifies epithelial cell abnormalities in the following manner: atypical squamous cells of undetermined significance (**ASCUS**); low grade squamous intraepithelial lesion (**LGSIL**) or **CIN I;** or high grade squamous intraepithelial lesion (**HGSIL**), which encompasses **CIN II** and **CIN III.** ASCUS can be due to inflammation or preinvasive lesions. Determination of CIN grade is dependent on the depth of epithelial involvement. In CIN I, the lower one third of cells are abnormal, while CIN II involves the lower two thirds, and CIN III is full-thickness involvement.

Approximately 80% to 85% of ASCUS and 30% of CIN I changes will resolve on follow-up Pap smear. As such, ASCUS and LGSIL Pap smears can be managed with repeat Pap testing every 4 to 6 months for 2 years, provided they remain normal, or with evaluation by colposcopy, endocervical curettage, and directed biopsy. **Colposcopy** is the microscopic evaluation of the transformation zone to identify abnormal areas that may display acetowhite epithelium, mosaicism, punctation, or atypical vessels. Additionally, HPV probes are currently used at some institutions to detect HPV serotypes and guide management in the presence of ASCUS Pap smear results.

While cervical cancer is typically a slowly progressing disease, taking approximately 7 years for CIN I and 4 years for CIN II to progress to invasive cervical cancer, occasional lesions can progress quite rapidly. Along with the above management of ASCUS and LGSIL Pap smear findings, current recommendations include treatment of CIN II and III with cryosurgery, laser surgery, loop electrosurgical excision procedure (LEEP), cervical conization, or hysterectomy depending on the severity of the lesion.

Approximately 80% of cervical cancer is squamous cell carcinoma, which can be subdivided into small cell, large cell keratinizing, and large cell nonkeratinizing. The remaining 10% to 20% of cases are mostly adenocarcinoma. Of note, clear cell carcinoma is a type of adenocarcinoma that is associated with in utero exposure to DES. Other rare types of cervical cancer are sarcoma and lymphoma.

While the classic presentation of cervical cancer is postcoital bleeding, other symptoms include watery discharge, rectal or urinary tract symptoms, abnormal vaginal bleeding, and pelvic pressure or pain. Findings consistent with cervical cancer on physical exam are an exophytic, ulcerative, papillary, or necrotic lesion involving the cervix and possibly vagina, and/or palpable lesions that extend from the cervix to the vagina, adnexa, or cul de sac. Suspicious lesions should be examined via biopsy for histologic diagnosis.

Staging of cervical cancer is clinical rather than surgical and is determined by the degree of invasion into adjacent structures and the presence of distant metastasis. Formal staging involves examination under anesthesia, chest x-ray, cystoscopy, proctoscopy, and occasionally IV pyelography, barium enema, or CT scan.

Stage IA1 (microinvasive disease) can be treated with cone biopsy excision, if the patient wishes to retain fertility, or with simple hysterectomy. **Cone biopsy** excision is the removal of a wedge-shaped portion of the cervical stroma and endocervical canal. Depending on the patient's medical status and age, hysterectomy or radiation can be performed if the cancer has not spread beyond the cervix, uterus, and vagina (stage IIA or less). With more advanced disease (stage IIB to IV), the treatment is chemoradiation, which involves weekly cisplatin and external beam radiation followed by brachytherapy (local application of radiation). Chemoradiation is also used for palliative purposes.

Prognosis of cervical cancer depends on lymph node metastases, tumor size, depth of invasion, and positive surgical margins. Five-year survival rates are as follows: stage I 85% to 90%; stage II 60% to 75%; stage III 35% to 45%; and stage IV 15% to 20%. While screening and treatment of preinvasive disease have led to a decrease in the incidence of cervical cancer, efforts continue to further improve current screening and treatment modalities as well as the development of a potential vaccine to human papillomavirus.

Case Conclusion   The patient is evaluated by gynecologic oncology and determined to have stage IIA disease. She subsequently undergoes radical hysterectomy with negative surgical margins and is scheduled for frequent follow-up appointments.

Thumbnail: International Federation of Gynecology and Obstetrics (FIGO) Staging for Cervical Cancer

Stage	Findings
Stage 0	Carcinoma in situ, intraepithelial carcinoma.
Stage I	The carcinoma is strictly confined to the cervix.
Stage IA	Invasive cancer identified only microscopically and limited to a maximum depth of 5 mm and no wider than 7 mm.
Stage IA1	Invasion ≤ 3 mm depth and no wider than 7 mm.
Stage IA2	Invasion 3–5 mm depth and no wider than 7 mm.
Stage IB	Clinical lesions confined to the cervix or preclinical lesions more extensive than stage IA.
Stage IB1	Clinical lesions ≤ 4.0 cm in size.
Stage IB2	Clinical lesions > 4.0 cm in size.
Stage II	The carcinoma extends beyond the cervix but has not extended to the pelvic wall. Vaginal involvement does not reach the lower third.
Stage IIA	No obvious parametrial involvement.
Stage IIB	Obvious parametrial involvement.
Stage III	The carcinoma has extended to the pelvic wall. No cancer-free space between tumor and pelvic wall on rectal exam. Lower one third of vagina involved. Hydronephrosis or nonfunctioning kidney.
Stage IIIA	No extension to the pelvic wall.
Stage IIIB	Extension to the pelvic wall and/or hydronephrosis or nonfunctioning kidney.
Stage IV	The carcinoma has extended beyond the true pelvis or involves the mucosa of the bladder or rectum.
Stage IVA	Spread to adjacent organs.
Stage IVB	Spread to distant organs.

Used with permission from the International Federation of Gynecology and Obstetrics.

Key Points

- Cervical cancer is the sixth leading cause of cancer death in the United States, and the leading cause of cancer death in undeveloped countries.

- Risk factors for cervical cancer include HPV infection, early age of first sexual activity, large number of sexual partners, cigarette smoking, and history of sexually transmitted infections.

- Pap smears are used to screen for cervical cancer and should be performed annually in all sexually active women or women over the age of 18.

- Without treatment, cervical dysplasia typically progresses slowly to CIN and finally to invasive cervical cancer.

- Treatment of cervical dysplasia and cancer varies depending on desired fertility and degree of invasion.

Questions

1. A 20-year-old woman presents for routine pelvic exam. She is sexually active and uses condoms occasionally. She began sexual activity at age 13 and has had seven lifetime partners. She has been treated for both chlamydia and gonorrhea over the past 3 years and experiences five to six urinary tract infections per year. She started menstruating at age 13 and continues to have irregular menses. Which of the following is not a risk factor for cervical dysplasia or cancer?

   A. Chlamydial infection
   B. Multiple sexual partners
   C. Recurrent urinary tract infections
   D. Cigarette smoking
   E. Early age of first sexual activity

2. In the process of performing an endometrial biopsy on a 56-year-old woman with postmenopausal bleeding, you notice an exophytic mass on the posterior portion of her cervix. A biopsy of this area shows squamous cell carcinoma. Which of the following is used to stage her disease?

   A. MRI
   B. Physical exam
   C. Margins from hysterectomy specimen
   D. Lymph node dissection
   E. All of the above

3. A 32-year-old woman is diagnosed with CIN II on Pap smear. Which of the following would not be appropriate management?

   A. Hysterectomy
   B. Cervical conization
   C. Loop electrosurgical excision procedure
   D. Cryotherapy
   E. Radiation

HPI: PM is a 61-year-old G2P0 woman who presents to your office complaining of increasing abdominal girth, bloating, and fatigue over the past 4 months. Her past medical history is significant for a tonsillectomy as a child and two first trimester miscarriages in her thirties. She reports regular menses until menopause at age 52.

PE: On physical exam, she is found to have a large abdomen with a demonstrable fluid wave. Rectovaginal exam reveals a left pelvic mass that is approximately 10 cm in diameter, nontender, and nonmobile. Suspecting ovarian cancer, you check a CA-125 level and send her for a pelvic ultrasound.

Thought Questions

- What is the epidemiology of ovarian cancer?
- How does ovarian cancer present?
- Discuss staging and treatment of ovarian cancer.
- Discuss the histologic types of ovarian neoplasms.

Basic Science Review and Discussion

Ovarian cancer is the fourth leading cause of cancer deaths in women, with approximately 15,000 deaths and 26,000 new cases diagnosed annually in the United States. The lifetime risk of developing ovarian cancer is roughly 1.5% in the general population. However, this risk is 10- to 20-fold higher in the 5% to 10% of ovarian cancers that are hereditary and due to *BRCA1* or *BRCA2* mutations. Ovarian cancer has a greater incidence in industrialized countries and women of low parity. Age appears to be the most important risk factor, with the median age of diagnosis being 61 years. Alternatively, factors that decrease the number of lifetime ovulations such as multiparity, breast-feeding, oral contraceptive use, and chronic anovulation appear to be protective against ovarian cancer.

Unfortunately, early signs of ovarian cancer are rare. As such, many women are diagnosed with advanced disease by the time they present with complaints of abdominal discomfort, increasing abdominal girth, and early satiety. Evaluation of suspected ovarian cancer should include a complete history and physical examination, as well as ultrasonography to characterize any pelvic masses and confirm the presence of ascites. Masses that are larger than 8 cm, solid, multilocular, and bilateral are suspicious for malignancy. In the case of advanced disease, CT scan is useful for treatment planning. Serum **CA-125** (a tumor marker) levels may be elevated, but are usually not useful in premenopausal women because other conditions can elevate CA-125 levels (e.g., endometriosis, pancreatitis).

Ovarian cancer is surgically staged (see Thumbnail). Complete staging includes obtaining pelvic washings, abdominal exploration of peritoneal surfaces, liver, bowel, and lymph nodes, biopsy of the omentum, possible appendectomy, and usually total abdominal hysterectomy and bilateral salpingo-oophorectomy (TAH-BSO). Removal of all gross disease should be attempted. Chemotherapy is usually recommended for stages IC and higher, with the typical regimen being six cycles of **carboplatin** and **paclitaxel.** Frequent follow-up evaluation during the first 2 years is critical, because the majority of recurrences will appear during this time. History, physical exam, and serial serum CA-125 levels should be evaluated. Signs and symptoms of recurrence can include small bowel obstruction, indigestion, ascites, or palpable pelvic mass. Additionally, CA-125 levels may be elevated. The most important prognostic factor is surgical stage, but other factors include patient age, extent of residual disease after debulking surgery, and volume of ascites. The overall 5-year survival rate for ovarian cancer is 35% (Table 42-1).

Many histologic subtypes of ovarian cancer exist (See Box 42-1). However, the majority (85%–90%) of ovarian cancers are epithelial in origin. The epithelial subtypes include **serous** (50%–70%), **mucinous** (10%–15%), **endometrioid, undifferentiated,** and **clear cell.** Additionally, there are tumors of low malignant potential known as **borderline ovarian tumors** that constitute 10% to 15% of epithelial ovarian cancers. These borderline tumors predominantly occur in young, premenopausal women and are mostly serous in origin. Treatment consists of unilateral oophorectomy to preserve fertility and complete surgical staging. These tumors rarely require adjuvant chemotherapy, and patients have an excellent 10-year survival rate of 95%.

Germ cell tumors (5%–7%) are the second group of ovarian cancers. They usually occur in young women and treatment involves unilateral oophorectomy if preservation of fertility

Table 42-1 Ovarian cancer: five-year survival rates

Stage	5-year survival (%)
I	75–95
II	45–65
III	20–40
IV	10–15

Box 42-1 Ovarian cancer histologic types

Epithelial Tumors (85%–90%)
Serous (50%–70%)
Mucinous (10%–15%)
Endometrioid (<5%)
Undifferentiated (<5%)
Clear cell (<5%)
Brenner tumor
Mixed mesodermal tumor

Germ Cell Tumors (5%–7%)
Dysgerminomas (3%)
Endodermal sinus tumor (<1%)
Embryonal carcinoma (<1%)
Immature teratoma (<1%)
Choriocarcinoma (<1%)

Sex Cord Stromal Tumors (5%–7%)
Granulosa cell tumors (3%–4%)
Sertoli-Leydig tumors (<1%)

Neoplasms Metastatic to Ovary
Gastrointestinal tract (Krukenberg)
Breast
Endometrium
Lymphoma

is desired. Otherwise, TAH-BSO and complete surgical staging can be performed. Radiation (for dysgerminomas only) and combination chemotherapy are also utilized. The subtypes of germ cell tumors include **dysgerminomas** (50%), which carry a long-term survival rate of 85% and can be followed by **lactate dehydrogenase** (LDH) as a tumor marker; **endodermal sinus tumors,** which can be followed by serum **alpha-fetoprotein** (AFP) levels; **embryonal carcinomas, choriocarcinoma,** and **immature teratomas.**

Sex cord stromal tumors (5%–7%) are the last group of ovarian cancers and include **granulosa cell tumors** (70%) and **Sertoli-Leydig tumors** (rare). Since these tumors produce hormones, signs and symptoms are often related to excess hormone production (e.g., virilism). Treatment is similar to that for germ cell tumors.

Case Conclusion Pelvic ultrasonography shows massive ascites and a 10-cm multiloculated mass that has both solid and cystic components. Additionally, her CA-125 level is very elevated. The patient is immediately referred to gynecologic oncology for further evaluation and subsequently undergoes exploratory laparotomy with complete surgical staging to reveal stage IIIC serous cystadenocarcinoma of the left ovary. She is scheduled for six cycles of carboplatin and paclitaxel.

Thumbnail: FIGO Staging of Ovarian Cancer

Stage	Findings
Stage I	Growth limited to the ovaries.
Stage IA	Growth limited to one ovary. No ascites. No tumor on the external surface, capsule intact.
Stage IB	Growth limited to both ovaries. No ascites. No tumor on the external surface, capsule intact.
Stage IC	Tumor either stage IA or IB but with tumor on surface of one or both ovaries; or with capsule ruptured; or with ascites containing malignant cells; or with positive peritoneal washings.
Stage II	Growth involving one or both ovaries with pelvic extension.
Stage IIA	Extension and/or metastases to the uterus and/or tubes.
Stage IIB	Extension to other pelvic tissues.
Stage IIC	Tumor either stage IIA or IIB, but with tumor on surface of one or both ovaries; or with capsule(s) ruptured; or with ascites containing malignant cells; or with positive peritoneal washings.
Stage III	Tumor involving one or both ovaries with peritoneal implants outside the pelvis and/or positive retroperitoneal or inguinal nodes. Superficial liver metastasis. Tumor is limited to true pelvis but with histologically proven malignant extension to small bowel or omentum.
Stage IIIA	Tumor grossly limited to true pelvis with negative nodes but with histologically confirmed microscopic seeding of peritoneal surfaces.
Stage IIIB	Tumor of one or both ovaries with histologically confirmed peritoneal implants < 2 cm in diameter. Negative nodes.
Stage IIIC	Abdominal implants > 2 cm in diameter and/or positive retroperitoneal or inguinal nodes.
Stage IV	Growth involving one or both ovaries with distant metastases. Parenchymal liver metastasis.

Used with permission from the International Federation of Gynecology and Obstetrics.

Key Points

- In the United States, ovarian cancer is the fourth leading cause of cancer death in women.

- The median age of diagnosis is 61 years.

- Protective factors for ovarian cancer include multiparity, breast-feeding, oral contraceptive use, and chronic anovulation.

- The majority (85%–90%) of ovarian cancers are epithelial in origin.

- Early symptoms of cervical cancer are rare, and diagnosis of disease in advanced stages is not uncommon.

- Ovarian cancer is surgically staged and treated with surgery and platinum-based chemotherapeutic agents.

- The overall 5-year survival rate for patients with epithelial ovarian cancers is 35%.

- Germ cell tumors comprise 5% to 7% of ovarian neoplasms and include dysgerminomas, immature teratomas, embryonal cell carcinomas, and endodermal sinus tumors.

- The overall 5-year survival rate for patients with germ cell tumors is 60% to 85%.

- Sex cord stromal tumors comprise 5% to 7% of ovarian neoplasms and typically occur in postmenopausal women.

- Sex cord stromal tumors produce hormones and include granulosa cell and Sertoli-Leydig tumors.

Questions

1. A 20-year-old virginal woman presents complaining of abdominal fullness and pain that started 2 months ago. Her menses are regular and she does not have any other medical problems. Your pelvic exam reveals a large right-sided mass that is suspicious for malignancy on ultrasonography. Which of the following tumor markers is matched to the correct neoplasm?

   A. Dysgerminomas—lactate dehydrogenase (LDH)
   B. Endodermal sinus tumor—CA-125
   C. Immature teratoma—hCG
   D. Embryonal carcinoma—LDH
   E. Choriocarcinoma—AFP

2. A 67-year-old woman undergoes exploratory laparotomy for a suspicious pelvic mass. During her surgery, a large amount of ascites is collected for evaluation. Additionally, a 12-cm mass encompassing the left ovary and tube with an intact-appearing capsule is removed in addition to the uterus and right adnexa. Her omentum, bowel, liver edge, and inguinal and retroperitoneal lymph nodes all appear grossly normal, but biopsy samples are still obtained. Her surgical pathology returns negative for malignant cells in the ascites or peritoneal and lymph node biopsy samples. Additionally, the tumor is confirmed to be serous adenocarcinoma but has not ruptured the ovarian capsule. What is the patient's stage?

   A. Stage IA
   B. Stage IC
   C. Stage IIA
   D. Stage IIC
   E. Stage IIIA

3. Which of the following correctly orders the types of ovarian neoplasms in order from most common to least common?

   A. Mucinous, serous, endometrioid, embryonal carcinoma
   B. Mucinous, endodermal sinus tumor, borderline tumors, dysgerminoma
   C. Serous, Sertoli-Leydig, choriocarcinoma, clear cell
   D. Serous, mucinous, granulosa cell, immature teratoma
   E. Dysgerminoma, immature teratoma, borderline tumors, mucinous

4. Which of the following is true of borderline (low malignant potential) tumors?

   A. They typically occur in young, premenopausal women.
   B. The majority are serous tumors.
   C. Treatment involves unilateral oophorectomy to preserve fertility and complete surgical staging.
   D. The 10-year survival rate is 95%.
   E. All of the above.

HPI: EC is a 60-year-old G0P0 woman who presents complaining of intermittent vaginal bleeding for the past month. She denies bladder or bowel symptoms, weight changes, or swelling. Her past gynecologic history is significant for infertility despite regular menses until menopause at age 53.

PE: On physical exam, she is found to have a small amount of blood in the vagina, a normal-appearing cervix, a mildly enlarged uterus, and no adnexal masses or tenderness. You perform an endometrial biopsy, which reveals a grade I adenocarcinoma. The patient is referred to gynecologic oncology for TAH, bilateral salpingo-oophorectomy, and complete surgical staging.

Thought Questions

- What is the epidemiology of endometrial cancer? How is it diagnosed?

- Discuss endometrial hyperplasia.

- What are the histologic types of endometrial cancer?

- Discuss the staging, treatment, and prognosis of endometrial cancer.

- Discuss uterine sarcomas.

Basic Science Review and Discussion

Ninety-five percent of uterine cancers are endometrial in nature, and the remaining 5% are uterine sarcomas. **Endometrial cancer** is the most common gynecologic cancer, with 36,100 new cases diagnosed in the United States each year. Despite being the most curable of the gynecologic malignancies, it still has a mortality rate of 6,500 women per year. Endometrial cancer is primarily a disease of post-menopausal women, with a median age at diagnosis of 60 years.

Risk factors for endometrial cancer tend to involve increased exposure to unopposed estrogen such as nulliparity, chronic anovulation, obesity, early menarche, late menopause, history of breast or ovarian cancer, or use of tamoxifen or exogenous estrogen. Additionally, women with hereditary nonpolyposis colorectal cancer syndrome (Lynch type II) are at increased risk for endometrial cancer. Conversely, factors that reduce exposure to estrogen or increase progesterone levels are protective, such as oral contraceptives, high parity, pregnancy, and smoking.

Fortunately, endometrial cancer tends to be diagnosed in its early stages because 90% of women will have abnormal vaginal bleeding. As a rule, vaginal bleeding of any type in a postmenopausal woman must be evaluated for malignancy. In premenopausal women, prolonged, heavy, or intermenstrual bleeding should be investigated. Evaluation of abnormal bleeding includes a thorough history and physical examination including a pelvic exam. Additionally, a Pap smear should be done because it will be abnormal in 30% to 40% of patients with endometrial cancer.

Finally, the endometrium must be sampled by endometrial biopsy or dilatation and curettage, the former of which is a simpler procedure yielding comparable results. **Endometrial biopsy** provides a tissue diagnosis and allows grading of tumor based on the percentage of solid (non-gland-forming) growth pattern. The percentage of tumor showing a solid growth pattern is 5% or less in **grade I**, 6% to 50% in **grade II**, and greater than 50% in **grade III** endometrial cancer. Eighty percent of endometrial cancers are adenocarcinoma. The remaining histologic types of carcinoma include adenosquamous (7%), clear cell (6%), uterine papillary serous (5%), and secretory (2%). Of note, although endometrial biopsy can identify malignancy, it has not been shown to be cost effective as a screening method.

Endometrial Hyperpasia   In addition to malignancy, endometrial biopsy can identify **endometrial hyperplasia,** which represents abnormal endometrial gland proliferation. Similarly to endometrial cancer, endometrial hyperplasia usually manifests as abnormal vaginal bleeding. It is usually a result of prolonged exposure to unopposed estrogen and is a premalignant lesion if atypia is present. Classification of endometrial hyperplasia as well as the risk for progression to malignancy depends on the type of glandular architecture as well as the presence of atypia (Table 43-1).

Table 43-1 Classification of endometrial hyperplasia

Architecture	Cytologic atypia	Progression to endometrial cancer
Simple hyperplasia	Absent	1%
Complex hyperplasia	Absent	3%
Atypical simple hyperplasia	Present	8%
Atypical complex hyperplasia	Present	29%

Glandular architecture is considered **simple** if the glands appear regular as opposed to irregular in the case of **complex** architecture. **Atypia** is identified in the presence of nuclear enlargement, hyperchromasia, or irregularities in nuclear shape. Treatment of endometrial hyperplasia should take into account the patient's desire for fertility and the existence of atypia. Hormonal treatment with oral contraceptives or cyclic progestins to convert the endometrium to a secretory state and stop proliferation can be utilized in women who wish to preserve fertility or do not have cytologic atypia. These women should undergo follow-up endometrial biopsy in 3 to 6 months. If atypia is present, hysterectomy is usually performed unless the patient wishes to preserve fertility, in which case hysterectomy can be postponed while endometrial curettage, long-term progestin treatment, and ovulation induction to assist the patient in becoming pregnant are carried out.

Endometrial cancer spreads primarily by direct extension, but also via lymphatic and hematogenous dissemination as well as transtubal passage of exfoliated cells. It is surgically staged (see Thumbnail) and treated with TAH-BSO, abdominal exploration, cytologic washings, and, depending on the extent of disease, lymph node dissection. Again, because endometrial cancer is usually diagnosed in early stages, approximately 75% of patients present with stage I disease. Postoperative pelvic radiation is given for patients with deep (greater than one third) myometrial invasion or a poorly differentiated cancer. Extended field radiation should be administered in cases of aortic or pelvic node metastases. Adjunctive hormonal therapy (e.g., Megace) is given for palliation in patients with extensive disease and high levels of progesterone receptors. If the tumor is receptor poor, chemotherapy (e.g., adriamycin) can be used, but has low efficacy.

Prognosis of endometrial cancer depends on histologic grade and type, surgical stage, depth of myometrial invasion, lymph/vascular invasion, and the patient's age. Survival rates vary by stage and grade of disease (Table 43-2).

Table 43-2 Five-year survival of endometrial cancer

Stage		Grade	
I	80%–95%	I	80%–90%
II	55%	II	65%–75%
III	40%–55%	III	55%–60%
IV	10%–15%		

Uterine Sarcomas **Uterine sarcomas** comprise 5% of uterine cancers. They include leiomyosarcomas, mixed mullerian tumors, and endometrial stromal sarcomas. In general, these tumors are aggressive, have a poor prognosis, and are treated surgically. **Leiomyosarcomas** are uterine smooth muscle tumors that must be differentiated from benign **leiomyomas,** otherwise known as fibroids, which are much more common. Unlike leiomyomas, leiomyosarcomas have a large number of cellular mitoses. **Mixed müllerian tumors** (MMTs) are composed of both carcinoma and sarcoma, and the malignant components can include bone, cartilage, or skeletal muscle. **Endometrial stromal sarcomas** (ESS) protrude into the endometrial cavity and can be low or high grade depending on the number of mitoses.

Case Conclusion The patient's surgery is uncomplicated, and she is found to have stage IB disease with invasion of less than one third of the myometrium. As such, she has an excellent prognosis and does not require adjuvant radiation therapy.

Thumbnail: FIGO Staging of Endometrial Cancer

Stage	Findings
Stage IA	Tumor limited to endometrium.
Stage IB	Invasion to less than half of the myometrium.
Stage IC	Invasion to greater than half of the myometrium.
Stage IIA	Endocervical glandular involvement only.
Stage IIB	Cervical stromal invasion.
Stage IIIA	Tumor invades serosa and/or adnexa, and/or positive peritoneal cytology.
Stage IIIB	Vaginal metastases.
Stage IIIC	Metastases to pelvic and/or para-aortic lymph nodes.
Stage IVA	Tumor invasion of bladder and/or bowel mucosa.
Stage IVB	Distant metastases including intra-abdominal and/or inguinal lymph nodes.

Used with permission from the International Federation of Gynecology and Obstetrics.

Key Points

- Endometrial cancer is the most common gynecologic malignancy and usually results from prolonged exposure to estrogen without progesterone (unopposed estrogen).
- The median age of diagnosis is 60 years, but any patient presenting with irregular bleeding, particularly postmenopausally, should be evaluated for endometrial cancer or hyperplasia.

- Approximately 80% of endometrial cancer is adenocarcinoma.
- Endometrial hyperplasia can be premalignant if atypia is present.
- Seventy-five percent of cancers are diagnosed at stage I because patients often present early with abnormal bleeding.

Questions

1. Rank the following types of cancer in women in the United States in order of decreasing incidence.
   - A. Breast cancer, endometrial cancer, cervical cancer, lung cancer, ovarian cancer
   - B. Breast cancer, lung cancer, endometrial cancer, ovarian cancer, cervical cancer
   - C. Breast cancer, lung cancer, endometrial cancer, cervical cancer, ovarian cancer
   - D. Lung cancer, endometrial cancer, breast cancer, cervical cancer, ovarian cancer
   - E. Lung cancer, ovarian cancer, breast cancer, endometrial cancer, cervical cancer

2. Rank the following cancers in decreasing order of annual deaths in women in the United States.
   - A. Breast cancer, lung cancer, ovarian cancer, endometrial cancer, cervical cancer
   - B. Breast cancer, lung cancer, cervical cancer, ovarian cancer, endometrial cancer
   - C. Lung cancer, breast cancer, endometrial cancer, cervical cancer, ovarian cancer
   - D. Lung cancer, breast cancer, ovarian cancer, endometrial cancer, cervical cancer
   - E. Lung cancer, breast cancer, cervical cancer, ovarian cancer, endometrial cancer

3. A 54-year-old G3P2 woman presents to your office complaining of vaginal bleeding for the past few months despite being menopausal for 3 years. Her medical history is significant only for HTN. On further history, the patient reveals that she stopped taking her replacement estrogen and progesterone several months ago because of concerns about heart disease. You perform an endometrial biopsy, which returns negative for cancer or hyperplasia. You reassure the patient that her bleeding is likely due to hormone withdrawal and advise her to return for repeat biopsy if the bleeding is persistent. Which of the following is a potential cause of postmenopausal bleeding?
   - A. Vaginal atrophy
   - B. Cervical cancer
   - C. Endometrial atrophy
   - D. Endometrial polyps
   - E. All of the above

4. A 63 year-old G0P0 woman presents for her first pelvic exam since becoming menopausal at age 55. On reviewing her history, you discover that she has been experiencing occasional vaginal bleeding for almost a year. On physical exam, she has a slightly enlarged uterus but no adnexal masses, although exam is limited by her obesity. You perform an endometrial biopsy, which returns grade 3 adenocarcinoma. The patient undergoes TAH-BSO and surgical staging, revealing stage IIIC endometrial cancer, for which she receives postoperative radiation treatment. Which of the following is not a risk factor for endometrial cancer?
   - A. Obesity
   - B. Nulliparity
   - C. Chronic anovulation
   - D. Early age of first intercourse
   - E. Late menopause

HPI: MP is a 15-year-old G1P0 girl at 9 5/7 weeks of gestation who presents to the ED complaining of severe nausea, vomiting, and inability to tolerate any oral intake for several days. She also reports that she has had vaginal spotting for the past week but was going to wait until her first prenatal appointment tomorrow to discuss it with a clinician. She denies fever, chills, pain, or loose stools.
She has no significant past medical history and is enrolled in the tenth grade at a local high school, where she is a "B" student and plays field hockey. She is sexually active with her boyfriend with occasional condom use. Although this was an unplanned pregnancy, they have decided to move into her parents' home and raise the child together.

PE: Her physical exam is significant for a moderate amount of blood in the vagina coming from the cervix. Her uterus is approximately 12 weeks size, and she has bilateral adnexal masses that are small and minimally tender to palpation. You check a quantitative β-hCG level and blood type and Rh. Pelvic ultrasonography reveals no identifiable fetus or cardiac motion. Instead, you see bilateral theca lutein cysts and a uterus filled with swollen chorionic villi resembling a "snowstorm" pattern.

Thought Questions

- What conditions are included in gestational trophoblastic disease (GTD)?

- Compare and contrast complete and partial hydatidiform moles.

- Discuss malignant GTD.

- Discuss the treatments for the various GTDs.

Basic Science Review and Discussion

Gestational trophoblastic disease is an umbrella term for a group of histologically distinct neoplastic diseases that arise from the placenta. Also referred to as gestational trophoblastic tumors (GTTs) and gestational trophoblastic neoplasia (GTN), GTD encompasses the following diseases: partial and complete hydatidiform moles, invasive moles, placental site trophoblastic tumors, and choriocarcinomas. While the latter three diseases are considered malignant GTD, the hydatidiform moles are considered benign unless they are invasive.

The incidence in the United States of the various GTDs varies, with hydatidiform moles being the most common (1:1200 pregnancies). The incidence of choriocarcinoma is approximately 1:20,000 to 40,000 pregnancies. Finally, placental site trophoblastic tumors are very rare. Approximately 80% of GTDs are hydatidiform moles. Invasive moles account for 10% to 15% of GTD, and choriocarcinoma represents 2% to 5% of GTD. Fortunately, GTD is exquisitely chemosensitive and considered to be the most curable gynecologic malignancy. In addition, β-hCG is a useful tumor marker to monitor disease in all the GTDs.

Benign GTD Hydatidiform moles, also referred to as molar pregnancies, can be either partial or complete. They vary in karyotype, clinical presentation, and pathology (Table 44-1). **Partial hydatidiform moles** usually contain 69 chromosomes from three haploid sets of chromosomes (two paternal and one maternal) and arise when a normal ovum is fertilized by two sperm at once. They also contain a nonviable fetus, a minimal amount of trophoblastic hyperplasia, and focally edematous chorionic villi. In contrast, **complete hydatidiform moles** contain 46 chromosomes that are paternally derived and arise when a single sperm fertilizes an empty ovum and then duplicates its chromosomes (90%), or when two sperm fertilize an empty ovum (10%). Complete moles do not contain fetal tissue and have severe trophoblastic hyperplasia in addition to diffusely edematous chorionic villi that are often described as "grape-like" vesicles and appear as a "snowstorm" pattern on ultrasonography (Figure 44-1). Clinically, complete moles tend to present with abnormal vaginal bleeding (85% of patients). Additional signs and symptoms of complete mole include excessive uterine size (28%), hyperemesis gravidarum (8%), anemia (5%), and preeclampsia before 24 weeks (1%). Patients may also report or be found to have expulsion of grapelike molar clusters into the vagina, bilateral theca lutein cysts, and hyperthyroidism. Additionally, β-hCG levels will be extremely elevated (>100,000 mIU/mL) and the characteristic snowstorm appearance may be evident on ultrasonography. While patients with partial moles can have similar signs and symptoms, they can also be asymptomatic and diagnosed with a missed abortion when fetal heart tones are not detectable and pathology specimen after suction curettage subsequently returns positive for molar gestation. The differential diagnosis for molar pregnancy includes multiple gestation pregnancy, erythroblastosis fetalis, fibroids,

Table 44-1 Partial and complete hydatidiform moles

Feature	Partial Mole	Complete Mole
Karyotype	69,XXX (20%) or 69,XXY (80%)	46,XX (90%) or 46,XY (10%)
Pathology		
Fetus	Often present	Absent
Amnion, fetal RBCs	Often present	Absent
Trophoblastic proliferation	Variable, focal, slight to moderate	Variable, slight to severe
Clinical presentation		
Ultrasound findings	Missed abortion, hydropic villi	Anembryonic molar gestation
Uterine size	Small for dates	50% are large for dates
Theca lutein cysts	Rare	Occur in 25%–30%
Medical complications	Rare	Frequent
Postmolar GTD	< 5%–10%	20%

threatened abortion, ectopic pregnancy, or normal intra-uterine pregnancy.

Both complete and partial moles can be 95% to 100% cured with suction evacuation and gentle curettage of the uterus. Additionally, IV oxytocin can be administered after uterine evacuation to stimulate contractions and minimize blood loss. Alternatively, if the patient has completed childbearing, hysterectomy can also be performed. Because the risk for persistent disease is 15% to 25% with complete moles and less than 4% with partial moles, close follow-up with weekly and then monthly β-hCG levels for 1 year is essential. Reliable contraception must also be provided to the patient during this time to prevent misinterpretation of β-hCG levels. After successful treatment of molar gestation,

the risk for developing GTD in subsequent pregnancies is less than 5%.

Malignant GTD There are three histologic types of malignant or persistent GTD: invasive moles, gestational choriocarcinoma, and placental site trophoblastic tumor. Prognosis is more dependent on clinical presentation than histologic type. Evaluation of metastases should include physical exam and chest x-ray at the minimum with possible CT scan of the head, chest, and abdomen. Multiple classification systems exist for malignant GTD. The World Health Organization's system allows the computation of a prognostic score based on the patient's age, the time interval between and type of antecedent pregnancy, β-hCG levels, size of tumor, sites and number of metastases, and prior chemotherapy used. The National Institutes of Health has a system that categorizes patients based on the presence of metastases because most nonmetastatic disease can be cured using single-agent chemotherapy (usually methotrexate) and, depending on fertility preferences, can also be treated with hysterectomy. Those patients with metastatic disease are further subdivided into low risk/good prognosis and high risk/poor prognosis disease. Patients with poor prognosis disease are treated initially with multi-agent chemotherapy (usually EMA/CO: etoposide, methotrexate, and dactinomycin alternating with cyclophosphamide and vincristine). Like the approach to benign GTD, follow-up should continue until serial β-hCG levels become undetectable, and concomitant reliable contraception is essential.

Invasive moles arise when villi and trophoblasts penetrate into the myometrium or even reach the peritoneal cavity. They result from persistent molar pregnancy (75%) or from recurrent GTD (25%) and are usually detected during the follow-up period when β-hCG levels plateau or rise after uterine evacuation. The incidence of invasive moles is approximately 1:15,000 pregnancies. Diagnosis is similar to

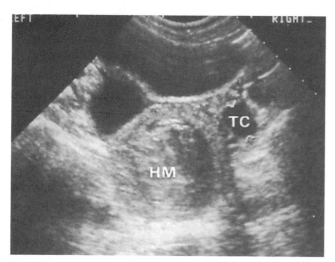

Figure 44-1 Complete molar pregnancy on ultrasonography. Note the hydropic villi (seen as black lucent areas) and the general snowstorm appearance. HM = hydatidiform mole, TC = theca lutein cyst. (Reprinted with permission from *Chamberlin G. Lecture Notes on Obstetrics*, 7th ed. Oxford: Blackwell Science, 1996.)

that for molar gestation. Fortunately, invasive moles rarely metastasize and are sensitive to single-agent chemotherapy, with a cure rate of 95% to 100%.

Gestational choriocarcinoma can arise weeks to years after molar gestations (50%), normal pregnancies (25%), or other gestations such as miscarriage or ectopic pregnancy (25%). It has an incidence of 1:40,000 pregnancies in the United States and is considered a pure epithelial neoplasm, consisting of syncytiotrophoblasts and cytotrophoblasts without chorionic villi. Early hematogenous spread to the lung, vagina, pelvis, brain, and liver can occur; therefore, patients should undergo thorough metastatic evaluation. Single- or

multi-agent chemotherapy is utilized depending on the presence of metastases. Surgery is not generally a part of choriocarcinoma treatment.

Placental site trophoblastic tumor (PSTT) is a variant of choriocarcinoma that arises from the placental implantation site and consists of cytotrophoblasts and no chorionic villi. Patients can present weeks to years after an antecedent pregnancy with bleeding. These tumors produce chronic low levels of β-hCG and human placental lactogen. Although PSTT is resistant to chemotherapy, it rarely metastasizes beyond the uterus and can be treated with hysterectomy.

Case Conclusion   The patient's β-hCG returns 256,000 mIU/mL and her blood type is B-negative. Given this and your ultrasound findings, you confirm the diagnosis of complete hydatidiform mole and treat the patient with suction curettage of uterine contents and administer RhoGAM to prevent Rh sensitization. A chest x-ray to evaluate for metastases is normal. The patient is also given oral contraceptives for birth control and subsequently undergoes regular monitoring of β-hCG levels until they go to zero.

Thumbnail: FIGO Staging for Gestational Trophoblastic Disease

Stage	Findings
Stage I	Disease confined to the uterus.
Stage IA	Disease confined to the uterus with no risk factors.
Stage IB	Disease confined to the uterus with one risk factor.
Stage IC	Disease confined to the uterus with two risk factors.
Stage II	GTT extends outside of the uterus but is limited to the genital structures (e.g., adnexa, vagina, broad ligament).
Stage IIA	GTT involving genital structures with no risk factors.
Stage IIB	GTT extends outside of the uterus but limited to the genital structures with one risk factor.
Stage IIC	GTT extends outside of the uterus but is limited to the genital structures with two risk factors.
Stage III	GTT extends to the lungs with or without known genital tract involvement.
Stage IIIA	GTT extends to the lungs with or without genital tract involvement and with no risk factors.
Stage IIIB	GTT extends to the lungs with or without genital tract involvement and with one risk factor.
Stage IIIC	GTT extends to the lungs with or without genital tract involvement and with two risk factors.
Stage IV	All other metastatic sites.
Stage IVA	All other metastatic sites with no risk factors.
Stage IVB	All other metastatic sites with one risk factor.
Stage IVC	All other metastatic sites with two risk factors.

*Risk Factors:

1. β-hCG > 100,000 mIU/mL

2. Duration from termination of antecedent pregnancy to diagnosis > 6 months.

Used with permission from the International Federation of Gynecology and Obstetrics.

Key Points

▶ GTD can be classified as benign (partial and complete moles) or malignant (invasive moles, choriocarcinoma, and PSTT).

▶ The GTDs tend to produce β-hCG, which is used to follow therapy and monitor for recurrence.

▶ Ninety percent of molar pregnancies are complete moles, which commonly have a 46,XX karyotype and no associated fetus.

▶ Malignant GTD is classified as nonmetastatic or metastatic; nonmetastatic GTD can often be treated with single-agent chemotherapy to preserve fertility, while metastatic GTD can be treated with either single- or multi-agent chemotherapy depending on the presence of risk factors.

▶ Invasive moles are diagnosed when β-hCG levels plateau or rise during the postmolar follow-up period, are generally not metastatic, and can be treated with single-agent chemotherapy, with a 95% to 100% cure rate.

Questions

1. Rank the following gestational trophoblastic diseases in order of decreasing incidence.
   A. Complete mole, partial mole, invasive mole, choriocarcinoma, placental site trophoblastic tumor
   B. Complete mole, invasive mole, partial mole, placental site trophoblastic tumor, choriocarcinoma
   C. Partial mole, complete mole, choriocarcinoma, invasive mole, placental site trophoblastic tumor
   D. Invasive mole, complete mole, partial mole, choriocarcinoma, placental site trophoblastic tumor
   E. Choriocarcinoma, complete mole, partial mole, invasive mole, placental site trophoblastic tumor

2. Which of the following are potential sites of metastases for choriocarcinoma?
   A. Vagina
   B. Liver
   C. Lungs
   D. Brain
   E. All of the above

3. Which of the following correctly matches the disease with its components?
   A. Complete hydatidiform mole—69,XXY
   B. Partial hydatidiform mole—46,XY
   C. Invasive mole—chorionic villi
   D. Choriocarcinoma—cytotrophoblasts and syncytiotrophoblasts
   E. Placenta site trophoblastic tumor—cytotrophoblasts and chorionic villi

4. A 42-year-old G3P1 presents with vaginal bleeding and is concerned she may have endometrial cancer. Her past gynecologic history is significant for a vaginal delivery of an infant with a neural tube defect 13 years ago, a first trimester miscarriage 10 years ago, and a ruptured ectopic pregnancy for which she underwent surgery 4 years ago. Her β-hCG level is elevated, but you cannot visualize a fetus or a snowstorm pattern on ultrasonography. The patient is diagnosed with PSTT and undergoes successful hysterectomy. Which of the following are considered risk factors for gestational trophoblastic disease?
   A. Age less than 20 or greater than 40 years
   B. Diets low in beta-carotene and folic acid
   C. History of prior molar pregnancy
   D. Women with blood type A married to men with blood type O
   E. All of the above

Case 30

1. A
2. D

Case 31

1. E
2. B

Case 32

1. C
2. E
3. C

Case 33

1. A
2. B

Case 34

1. E
2. B
3. D

Case 35

1. A
2. B
3. D

Case 36

1. E
2. D

Case 37

1. B
2. D

Case 38

1. B
2. B
3. E
4. C

Case 39

1. D
2. C

Case 40

1. A
2. E
3. E

Case 41

1. C
2. B
3. E

Case 42

1. A
2. C
3. D
4. E

Case 43

1. B
2. D
3. E
4. D

Case 44

1. A
2. E
3. D
4. E

Answers

Case 1

1. C Concentric hypertrophy is the result of pressure overload, which is usually the result of AS or uncontrolled, long-term HTN. Eccentric hypertrophy and subsequent chamber dilatation are secondary to long-term volume overload. Severe aortic and MR impose a volume overload on the LV. A VSD or ASD with a large left-to-right shunt would also result in volume overload and eccentric hypertrophy.

2. D Nitrates result in vascular smooth muscle relaxation and produce greater dilatation of the veins than the arterioles. The resulting venodilation induces venous pooling and decreased preload because of diminished venous return. At higher doses, nitrates can also cause increased arteriolar dilatation and afterload reduction. Choices A, B, C, and E are all effective treatments for CHF, but all four choices are pure afterload reducing agents.

Case 2

1. B Treatment of heart failure secondary to diastolic dysfunction is similar to that for heart failure secondary to systolic dysfunction, except for the use of positive inotropic drugs (digoxin, dobutamine, dopamine, milrinone). Positive inotropic drugs can worsen diastolic dysfunction by (1) promoting tachycardia, (2) decreasing diastolic filling time, (3) increasing myocardial oxygen requirements, and (4) worsening underlying myocardial ischemia.

2. E Beta-blockers improve diastolic filling via choices A through D. Choice E is incorrect because beta-blockers decrease the LV outflow gradient.

In addition to diastolic dysfunction, beta-blockers are also used to treat patients with elevated subaortic valve gradients secondary to LV hypertrophy (asymmetric septal hypertrophy/hypertrophic obstructive cardiomyopathy). With severe septal or LV hypertrophy, the LV outflow tract is narrowed. With increased contractility (as seen with increased physical activity) the LV outflow tract narrows and obstruction increases further. This dynamic narrowing (or dynamic outflow obstruction) increases the LV outflow gradient and LV end-diastolic pressure with resultant pulmonary edema. Beta-blockers therefore can decrease this narrowing, decrease the LV outflow gradient, improve LV outflow, and decrease pulmonary edema.

Case 3

1. C All five of these biochemical markers increase in MI, but troponin is the most specific and has the longest duration of elevation. Myoglobin and creatinine kinase decrease to baseline within 24 to 36 hours. SGOT peaks in 2 days but returns to baseline within 5 days. LDH can remain elevated for up to 6 days but is a relatively nonspecific marker. Troponin I can remain elevated for up to 10 days and is very specific for myocardial necrosis.

2. D Approximately one third of patients with inferior MI develop RV necrosis because the right coronary artery (RCA) supplies both the LV inferior wall and RV. Patients with RCA occlusion often present with severe bradycardia and heart block because the AV node receives its blood supply from the RCA. Occlusion of the RCA results in poor RV contractile function, but LV systolic function remains relatively unimpaired. As a result, signs of right-sided heart failure (elevated JVP, pulsatile liver) are out of proportion to signs of left-sided heart failure (lack of CHF and clear lungs). The impairment of LV filling due to poor RV contractile function is the main cause for the hypotension, and the treatment of choice is IV fluid resuscitation.

Case 4

1. C Studies have demonstrated that a 60% to 70% stenosis is necessary before the coronary blood flow is diminished enough to provoke stable angina. However, this critical narrowing decreases to 45% when unrestricted flow is increased up to fourfold with peak exercise. Several studies have demonstrated that although angina becomes more severe with the severity of the stenosis, many of the fibrous plaques that rupture to form the complicated lesion are the plaques that do not form the most severe stenosis.

2. D A TNF-α epitope analogue would actually increase the local proinflammatory effect and attract additional macrophages to form foam cells. An oxidized LDL scavenger could potentially decrease the release of vascular adhesion molecules. Inhibition of the matrix metalloproteinase activity could prevent fibrous cap rupture. Smooth muscle proliferation of the media layer could be reduced with decreasing PDGF activity. Finally, the antiplatelet and anti-inflammatory effects of an enhanced aspirin would be beneficial in preventing atherosclerosis.

Case 5

1. C This patient presents with mitral stenosis secondary to rheumatic heart fever. As a result of her mitral stenosis, she has LA HTN, which induces LA enlargement, atrial fibrillation, and pulmonary congestion. The elevated left-sided pressures are then transmitted to the right-sided chambers, resulting in RV dilatation and hypertrophy and peripheral edema. She also presents with the prototypical malar erythema and OS secondary to the sudden tensing of the chordae upon opening. The cardiac catheterization tracing for mitral stenosis is choice C, with the solid line representing the LV pressure and the dotted line representing the LA pressure. A pressure gradient is present throughout diastole.

2. D After mitral valvuloplasty, one of the most common complications is acute MR. The hemodynamic profile of MR is best characterized by choice D, with a large C-V wave noted in the LA tracing, corresponding to the large regurgitant pressure wave transmitted retrograde from the LV to the LA through the incompetent mitral valve.

Case 6

1. B This patient presents with syncope secondary to critical AS. The median survival for severe AS patients is 5 years for angina, 3 years for syncope, and 2 years for CHF. His exam is notable for the prototypical systolic murmur radiating upward. The apical component of the murmur is the Gallavardin phenomenon. The second heart sound (composed of an aortic and pulmonic component) is paradoxically split (P_2 occurs before A_2) because LV ejection is prolonged in severe AS. Unlike MR, handgrip does not change the AS murmur. The cardiac catheterization tracing consistent with AS is that shown in B, with the solid line representing the LV pressure and the dotted line representing the aortic pressure. The difference between the two lines at mid-systole is the peak-to-peak gradient generated by the stenotic valve. Choice A is the pressure tracing for a normal aortic valve. Choice C is the pressure tracing for severe aortic insufficiency when there is a rapid decrease in aortic pressure during diastole and a concomitant rise in LV pressure from the regurgitant volume.

2. E This patient presents with chronic decompensated aortic insufficiency and CHF secondary to increased LVEDP and pulmonary congestion. The primary treatment for decompensated aortic insufficiency is afterload reduction (with ACE inhibitors, angiotensin receptor blockers, or hydralazine) to improve forward cardiac output, diuresis to decrease the LVEDP, and increased inotropy with digoxin. Although the patient presents with angina, it is unlikely secondary to coronary artery disease, and beta-blockers are therefore unlikely to improve his angina. With aortic insufficiency, relative bradycardia actually worsens the clinical symptoms and can precipitate angina. Bradycardia causes an increase in the diastolic filling period and regurgitant volume with a resultant increase in LVEDP and a decrease in diastolic coronary perfusion.

Case 7

1. C *Streptococcus bovis* is almost always associated with GI tumors, interventions on the GI tract, or digestive infectious diseases. Genitourinary tumors such as transitional cell carcinoma of the bladder would be more commonly associated with enterococci, gram-negative bacilli, or *Staphylococcus aureus*. Endocarditis associated with infections of the respiratory tract would include penicillin-sensitive streptococci.

2. C Mitral valve prolapse without MR is associated with no risk of IE and does not require antibiotic prophylaxis. However, mitral valve prolapse with mitral valve regurgitation is associated with a risk of IE 6 to 14 times greater than normal and does require antibiotic prophylaxis. Bicuspid aortic valve also requires antibiotic prophylaxis and is found in up to 25% of cases of aortic endocarditis. A patent DA also requires antibiotic prophylaxis, but risk is greatly decreased with correction. Prosthetic heart valves carry a risk 5 to 10 times greater for IE than patients with native valves and therefore require antibiotic prophylaxis.

Case 8

1. B Factors that contribute to coronary artery spasm include (1) cigarette smoking, (2) hypomagnesemia, (3) cocaine use, (4) sumitriptan migraine medication, and (5) cold stimulation. Variant angina attacks are more common at night or in the early morning. Silent ischemia is asymptomatic ischemia that is most often seen in diabetic patients who experience decreased pain sensation from myocardial ischemia.

2. A Although choices B, D, and E could cause recurrent chest pain, it is unlikely that these pathologies developed in such a short time since the last angiogram. A negative ergonovine challenge for vasospasm also decreases the likelihood of vasospasm. Myocardial ischemia may occasionally occur in the presence of normal arteries and in the absence of vasospasm. Conditions associated with this clinical presentation include (1) coronary artery embolization, (2) coronary artery thrombosis with spontaneous thrombolysis, (3) increased blood viscosity, (4) marked increase in myocardial oxygen demand, and (5) small vessel coronary artery (microvascular) disease.

3. C Other clinical conditions can resemble myocardial ischemia. Pericarditis is difficult to differentiate from myocardial ischemia because it can often present with diffuse ECG changes. However, pericarditis is usually pleuritic, sharp, positional in nature, and associated with a friction rub. Pericarditis is often associated with postviral syndromes and renal failure. GI disorders such as esophageal spasm, reflux disease, and duodenal or gastric ulcers can also mimic angina, but differentiating aspects include relief with antacids, association with acid taste in mouth, or aggravation with certain foods. Biliary colic and pancreatitis can also mimic ischemic heart disease but they are often temporally related to meals and associated with focal tenderness in the abdomen. Cervical or thoracic radiculitis and intercostal neuritis can be differentiated based on the dermatomal distribution of pain. Finally, costochondritis and chest wall pain is usually pleuritic, localized, and point tender.

Case 9

1. E ACE inhibitors are particularly well suited for the treatment of HTN in diabetic patients because they can reduce the degree of proteinuria and forestall the development of diabetic nephropathy. Recent trials have also shown that a particular ACE inihibitor, ramipril, can actually decrease the risk for MI, death, and CVA in diabetic patients without a history of heart failure or low ejection fraction (HOPE trial, 2000).

2. D ACE inhibitors are contraindicated in patients with bilateral renal artery stenosis. Her presentation with refractory HTN and abdominal bruits suggests that her HTN is secondary to renal artery stenosis. In bilateral renal artery stenosis, ACE inhibitors can precipitate acute renal failure by depleting the glomeruli of blood flow (efferent arterioles are vasodilated while afferent inflow is limited by the stenosis). ACE inhibitors are also contraindicated in hyperkalemia because they can cause elevated potassium levels.

Case 10

1. E The patient's postoperative state increases his risk for all SVTs. However, the prompt resolution of the tachycardia with IV adenosine suggest that the tachycardia circuit involves the AV node and is most likely to be either AVNRT or AVRT. Although adenosine decreases the rate of conduction through the AV node and can slow the ventricular rate of non-AV node-dependent tachycardia circuits (sinus tachycardia, atrial flutter, atrial fibrillation, multifocal atrial tachycardia), the inhibition of the AV node usually does not terminate the tachycardia.

2. C The most straightforward arrhythmia for ablation is typical flutter. In typical flutter, the reentrant circuit is usually located in a defined anatomic location within the RA (the circuit passes along a narrow isthmus of tissue between the tricuspid valve annulus and entrance of the inferior vena cava) and is easily interrupted. Atypical atrial flutter is much more difficult to locate because the flutter circuit can exist anywhere within the RA or LA. Although experimental protocols are now available, multifocal atrial tachycardia and atrial fibrillation are not typically amenable to ablation because of their multiple foci. Sinus tachycardia is a physiologic response to a stressor, and the treatment is correction of the underlying stressor (pain, dehydration, fever, etc.), not ablation.

Case 11

1. D Patients with MI secondary to proximal RCA occlusion are most likely to present with severe bradycardia. Although the SA node receives its blood supply only 60% of the time from the RCA, the AV node receives blood from the RCA 90% of the time. Patients with severe right coronary infarcts often require temporary electronic pacing.

2. E A patient with any bundle branch block has a disturbance in impulse conduction. Clinical scenarios A and B are the least impaired. Clinical scenarios C and D have a higher degree of impaired impulse conduction because only one branch of the left bundle is fully functional. Choice E is the most likely to receive a pacemaker because right bundle branch block with alternating hemiblock implies there is severe intraventricular conduction disease. Choice E usually presents with second degree Mobitz type II impaired conduction.

Case 12

1. E Polymorphic VT suggest that the underlying etiology for the recurrent arrhythmia is ongoing ischemia. Although IV magnesium replacement and IV antiarrhythmics may temporize the situation, these steps will not address the underlying ischemia. An AICD will correct the VT but will defibrillate incessantly for recurrent VT until the underlying ischemia is corrected. Thrombolysis could potentially address the occluded coronary artery, but given the patient's presumed cardiogenic shock, cardiac catheterization and angioplasty would be the most reasonable option.

2. D Supraventricular arrhythmias such as atrial fibrillation, atrial flutter, and AVRT rarely present with loss of consciousness. The loss of cardiac contractile function in ventricular fibrillation is usually so severe that no pulse can be discerned. She most likely has the torsade de pointes ("twisting of points" in French) form of VT that is distinguished by varying amplitudes and undulating sinusoidal appearance. It is most often associated with prolonged QT intervals, drugs (quinidine), and electrolyte abnormalities such as hypocalcemia and hypokalemia.

Case 13

1. D With TGA, it is imperative to maintain DA patency to allow for right-to-left shunting of oxygenated blood. Prostaglandin infusion allows for the DA to remain patent until a definitive surgical procedure is performed. Balloon atrial septostomy is another palliative procedure to establish shunting at the interatrial level. Supplemental oxygen would have little effect since the increasingly oxygenated blood would remain isolated within the LV circuit. Inotropic support would not increase oxygenation due to persistent shunting. Indomethacin would actually hasten DA closure. Finally, TGA patients are already polycythemic from hypoxia, and additional blood transfusion can exacerbate symptoms.

2. E In TOF, deoxygenated blood is routed from the RV, through a VSD, and into the systemic circulation. Therefore, any condition causing (1) lower SVR, (2) increased venous return, or (3) worsened pulmonic stenosis can exacerbate the baseline hypoxemia. Although hydralazine is an afterload-reducing agent often used in systolic heart failure, this medication could potentially worsen the clinical situation because right-to-left shunting would increase, resulting in increased hypoxia. TOF patients are at risk for endocarditis, and prophylactic antibiotics are appropriate. Supplemental oxygen would improve their baseline hypoxia. Supplemental iron will prevent anemia by providing the iron reserves for the adaptive polycythemia. Beta-blockers are also considered standard of care for TOF because they decrease the degree of dynamic RV outflow obstruction/pulmonic stenosis during ventricular systole.

Case 14

1. B The usual oxygen saturation in the vena cava, right-sided heart chambers, and pulmonary arteries is approximately 70%, while the oxygen saturation in the left-sided heart chambers is 96% to 98%. If there is a left-to-right shunt, oxygenated blood from the left heart will cross over into the right-sided heart chambers and increase the oxygenation level on the right side. When oxygen saturation samples are drawn, there will be a "step up" in oxygenation at the level of the shunt. Answer A is a normal saturation run with no shunting. Answer B demonstrates normal right-sided saturations of 70% until oxygenated blood from the aorta crosses over via PDA into the pulmonary artery with a resultant rise in oxygenation to 90%. Answer C is the result of a left-to-right shunt at the atrial level (ASD). Answer D is secondary to left-to-right shunting at the ventricular level (VSD). Answer E is the result of a shunt between the common femoral artery and vein.

2. D In a typical small PDA, the amount of left-to-right shunt flow is limited by the actual size of the orifice. In a very large PDA, the amount of shunting is determined by the degree of pulmonary vascular resistance. A decrease in the pulmonary vascular resistance by inhaled nitric oxide would increase the amount of shunting from the systemic circulation into the pulmonic circulation. The result of this increased flow is pulmonary edema and LV failure from fluid overload. Supplemental oxygen and inhibition of prostaglandin synthesis with indomethacin and aspirin would potentially accelerate physiologic ductal closure. Although not standard of care, phenylephrine within the pulmonary circulation would theoretically raise the pulmonary vascular resistance and decrease the amount of left-to-right shunting.

Case 15

1. D Elevated blood keto acids are responsible for the increased anion gap metabolic acidosis seen in DKA. These acids are utilized by the brain for energy when glucose is unavailable, as in a low insulin state. Anion gap is calculated using the following formula:

$$AG = (Na^+ + K^+) - (Cl^- + HCO_3^-)$$

Normal anion gap values are usually 8 to 12. In this case, the anion gap is elevated at 35. Other causes of anion gap acidosis include methanol ingestion, uremia from chronic renal failure, lactic acidosis, and ethanol intoxication.

2. B In endogenous pancreatic insulin production, the insulin molecule is first produced in its precursor form, a molecule known as proinsulin. This proinsulin molecule consists of an α and a β chain linked by two disulfide bonds and a C-peptide region. This C-peptide must be cleaved off the proinsulin molecule before it becomes insulin. Serum C-peptide levels can thus be used as a marker for endogenous insulin production. With exogenously administered insulin, the insulin is injected in its active form, without the C-peptide portion. Measurement of C-peptide levels in the blood of patients who are on exogenous insulin therapy will be decreased compared with people who are not on insulin.

Case 16

1. C The HbA_{1c} test documents the average blood glucose levels in the 3 months immediately prior to testing. The reported value is directly proportional to the average blood glucose concentration over the life span of the patient's circulating RBCs (120 days). The glucose tolerance test, fasting serum glucose, and urinalysis can all be used to help diagnose DM and may reflect immediate glycemic status, but are not indicative of long-term diabetic control. CBC is also not indicated for this purpose.

2. B Insulin may be required for treatment of type 2 DM, but is usually considered a second-line agent, after several of the other

diabetes medications have failed to achieve glucose homeostasis. Because type 2 diabetics have some insulin secretion, but not enough to overcome their resistance, pharmacologic treatment of type 2 DM aims to change insulin secretion/action or alter the absorption of glucose. Glyburide is a sulfonylurea that lowers blood glucose by stimulating insulin secretion from the pancreas and increasing tissue sensitivity to insulin. The most common side effect of the sulfonylureas is hypoglycemia. Metformin is a biguanide drug often used in combination with the sulfonylureas. Its actions are to decrease hepatic gluconeogenesis and increase peripheral glucose utilization. While metformin does not induce hypoglycemia, it does inhibit lactate metabolism and can cause rare lactic acidosis. Acarbose is an α-glucosidase inhibitor that delays the digestion and absorption of complex carbohydrates in the small intestine. This class of medications is primarily used as an adjunct in type 2 patients, but many patients complain of increased GI effects such as nausea, diarrhea, bloating, and flatulence. Pioglitazone is a thiazolidinedione that decreases peripheral insulin resistance in skeletal muscle and adipose tissue without increasing insulin secretion. Because of concerns for hepatitis and liver failure, these medications have currently been removed from the market. At the very least, patients must have liver function tests measured regularly, because increased liver transaminases are a common occurrence.

3. D All of the choices except smoking are risk factors for the development of type 2 diabetes. Diabetes results from a combination of genetic and environmental factors. While genetic factors cannot be altered, environmental influences are modifiable and should be altered toward the prevention and treatment of diabetes. In this case, the patient should be encouraged to exercise, lose weight, and eat sensibly. Smoking cessation is not a bad idea either, since smoking is a known risk factor for other multiple conditions. Since these recommendations require major lifestyle changes, the patient should receive as much lifestyle support and diabetes education as possible. This may include diabetes classes for the patient and encouraging family members to assist with her health management.

Case 17

1. C Levothyroxine is used to treat lifelong hypothyroidism, not hyperthyroidism. All of the other methods are potential treatments for hyperthyroidism. The thioamides (PTU and methimazole) are drugs that decrease thyroid hormone synthesis by binding to and inhibiting all steps of thyroid hormone synthesis catalyzed by thyroid peroxidase. Skin rash is a common side effect of these medications. Aplastic anemia and agranulocytosis can also occur on rare occasions. Beta-blockers such as propranolol are sometimes used as symptomatic therapy to decrease the peripheral manifestations of hyperthyroidism such as increased heart rate, arrhythmias, and excess sweating. Surgery is the definitive therapy for all patients with thyrotoxicosis, but patients must be supplemented with exogenous thyroid hormone for the rest of their lives.

2. E TSH is the best test for assessing thyroid function because changes in TSH can be detected before alterations in the levels of

T_4. Free T_4 is a more accurate measurement than total T_4 because total T_4 includes all the T_4 that is bound to thyroid-binding proteins. Although the total T_4 may rise or fall secondary to changes in serum binding protein levels, the free T_4 value remains normal if the patient is healthy. A pattern of increased TSH and low free T_4 and T_3 is consistent with hypothyroidism, while decreased TSH and increased free T_4 and T_3 suggest a hyperthyroid state.

Case 18

1. B Hypothyroidism following recovery from a URI is consistent with **subacute thyroiditis** (also known as de Quervain's thyroiditis). The cause of the thyroiditis appears to be related to a postviral syndrome complete with positive viral antibody titers. Characteristically, patients complain of ear tenderness in combination with a diffusely enlarged and tender thyroid gland. The typical pattern of illness presents clinically 2 to 3 weeks after URI has resolved. First, there is a hyperthyroid phase, which lasts from 0 to 4 weeks. A hypothyroid phase follows from weeks 4 to 12. The recovery phase occurs after 12 weeks with return of normal thyroid function. Symptoms during both hyper- and hypothyroid phases are usually mild. Because the disease process is self-limited to roughly 6 months, treatment is symptomatic. Glucocorticoids have proved to be most effective at reducing thyroid inflammation. Beta-blockers such as propranolol can be used to treat the stage of thyrotoxicosis. Hashimoto's thyroiditis is not likely because the thyroid gland should be painless and symptoms of hypothyroidism are usually not present until middle age. Iodine deficiency became rare in the United States following the introduction of iodized salt. At least 100 μg of iodide is required to maintain normal function of the thyroid. Thyroid function is usually normal in people with iodine-deficient goiter. The goiter is simply a compensatory hypertrophy of the gland to increase production of hormone. Long-standing iodine deficiency may ultimately result in hypothyroidism, but the symptoms would not present with such acuity. Neoplasms are usually painless, fixed, and localized. They would be more common in males with a history of radiation exposure. Finally, pituitary adenomas are often hyperfunctioning nodules that would most likely cause visual changes, headache, hyperthyroidism, or other associated endocrine abnormalities.

2. D This patient presents with hypothyroidism, confirmed by the low levels of serum free T_4. Normochromic, normocytic anemia is a common finding in hypothyroidism due to the decrease in metabolic rate. Hypothyroidism can be classified as primary or secondary, depending on the location of the defect. Primary hypothyroidism is caused by a defect within the thyroid gland itself, whereas secondary hypothyroidism is caused by a defect in the pituitary gland or the hypothalamus. The best test to determine the cause of this patient's hypothyroidism is to check the serum TSH level. TSH will be increased in primary thyroid diseases, but normal or low in secondary conditions. Pituitary or hypothalamic causes are often accompanied by associated physical exam findings. Pituitary tumors, for example, commonly present with bitemporal visual field deficits due to increased pressure on the optic chiasm secondary to the enlarging mass.

Case 19

1. B The most specific test to screen for glucocorticoid excess is **24-hour urinary cortisol** production. The patient's urine is collected over a 24-hour period and tested for the amount of cortisol. Levels higher than 50 to 100 μg a day in an adult suggest Cushing's syndrome. An elevated urinary cortisol confirms excess cortisol production; however, it does not distinguish one cause from another. Subsequent evaluation to localize the source of ACTH or cortisol is usually required. Pituitary MRI can be used if a pituitary adenoma is suspected; the pituitary fossa will be enlarged or the tumor may be visualized. CT scan can be used to evaluate the possibility of adrenal adenoma or carcinoma; the CT scan may show a mass in the affected gland. Low- and high-dose dexamethasone suppression tests help distinguish patients with excess production of ACTH due to pituitary adenomas from those with ectopic ACTH-producing tumors. Dexamethasone is a synthetic glucocorticoid that should suppress endogenous cortisol and ACTH secretion. Ectopic ACTH production will not respond to dexamethasone suppression. Low doses are given first to confirm Cushing's syndrome. A high dose can subsequently be given to localize the etiology to the pituitary or adrenal gland. A drop in blood and urine cortisol levels is consistent with Cushing's syndrome, but the dexamethasone suppression test can produce false-positive results in patients with depression, alcohol abuse, high estrogen levels, acute illness, and stress. Conversely, drugs such as phenytoin and phenobarbital may cause false-negative results in response to dexamethasone suppression (Figure A-1).

2. E All of the choices provided are actions of cortisol, but it is cortisol's anti-inflammatory properties that decrease airway edema and inflammation in asthma. This anti-inflammatory action is mediated through the inhibition of prostaglandin formation.

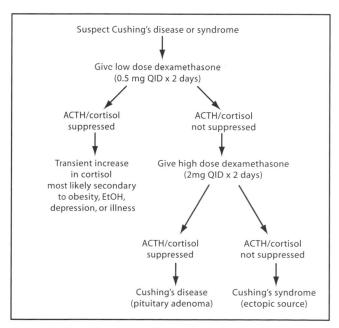

Figure A-1 Algorithm for the dexamethasone suppression test.

Specifically, glucocorticoids inhibit phospholipase A2, the enzyme that liberates arachidonic acid from cell membranes. Arachidonic acid is the precursor to prostaglandin, prostacyclin (PGI_2), thromboxane, and leukotriene synthesis. Without prostaglandins, prostacyclins, and leukotrienes, the inflammatory response that accompanies airway hyperreactivity in asthma is blunted. Although quite effective in controlling inflammation, chronic oral steroid therapy is associated with numerous side effects that must be weighed against the benefits of treatment. Specifically, patients can develop cushingoid features, including excess fat deposition, moon facies, and striae. Chronic complications from glucocorticoid excess can also develop, such as osteoporosis, HTN, and diabetes. Interestingly, exogenous steroid intake is the most common cause of Cushing's syndrome.

Case 20

1. B **Craniopharyngeomas** are pituitary gland tumors derived from remnants of Rathke's pouch oral ectoderm. Craniopharyngiomas are the most common cause of panhypopituitarism in adolescents. With panhypopituitarism, patients are deficient in LH, FSH, TRH, PRL, ACTH, and GH. The lack of gonadotropins and GH explains this patient's delayed puberty and short stature. In addition, secondary adrenal insufficiency will result from the lack of ACTH stimulation to the adrenal cortex. Because ACTH regulates secretion from the zona fasciculata and the zona reticularis, cortisol and androgen production will be decreased. Aldosterone secretion from the zona glomerulosa will not be affected. Secondary insufficiency differs in presentation from primary insufficiency (Addison's disease) in that the patients do not present with hypotension or hyperpigmentation.

2. A Autoimmune adrenalitis is the most common cause of primary adrenal insufficiency in the United States. An autoimmune cause is also most likely in this patient because she has a history of Graves' disease, an autoimmune mediated thyroiditis. Patients with autoimmune diseases tend to have other simultaneous autoimmune-mediated conditions. Although skin hyperpigmentation is characteristic of Addison's disease secondary to increased MSH, this patient presents with patches of depigmentation. This depigmentation is known as vitiligo and is also common in patients with autoimmune disease. The vitiligo occurs through an autoimmune-mediated attack on melanocytes. The diagnosis of Addison's disease can be confirmed with laboratory findings of low morning cortisol levels (<3 μg/dL) and high plasma ACTH levels (≥100 pg/mL).

Case 21

1. A Early osteoporosis is a potential complication of hyperparathyroidism. Because PTH functions to increase bone resorption by osteoclasts, this process is accelerated in hyperparathyroidism. Osteoporosis results in a decrease in the amount of normal trabecular bone; patients with osteoporosis are thus more easily prone to fracture and bone injury, even with minimal trauma. Osteoarthritis is not likely in this patient due to her young age. Rheumatoid arthritis is also unlikely due to the lack of typical joint symptoms and the lack of systemic symptoms. Patients with osteo-

genesis imperfecta would present in childhood with multiple fractures, lax ligaments, and blue sclera, resulting from an autosomal-dominant defect in collagen synthesis. Finally, fibromyalgia would present with a more chronic history of muscle aches and pains; it would not explain her hypercalcemia or tendency to fracture easily.

2. E All of the choices are mediators that cause hypercalcemia associated with malignancy. The primary cause of hypercalcemia in this instance is paraneoplastic release of PTHrP from the small cell lung carcinoma. PTHrP functions by binding to the PTH receptor in the bone and kidney, causing increased bone resorption and increased renal tubular calcium reabsorption. When skeletal metastases are present, there is also release of prostaglandin E_2 and numerous growth factors such as TGF-α and PDGF that contribute to the hypercalcemia.

Case 22

1. E This patient presents with infertility and the typical features associated with GH excess. Because pituitary adenomas can often crowd out normal functioning pituitary tissue, other pituitary hormones may be affected. The diagnosis of acromegaly is most readily confirmed with a serum IGF-1 measurement. Unless the patient is pregnant, an elevated IGF-1 is diagnostic of acromegaly. Measurements of serum LH, FSH, and testosterone may be ordered concurrently for the workup of infertility, but are not diagnostic. In addition, an MRI of the head should be ordered after IGF-1 measurement to confirm the presence of an adenoma. GH is not a reliable diagnostic test due to its oscillating pattern of secretion. GHRH is also not routinely measured.

2. D Delayed puberty is a consequence of dwarfism, caused by GH deficiency prior to closure of the epiphyseal growth plates. In contrast, acromegaly is GH excess that occurs after puberty. Hypersecretion of GH stimulates diabetogenic changes in sugar and lipid metabolism. Specifically, there is decreased glucose utilization and increased lipolysis, resulting in DM. Patients can also be hypertensive secondary to the systemic edema and have overgrowth of colonic polyps resulting in colon cancer. Finally, overgrowth of bone and cartilage often leads to arthritis.

Case 23

1. A Metabolic alkalosis, not acidosis, is a primary feature of Conn's syndrome, occurring as a result of elevated aldosterone levels stimulating H^+ secretion from the renal distal tubule. In addition, the excess aldosterone increases K^+ excretion and Na^+ reabsorption. The sodium and water retention elevates systemic BP, which is usually not responsive to antihypertensive medications. Plasma renin levels are low in primary hyperaldosteronism because the elevated aldosterone feeds back upon the renin-angiotensin system in the form of increased Na^+ to the JGA. The JGA senses increased renal perfusion and decreases renin secretion from the JG cells.

2. E Both spironolactone and ACE inhibitors can be used for medical treatment of primary hyperaldosteronism due to bilateral adrenocortical hyperplasia. This is the most common cause of primary hyperaldosteronism in children, although the cause of hyperplasia remains unknown. The adrenal glands start to grow excessively to produce nodules, either large (macronodular) or small (micronodular), that secrete aldosterone. Since these nodules are usually responsive to angiotensin II, ACE inhibitors have been effective in decreasing aldosterone secretion from the nodules. In addition, spironolactone, an aldosterone antagonist, can be used to block aldosterone's actions. In high doses, however, spironolactone can inhibit testosterone production, causing gynecomastia, reduced libido, and impotence in men or irregular menstrual cycles in women. To improve the hypokalemia associated with hyperaldosteronism, potassium-sparing diuretics such as amiloride can be used. Loop diuretics are actually contraindicated with hyperaldosteronism because they cause potassium wasting from the loop of Henle and can aggravate the hypokalemia. Surgery is the definitive therapy for hyperaldosteronism due to discreet lesions such as an adrenal adenoma or carcinoma, but not for bilateral zona glomerulosa hyperplasia.

Case 24

1. B Dopamine is a precursor molecule in the production of the catecholamines, norepinephrine and epinephrine; it is not a possible treatment option for pheochromocytoma. All of the choices listed with the exception of dopamine can be used in the management of pheochromocytoma. However, surgical removal of the tumor is the only definitive form of treatment. Preoperative administration of α-adrenergic blocking drugs decreases the risk for a life-threatening hypertensive crisis, which can occur when catecholamines are released into the circulation during surgical manipulation of the tumor. This alpha-blockade can be achieved with phenoxybenzamine, an irreversible nonselective $\alpha_1\alpha_2$-blocker, or phentolamine, a reversible nonselective $\alpha_1\alpha_2$-blocker. Once BP control is achieved, the beta-blocker propranolol is an effective means of controlling tachycardia or arrhythmias. Patients should be closely monitored during surgery for sudden changes in BP or cardiac abnormalities.

2. C This patient is experiencing a paroxysmal hypertensive crisis most likely initiated by the presence of a pheochromocytoma. The release of excess catecholamines into the circulation is responsible for sudden, unprovoked overactivation of the sympathetic nervous system, resulting in attacks of HTN, abdominal pain, palpitations, headache, and visual changes. Often the attacks are mistaken for thyrotoxicosis, an anxiety attack, or even acute abdomen. To confirm the diagnosis of a pheochromocytoma, the best test at this time is a 2-hour timed urine collection for metanephrines (VMA, HMA) because the patient is in the midst of a hypertensive crisis. Urinary levels of VMA and HMA will be elevated if measured at this time. Concomitant thyroid function tests can rule out thyrotoxicosis, but will not confirm a pheochromocytoma. Abdominal CT can help identify the location of the tumor, especially if it is in the adrenal glands. If the patient is not experiencing an acute attack but pheochromocytoma is suspected, a 24-hour timed urine collection is warranted for detection of urinary catecholamines and metanephrines. Repeat BP measurement can confirm elevated BPs, but is not diagnostic of any particular cause for the HTN.

Case 25

1. C DHEA levels are most likely elevated in this young girl who presents with hirsutism and growth abnormalities secondary to a mild form of CAH. DHEA is a mild androgen that can cause virilization in a female infant if present in excess amounts. Patients with nonclassical CAH have enough enzyme function to spare them from virilization and salt-wasting, but can present later in life with evidence of androgen excess from the shunting of cortisol and aldosterone precursors. In this case, androgen excess has resulted in an abnormal growth pattern, delayed menarche, obesity, and hirsutism. Women with unrecognized CAH often present with infertility. The most commonly involved enzyme deficiency in CAH is 21-hydroxylase, followed by 11β-hydroxylase. These enzymes are necessary for the biosynthesis of cortisol and aldosterone from cholesterol. Patients with CAH will have decreased levels of serum cortisol and aldosterone, which can lead to secondary electrolyte abnormalities and an inability to mount an appropriate stress response. ACTH levels will be increased in these patients as well due to the loss of negative feedback on the pituitary gland. These patients may complain of increased skin pigmentation secondary to the chronically elevated levels of ACTH.

2. B Of the choices listed, the hormone most likely to account for this child's symptoms is aldosterone. Aldosterone is a mineralocorticoid produced by the zona glomerulosa of the adrenal cortex. Aldosterone functions to maintain BP by increasing renal tubular absorption of sodium and thus facilitating excretion of potassium. Aldosterone secretion is regulated by the RAS system; angiotensin II directly stimulates its secretion from the adrenal cortex. Patients classically CAH present with both cortisol and aldosterone deficiency at birth. In female infants, it is often recognized early because of the presence of ambiguous genitalia secondary to androgen excess. Male infants, however, usually present a few weeks after birth because their external genitalia appear normal. These infants are diagnosed with CAH after they present with acute symptoms of glucocorticoid and mineralocorticoid deficiency, including failure to thrive, dehydration, vomiting, and severe hyponatremia with hyperkalemia. Lifelong treatment with exogenous mineralocorticoid and glucocorticoid therapy is required for these infants to survive. Deficiencies in the other hormones listed would not present in the first few weeks of life with dehydration and failure to thrive.

Case 26

1. D This patient presents with the classical description of Sheehan's syndrome. Panhypopituitarism occurs as a result of ischemia in the pituitary gland secondary to hypovolemic shock from postpartum hemorrhage. The cells that are most affected are those that lie in the pars distalis portion of the anterior pituitary. Atrophy of thyrotrophs will result in failure to synthesize TSH and the signs and symptoms of hypothyroidism. These include cold intolerance, dry skin, and constipation. If unrecognized, secondary hypothyroidism is a life-threatening event because of the possibility of myxedema coma. Failure to lactate occurs as a result of PRL deficiency. Stress intolerance occurs as a result of glucocorticoid deficiency and may make the patient susceptible to a variety of infections. Loss of gonadotrophs will cause loss of secondary sex characteristics such as axillary and pubic hair. Women may also describe amenorrhea and decreased libido. ACTH in excess amounts causes increased skin pigmentation because ACTH and MSH are formed from the same precursor. Because ACTH secretion is low or absent in Sheehan's syndrome, skin pigmentation is decreased, not increased.

2. A This child most likely has a craniopharyngioma. These tumors are derived from pituitary development, specifically oral ectoderm cells that give rise to the anterior pituitary. Craniopharyngeomas are problematic due to their location within the CNS. Because the pituitary gland is located immediately beneath the optic chiasm, headache and visual field defects are common when the gland enlarges secondary to compression of the optic nerves or chiasm. Classically, pituitary tumors cause a bitemporal hemianopsia. Craniopharyngeomas are rarely functioning or secretory. Instead, patients can present with symptoms of pituitary insufficiency if the tumor outgrows the natural blood supply of the gland. Increased pituitary volume can also activate osteoclasts, enlarging the sella turcica. Dwarfism is caused by isolated GH deficiency. Prolactinomas are PRL-secreting tumors commonly seen in women. Cushing's disease is a pituitary ACTH-producing tumor resulting in glucocorticoid excess. Addison's disease is primary adrenal insufficiency resulting in absence of both glucocorticoids and mineralocorticoids. While these alternative syndromes can present with isolated endocrine dysfunction and an enlarging pituitary gland, a craniopharyngeoma best accounts for the symptoms of panhypopituitarism.

Case 27

1. D This infant most likely has nephrogenic diabetes insipidus, a condition characterized by nephrogenic unresponsiveness to ADH and the inability to concentrate urine. In infants, this condition is likely inherited, rather than acquired, and presents shortly after birth with failure to thrive, poor feeding, and irritability. Often, the baby's diapers are dripping wet with excessive urination. Polyuria, polydipsia, and hypotonic urine occur, but since the baby is unable to communicate thirst, symptoms of dehydration rapidly develop. Signs of dehydration include the absence of tears, dry mucous membranes, hypotonia, and poor skin turgor. One of the most severe complications of NDI in infants is permanent brain damage with mental retardation if treatment is not started early. Patients with NDI will not respond to DDAVP, but rapid rehydration therapy is essential. Ensuring adequate free-water intake will prevent symptoms and serious sequelae. Thiazide diuretics may also be helpful. Central pontine myelinosis is a rare complication of overly rapid correction of hyponatremia. It can occur following aggressive treatment for SIADH. Psychosis is also a complication of SIADH that can occur secondary to brain edema. CHF and diarrhea are not symptoms of DI or SIADH.

2. B All of the choices except B are correct associations between malignancy and ectopic hormone production. Small cell lung carcinoma produces ADH, not squamous cell carcinoma. These paraneoplastic syndromes can imitate actual endocrine gland disturbances. For example, ectopic ACTH production causes Cushing's syndrome, while PTHrP production causes symptoms of hypercal-

cemia. Renal cell carcinoma can produce ectopic erythropoietin, which results in polycythemia. Although there are numerous causes of SIADH, the initial treatment of choice is water restriction until the underlying cause is identified. In the case of a paraneoplastic overproduction of ADH, the definitive treatment lies in removal of the hormone-producing tumor.

Case 28

1. B Autosomal-dominant mutations in the *menin* tumor suppressor gene on chromosome 11 are responsible for MEN type I, described in this patient's mother. MEN I consists of parathyroid hyperplasia, pituitary adenoma, and pancreatic islet cell neoplasm. The history of DM implies hyperglycemia secondary to a pancreatic glucagonoma, while kidney stones suggest symptomatic hypercalcemia. In addition, the presence of a pituitary neoplasm is a likely explanation for her mother's chronic headaches. Parathyroid hyperplasia is the most common finding in MEN I, consistent in up to 90% of patients. It is also present in MEN IIa. While the other choices are helpful screening tests for the diagnosis of MEN II syndromes, they would not contribute to the diagnosis of MEN I. Serum Ca and intact PTH measurement may be helpful for both MEN I and MEN IIa, but only *menin* germline mutation evaluation is specific for MEN I.

2. E This patient most likely has MEN IIb, as suggested by attacks of paroxysmal HTN secondary to pheochromocytoma and a distinctive marfanoid appearance. Because MEN IIb consists of medullary thyroid carcinoma, pheochromocytoma, and mucosal neuromas, this patient is most at risk for thyroid carcinoma. Derived from C cells within the thyroid gland, medullary carcinoma often causes elevated calcitonin levels. In MEN IIb patients, this type of cancer is extremely aggressive and is responsible for the major morbidity and mortality arising from the syndrome. Peptic ulcer disease, osteoporosis, and galactorrhea are features of MEN I. Hyperthyroidism is not associated with the multiple endocrine neoplasias.

Case 29

1. C Any young patient with recurrent hepatic disease and unexplained neurologic symptoms should be suspected to have Wilson's disease. Wilson's disease is an autosomal recessive disorder that results in the excess deposition of copper in the brain, liver, kidney, and cornea. Kayser-Fleischer rings are pathognomonic for the condition, but not essential for diagnosis. Copper chelation therapy with penicillamine is an effective treatment option for Wilson's disease. Hereditary hemochromatosis is also an autosomal recessive metabolic disorder that results in multi-system organ dysfunction. In contrast to Wilson's disease, hemochromatosis involves excess iron accumulation. Although weekly phlebotomy is the treatment of choice for hemochromatosis, chelation therapy with deferoxamine is another option. Both Wilson's disease and hemochromatosis patients are at greatly increased risk (>200 times) for hepatocellular carcinoma.

2. A Hemochromatosis is best diagnosed with a serum transferrin saturation level. Levels greater than 50% are highly sensitive for iron overload, but do not distinguish hereditary etiology from chronic transfusion therapy or exogenous iron overload. While elevated serum ferritin and hepatic iron concentration obtained through liver biopsy are also consistent with iron overload, these tests are not considered the initial tests of choice. Serum ferritin is not as sensitive as transferrin saturation, while liver biopsy is an overly invasive initial procedure. With the finding of elevated transferrin saturation levels, the diagnosis of hereditary hemochromatosis can be confirmed with genetic testing for the *C282Y* mutation. A 24-hour urine iron level is not a diagnostic test for hemochromatosis.

Case 30

1. A Normal male gonadal development is dependent on the sex-determining region of the Y chromosome (SRY) and also depends on the presence of an X chromosome. Interestingly, the testes do not form properly if more than one X chromosome is present (as in the case of Klinefelter's syndrome 47,XXY). While MIS is necessary to prevent differentiation of female internal genitalia, the testes will still form in the absence of MIS. Testes will still form in the absence of adrenal androgens, but normal male sexual development will not proceed normally in that setting.

2. D This individual has bilateral dysgenesis of the testes (Swyer's syndrome) and is a male pseudohermaphrodite; that is, genetically male, but phenotypically female. Failure of testicular development occurs prior to internal duct and external genitalia development, and is presumed to be a result of a mutation in the *SRY* gene. The testes do not develop and are replaced by fibrous bands. As such, local testosterone production is absent, preventing the embryo from developing male internal and external genitalia. Additionally, MIS normally secreted by Sertoli cells will be absent, and development of female internal genitalia, including fallopian tubes, uterus, and upper vagina, will not be suppressed. Affected individuals usually present with primary amenorrhea and a failure to develop secondary sexual characteristics at puberty. There will be minimal breast development and no male genitalia or secondary sexual characteristics.

Case 31

1. E In testicular feminization syndrome, also known as androgen insensitivity, genetically male fetuses (46,XY) develop phenotypically female external genitalia due to an intrinsic inability to respond to testicular androgens. This is an example of male pseudohermaphroditism. The presence of a Y chromosome in these individuals leads to development of testes as well as MIS. Thus, these individuals do not develop female internal genitalia despite their outward appearance. In addition, the testes are often undescended and should be surgically removed because they have an increased rate of malignancy.

True hermaphroditism occurs very rarely and is the simultaneous presence of both ovarian and testicular tissue in an individual. The external genitalia are often ambiguous. As above, pseudohermaphroditism occurs when the phenotypic sex does not correspond to the genotypic sex. Female pseudohermaphroditism is usually due to abnormalities in adrenal steroid synthesis, result-

ing in the development of clitoromegaly and hypertrophied labia majora that may be partially fused and resemble a scrotum in genetic females. Turner's syndrome occurs when an X chromosome is either absent or abnormal (45,XO or mosaicism in 46,XX or 46,XY), resulting in rudimentary or streak gonads. These individuals are phenotypically female and possess characteristic features that are discussed in the Turner's syndrome case. Klinefelter's syndrome is another disorder of gonadal development resulting from an XXY karyotype. Clinically, it is characterized by small, firm testes, azoospermia, gynecomastia, and mental retardation.

2. B The wolffian ducts give rise to the epididymis, vas deferens, and seminal vesicles. The müllerian ducts give rise to the fallopian tubes, uterus, and upper one third of the vagina. The gubernaculum is a mesenchymal condensation attached to the caudal portion of each testis and assists in testicular descent. Bartholin's glands are mucous glands that form at the base of the labia majora.

Case 32

1. C In addition to an increased risk for gynecologic malignancies, patients exposed to DES in utero are also at increased risk for infertility due to mullerian anomalies or idiopathic etiologies (see Case 31). Women who have undergone one therapeutic abortion, used OCPs, or are young are not at increased risk for infertility. Early menarche is not a risk factor for infertility.

2. E Testicular androgens are important for spermatogenesis to occur. Many body builders and competitive athletes are known to take exogenous androgens, which can lead to testicular atrophy and diminished or absent spermatogenesis. While the other answer choices are possible causes of male factor infertility, they are unlikely to be the cause in this male in good health. Additionally, although diminished androgen secretion can occur with very advanced age, it is unlikely to be a factor in this middle-aged man.

3. C Nondisjunction is the failure of a pair of chromosomes to separate during meiosis and can occur during either meiosis I or II. The most likely time for this to occur in a woman of advanced maternal age is during metaphase I, where chromosomes have been released from prolonged suspension in prophase I. Of note, while meiosis is divided into discrete phases for descriptive purposes, it is actually a continuous process.

Case 33

1. A Estrogen leads to a number of changes, including effects on the secondary sexual characteristics, bone growth, and an increase in hepatic enzymes. This can be seen in pregnancy when the increased levels of estrogen lead to greater release of hepatically produced binding proteins and clotting factors. While DHEAS does lead to axillary and pubic hair production in females, it is generally converted to DHT in males. LH and FSH act primarily on the gonads to both foster maturation and produce hormones and gametes. GnRH's effects are mediated in part because of its pulsatile effect. If it is released in a continuous fashion, its receptors are down-regulated, and its effect is minimized.

2. B The most common order of the stages of puberty is adrenarche, gonadarche, thelarche, pubarche, and menarche. Of note, the latter three events can vary in timing with respect to one another. In fact, some girls will start menstruating prior to thelarche.

Case 34

1. E Because most women have two functioning ovaries, the loss of one does not generally disrupt the onset of puberty in any significant way. Patients with the surgical removal of one ovary may have the onset of menopause approximately 1 year sooner. However, this has never been addressed in a prospective, randomized trial. Intense physical activity can lead to hypogonadotropic hypogonadism. Disruptions in the genital tract such as transverse vaginal septum and imperforate hymen result in the collection of menses behind these obstructions and backflow of menses into the pelvis. These patients often have monthly menstrual symptoms and can develop severe endometriosis. Patients with testicular feminization are actually genetically male, but because of a failure to respond to testosterone, they are phenotypically female. However, they lack a uterus, fallopian tubes, and ovaries.

2. B In this patient with excessive weight gain during college making her morbidly obese, the most likely etiology of her secondary amenorrhea is elevated estrogen disrupting her hypothalamic-pituitary-ovarian feedback loop and resulting in anovulation. These patients will often have breakdown of their endometrium leading to heavy menses every few months (anovulatory bleeding), but they can also present with frank amenorrhea. The weight loss and exercise since college are unlikely to lead to amenorrhea since the weight loss is bringing her back to her optimal weight and the exercise is not particularly excessive. While pregnancy is the leading cause of secondary amenorrhea and should be ruled out in this patient, it is less likely given another etiology and complaints of amenorrhea for 2 years. Because this patient had normal menses throughout adolescence, testicular feminization is not a feasible diagnosis.

3. D This patient has premature ovarian failure. A lack of response to progestin-only challenge in a previously menstruating woman indicates that she is now estrogen deficient. This is confirmed when she has a withdrawal bleed to estrogen/progestin challenge. The differential diagnosis is now dependent on an FSH level, which if elevated will indicate a diagnosis of hypergonadotropic hypogonadism or premature ovarian failure. If the FSH level is low, the patient has hypogonadotropic hypogonadism as a result of either severe hypothalamic dysfunction or brain lesion (e.g., empty sella syndrome, Sheehan's syndrome). These can be distinguished by clinical findings as well as head MRI. Asherman's syndrome (development of intrauterine synechiae) is usually the result of intrauterine instrumentation or infection. Additionally, a patient with Asherman's would not have a response to progestin or estrogen/progestin challenge because the abnormality is not hormonal in nature but rather outflow obstruction. Patients with PCOS will often have a withdrawal bleed to progestin alone because they are not estrogen deficient. Additionally, patients with PCOS will have other clinical findings consistent with the syndrome such as abnormal hair growth or insulin resistance. Patients

with testicular feminization syndrome will present with primary rather than secondary amenorrhea.

Case 35

1. A This woman's history of depression and tobacco use make hormonal contraceptives unsuitable for her because they can worsen her depression and put her at increased risk for thromboembolic disease. Given this, the copper IUD is an appropriate contraceptive. Additionally, IUDs are easier to insert and have a lower likelihood of spontaneous expulsion in women who have had children before.

2. B Condoms are the only method of contraception that can help prevent the passage of sexually transmitted diseases (STDs) because they minimize the exchange of bodily fluids. Other barrier methods such as the diaphragm and cervical cap also decrease the exchange of bodily fluids, but are not as effective as condoms in preventing STDs and subsequent PID. Hormonal contraceptives do not prevent transmission of STDs. IUDs can actually exacerbate pelvic infections because they are foreign bodies.

3. D Combination oral contraceptives function by preventing ovulation, thickening cervical mucus, and making the endometrium unsuitable for implantation. The diaphragm is a barrier method that prevents sperm from entering the uterus and reaching the egg. Depo-Provera and Norplant are hormonal contraceptives that function similarly to OCPs.

Case 36

1. E Mifepristone is a progesterone antagonist that blocks the stimulatory effects of progesterone on endometrial growth. Methotrexate is a folic acid antagonist that stops embryonic cell division. Both are used in conjunction with a prostaglandin such as misoprostol to induce contractions and expel the uterine contents.

2. D Approximately 1.2 million elective pregnancy terminations are performed each year in the United States. Abortion is not illegal in Utah. Prior to 1973, abortion was legal in New York. One third of abortions are performed on women under 20, one third in women ages 20 to 24, and the remaining one third in women over the age of 25.

Case 37

1. B Cardiac output increases 30% to 50% in pregnancy. SVR decreases secondary to the increased levels of progesterone that lead to relaxation of smooth muscle. The decrease in SVR leads to decreased BPs, which persist until term in the normal patient. Because of the blood volume expansion that outpaces production, both erythrocytes and platelets are more dilute, leading to a decreased hematocrit and platelet count.

2. D BUN and serum creatinine both decrease in pregnancy as a result of increased GFR. Tidal volume and minute ventilation both increase, while respiratory rate remains unchanged. This increased minute ventilation actually leads to a decrease in P_{CO_2} and an increase in pH.

Case 38

1. B Not all Rh D-negative women need to receive RhoGAM (anti-D immune globulin) after delivery. If the fetus is found to be Rh D-negative following delivery, administration of anti-D immune globulin is not indicated. However, if determination of fetal Rh status is delayed for any reason, RhoGAM should be administered to all nonimmunized mothers within 72 hours after delivery. Women who are Rh D-negative are given prophylactic RhoGAM in the setting of a spontaneous or elective termination of pregnancy, ectopic pregnancy, invasive procedure such as amniocentesis or CVS, routinely at approximately 28 weeks of gestation, and anytime in the third trimester when the antibody screen is negative despite having already received a prophylactic dose.

2. B When following ΔOD_{450} values for fetal hemolysis, Liley zone 1 is reassuring, but fetuses with values in zone 3 and high zone 2 are at risk for fetal anemia. Once these values are attained, direct fetal blood sampling via PUBS to determine fetal hematocrit and transfuse cross-matched Rh-negative blood is necessary. Because of the risk for delivery either shortly after or during the PUBS, patients are often given a course of antenatal corticosteroids. If the measurement were just in the middle to low area of zone 2, it would be reasonable to continue fetal assessment with ultrasound and more frequent amniocentesis every 7 to 10 days.

3. E While ultrasonography is not the most sensitive test for fetal hemolysis, the presence of ascites and pleural and pericardial effusions is particularly specific for fetal hemolysis in Rh-positive fetuses with Rh-negative moms. The Liley curve is used to predict severity of fetal disease. Values in zone 3 are suggestive of severe fetal disease.

4. C The various fetal structures allow maximum fetal oxygenation. The foramen ovale is located between the two atria and shunts blood from the RA to the LA to bypass the pulmonary circulation. The DA also bypasses the pulmonary system by shunting blood from the pulmonary artery to the aorta. Blood is shunted from the liver by the ductus venosus. The umbilical vein transports oxygenated blood to the fetus while the umbilical arteries transport deoxygenated blood back to the placenta.

Case 39

1. D Masters and Johnson initially described the sexual response cycle as four phases: excitement, plateau, orgasm, and resolution. The phase of sexual attraction or arousal was later described and logically is the start of the human sexual response cycle.

2. C Although the use of H2 blockers can cause erectile dysfunction, acid reflux in itself is not a known cause. However, stroke, depression, atherosclerosis, and hyperthyroidism are all potential

causes of erectile dysfunction, with vascular causes being the most common.

Case 40

1. A Two proven benefits of HRT are decreased risks of colon cancer and bone fractures. However, HRT has been associated with increased risks of heart disease, stroke, blood clots, breast cancer, and uterine cancer.

2. E Menopause is associated with characteristic signs and symptoms, including vaginal atrophy and drying, decrease in breast size or change in texture, hot flushes, and night sweats (hot flushes that occur at night).

3. E All of the answer choices are risk factors for osteoporosis, which is defined as 2.5 standard deviations or more below the adult peak mean. Treatment options include weight-bearing exercises, calcium and vitamin D supplementation, hormone replacement, bisphosphonates, SERMs, and calcitonin.

Case 41

1. C Recurrent urinary tract infections have not been shown to increase the risk for cervical dysplasia or cancer. However, HPV and HIV infection, early age at onset of sexual activity, large number of sexual partners, history of sexually transmitted infections, and cigarette smoking are all risk factors for cervical dysplasia and cancer.

2. B Cervical cancer is clinically staged. As such, physical exam, including pelvic examination under anesthesia, is the main staging modality. MRI is not used, but CT scan is occasionally used to assess for hydronephrosis. Because cervical cancer is not surgically staged, hysterectomy specimen and lymph node dissection are not used to assign stage of disease.

3. E All of the answer choices would be appropriate treatment for CIN II except for radiation, which is reserved for early to advanced cervical cancer. Although cryotherapy and laser surgery could both be used, cold knife conization and LEEP are preferable because they would provide a specimen for evaluation of margins. Of note, conization must be performed in the operating room, and thus is more costly than LEEP.

Case 42

1. A Serum tumor markers can be useful aids in determining response to therapy with germ cell tumors. Dysgerminomas produce LDH and CA-125. Embryonal carcinomas produce hCG, AFP, and CA-125. Endodermal sinus tumors produce AFP. Immature teratomas produce CA-125. Choriocarcinomas produce hCG.

2. C Because the patient's tumor was confined to the ovary and tube but did not rupture the ovarian capsule or seed her abdomen, she is considered stage IIA; that is, disease extension from the ovary to the pelvis but confined to the uterus or fallopian tube and without evidence of malignant ascites or peritoneal cytology. Had the tumor been limited to the ovary only, she would have been stage I. Fortunately, the patient did not have abdominal or lymph node metastases, and therefore was not stage III.

3. D Epithelial ovarian neoplasms are the most common, and among them, the majority are serous, then mucinous. The remaining epithelial subtypes (with the exception of borderline tumors, which comprise 10%–15%) each represent less than 5% of ovarian neoplasms. The germ cell and sex cord stromal tumors each comprise 5% to 7% of ovarian neoplasms, and among them, the granulosa cell tumors and dysgerminomas are the more common.

4. E Borderline tumors are considered epithelial in origin and tend to occur in premenopausal women. They are treated surgically, and patients have an excellent prognosis. However, they have been found to recur as many as 20 years after excision.

Case 43

1. B There are approximately 182,800 new cases of breast cancer diagnosed annually in the United States. This exceeds the total incidence of lung, endometrial, ovarian, and cervical cancers combined. The incidence of lung cancer is 74,600; endometrial cancer 36,100; ovarian cancer 23,100; and cervical 12,800.

2. D Lung cancer accounts for approximately 67,600 deaths annually in the United States. Breast cancer follows with 40,800 deaths annually. Of the gynecologic cancers, ovarian cancer tends to be diagnosed in later stages, and thus accounts for 14,000 deaths per year. Endometrial cancer causes 6,500 deaths and cervical cancer 4,600 deaths per year.

3. E The differential diagnosis for postmenopausal bleeding includes endometrial cancer, endometrial hyperplasia or atrophy, endometrial polyps, exogenous estrogens, cervical polyps or cancer, uterine sarcoma, and trauma.

4. D Factors that increase exposure to estrogen, particularly unopposed estrogen, are risk factors for endometrial cancer. These include nulliparity, chronic anovulation, late menopause, and exogenous estrogen use. Additionally, obesity increases peripheral conversion of adrenal androgens to estrogens by aromatase activity in adipose tissue. Combined with the lower concentration of sex hormone binding globulin found in obese women, these factors account for the increased bioavailability of estrogen and make obesity an important risk factor for endometrial cancer. Early age of first intercourse is not associated with endometrial cancer, but is associated with cervical cancer.

Case 44

1. A Eighty percent of GTD is molar pregnancy, with 90% of molar pregnancies being complete moles. Invasive moles account for 10% to 15% of GTD, while choriocarcinoma accounts for 2% to 5%. Placental site trophoblastic tumors are exceedingly rare.

2. E Choriocarcinoma can metastasize to many locations. In fact, it often presents as metastatic disease and is known as the great imitator because its signs and symptoms are very similar to other diseases. Given this potentially confusing presentation and the fact that it can arise weeks to years after any gestation, diagnosis of choriocarcinoma is often delayed.

3. D Choriocarcinoma consists of cytotrophoblasts and syncytiotrophoblasts only. There are no chorionic villi present. PSTTs also lack chorionic villi. Complete moles have a 46,XY or 46,XX karyotype, while partial moles are either 69,XXY or 69,XXX. Invasive moles contain chorionic villi and trophoblasts.

4. E Reported risk factors for GTD vary but include all of the following: maternal age under 20 or over 40 years; history of prior molar pregnancy or miscarriage; diets low in beta-carotene, folic acid, and vitamin A; women with blood type A married to men with blood type O; and use of oral contraceptives.

Index